Congenital Malformations of the Head and Neck

Lisa M. Elden • Karen B. Zur
Editors

Congenital Malformations of the Head and Neck

Springer

Editors
Lisa M. Elden
Pediatric Otolaryngology
The Children's Hospital of Philadelphia
Philadelphia, PA, USA

Karen B. Zur
Pediatric Otolaryngology
The Children's Hospital of Philadelphia
Philadelphia, PA, USA

ISBN 978-1-4419-1713-3 ISBN 978-1-4419-1714-0 (eBook)
DOI 10.1007/978-1-4419-1714-0
Springer New York Heidelberg Dordrecht London

Library of Congress Control Number: 2013952919

Printed on acid-free paper

Springer is part of Springer Science+Business Media (www.springer.com)

Preface and Acknowledgements

This book was designed to provide the reader with a conceptual and visual approach to children with congenital malformations of the head and neck. We are indebted to our contributors, who not only wrote thoughtful chapters but also searched their photo collections, radiology images, and libraries of endoscopic images to obtain many never previously published examples of these malformations. We are grateful to our partners at the Children's Hospital of Philadelphia, including Drs. Bill Potsic, Ralph Wetmore, Steve Handler, Larry Tom, Ian Jacobs, Ken Kazahaya, John Germiller, Brian Dunham, Mark Rizzi, Luv Javia, and Steve Sobol. As a team, this group has continued to contribute their best photographs to a large, shared database over the years. We also thank their patients who agreed to pose for these photographs. We personally thank Donna McDonald-McGinn, Diana Sweeney, David Low, and Scott Bartlett for providing many photographs related to Genetics and Plastic/Reconstructive Surgery. We thank our Developmental Editor, Flora Kim, for her patience and guidance throughout the writing of this book. We are especially grateful to our academic coordinator, Beth McCullough, who reviewed each chapter and photograph to ensure they were ready for publication. Finally, we thank our families for their patience while we completed this project. Thanks to Pat, Maddy, and Nick from their wife and mom, Lisa and to Rob, Ellie, and Arielle from their wife and mom, Karen.

Philadelphia, PA, USA

Lisa M. Elden
Karen B. Zur

Contents

Contributors

Daniel I. Choo, M.D. Division of Pediatric Otolaryngology, Department of Otolaryngology Head and Neck Surgery, Cincinnati Children's Hospital Medical Center, Cincinnati, OH, USA

J. Matthew Dickson, B.Sc., M.D., F.R.C.S.(C) Division of Otolaryngology, Department of Surgery, Surrey Memorial Hospital, University of British Columbia, Surrey, BC, Canada

Brian P. Dunham, M.D. Division of Pediatric Otolaryngology, The Children's Hospital of Philadelphia, Philadelphia, PA, USA

Department of Otolaryngology: Head and Neck Surgery, Perelman School of Medicine at the University of Pennsylvania, Philadelphia, PA, USA

Lisa M. Elden, M.S., M.D. Division of Pediatric Otolaryngology, Department Surgery The Children's Hospital of Philadelphia, Philadelphia, PA, USA

Otolaryngology: Head and Neck Surgery, Perelman School of Medicine at the University of Pennsylvania, Philadelphia, PA, USA

Richard E. Kirschner, M.D., F.A.C.S., F.A.A.P. Section of Plastic and Reconstructive Surgery, Nationwide Children's Hospital, Columbus, OH, USA

Jonathan A. MacLean, M.D. Department of Otolaryngology–Head and Neck Surgery, Emory Children's Center, Emory University School of Medicine, Atlanta, GA, USA

Donna M. McDonald-McGinn, M.S., C.G.C. Department of Clinical Genetics, The Children's Hospital of Philadelphia, Philadelphia, PA, USA

Gregory D. Pearson, M.D. Department of Plastic and Reconstructive Surgery, Nationwide Children's Hospital, Columbus, OH, USA

Mark D. Rizzi, M.D. Division of Pediatric Otolaryngology, The Children's Hospital of Philadelphia, Philadelphia, PA, USA

Department of Otolaryngology: Head and Neck Surgery, Perelman School of Medicine at the University of Pennsylvania, Philadelphia, PA, USA

Michael J. Rutter, M.D., F.R.A.C.S. Department of Otolaryngology, Cincinnati Children's Hospital Medical Center, Cincinnati, OH, USA

Ravi N. Samy, M.D. Department of Otolaryngology Head and Neck Surgery, University Hospital/University of Cincinnati, Cincinnati, OH, USA

Nael M. Shoman, M.D., F.R.C.S.(C) Division of Otolaryngology–Head and Neck Surgery, Department of Surgery, St. Paul's Hospital, Saskatoon, SK, Canada

Steven E. Sobol, M.D., M.Sc. Division of Pediatric Otolaryngology, The Children's Hospital of Philadelphia, Philadelphia, PA, USA

Department of Otolaryngology: Head and Neck Surgery, Perelman School of Medicine at the University of Pennsylvania, Philadelphia, PA, USA

Tara L. Wenger, M.D., Ph.D. Department of Clinical Genetics, The Children's Hospital of Philadelphia, Philadelphia, PA, USA

Elaine H. Zackai, M.D. Department of Clinical Genetics, The Children's Hospital of Philadelphia, Philadelphia, PA, USA

Karen B. Zur, M.D. Division of Pediatric Otolaryngology, Center for Pediatric Airway Disorders, The Children's Hospital of Philadelphia, Philadelphia, PA, USA

Department of Otolaryngology: Head and Neck Surgery, Perelman School of Medicine at the University of Pennsylvania, Philadelphia, PA, USA

1 Genetics of Common Congenital Syndromes of the Head and Neck

Tara L. Wenger, Donna M. McDonald-McGinn, and
Elaine H. Zackai

Abstract

This chapter introduces the reader to the more common congenital syndromes of the head and neck. The chapter begins with a general overview of genetic sequences, associations, and syndromes. In-depth descriptions and photographs of patients with the more common syndromes are then presented including Pierre Robin sequence, CHARGE association, 22q11.2 deletion syndrome, Treacher Collins syndrome, craniosynostosis syndromes, and oculo-auriculo-vertebral spectrum (Goldenhar, hemifacial microsomia).

Keywords

Pierre Robin sequence • CHARGE association • 22q11.2 Deletion syndrome • Treacher Collins syndrome • Craniosynostosis syndromes • OAVS (Goldenhar, hemifacial microsomia)

General Information and Definitions

General Information

When approaching a patient with congenital malformations, it is important to take a detailed family history and pregnancy history and perform a detailed physical examination observing associated abnormal features. Pregnancy history should include any illnesses, environmental exposures, medications, and use of illicit drugs as well as any complications of chronic medical illnesses (e.g., gestational diabetes). Taking note of both major structural defects and minor dysmorphic features may help to establish a unifying diagnosis. Birth defects can be isolated or can occur as part of a set of features which can be broken down by embryologic etiology into the following groups: syndrome, sequence, deformation, malformation, dysplasia, and disruption. There are important implications for etiology and inheritance for each category.

Multiple abnormalities can be caused by genetic defects, environmental exposures, or

T.L. Wenger, M.D., Ph.D. (✉)
• D.M. McDonald-McGinn, M.S., C.G.C. •
E.H. Zackai, M.D.
Department of Clinical Genetics,
The Children's Hospital of Philadelphia,
8th Floor Main Building, 3400 Civic Center
Boulevard, Philadelphia, PA 19106, USA
e-mail: wengert@email.chop.edu;
mcginn@email.chop.edu; zackai@email.chop.edu

L.M. Elden and K.B. Zur (eds.), *Congenital Malformations of the Head and Neck*,
DOI 10.1007/978-1-4419-1714-0_1,

disruptions of embryologic development. Abnormal embryologic development may occur because of (a) malformation of a precursor structure, (b) damage to a properly formed structure (e.g., amniotic band sequence), or (c) abnormal fetal movement resulting in structural differences (e.g., high arched palate and micrognathia in neuromuscular disorders due to limited chin movement *in utero*).

Definitions

Major dysmorphic feature: A structural difference noted at birth that (a) will cause significant effect, (b) may require immediate medical or surgical intervention, and (c) is not considered to be part of normal variation. Examples include congenital heart disease, cleft palate, and hypospadias.

Minor dysmorphic feature: A physical difference that is not common in the general population but may be seen at a higher rate in individuals with identifiable syndromes. Examples include transverse palmar crease, clinodactyly (medially curved finger of the fifth digit), and hypertelorism.

Syndrome: A collection of well-defined major and minor anomalies that occur because of a common underlying cause often due to genetic causes or exposure to teratogenic agents. The anomalies are independent in that they arise in embryologically distinct structures.

Sequence: A group of abnormal features that result from a single embryologic major anomaly and affects the development of adjacent or related structures.

Deformation: An extrinsic physical force that impairs proper embryologic development. Multiple gestation, oligohydramnios, and uterine structural defects such as fibroids can impose physical developmental constraints.

Malformation: An abnormal formation of an embryologic structure due to genetic, environmental, or epigenetic causes.

Dysplasia: Defects attributed to abnormal cellular architecture in underlying tissue (e.g., skeletal dysplasia resulting from defect of collagen formation).

Disruption: A normally developing structure that has been damaged by an extrinsic force (i.e., amniotic band syndrome is the result of an appropriately forming limb, which became severed by a piece of amion).

Associations: Abnormal features that often occur together perhaps as the result of an insult at a specific time during embryogenesis.

Specific Disorders

Sequences

Pierre Robin Sequence

Definition

Pierre Robin sequence is described as the association of micrognathia, wide U-shaped cleft palate, and upper airway obstruction [1, 2]. The diagnosis of Pierre Robin is sometimes made when only two out of three features are present, micrognathia and glossoptosis, which represent a common final phenotype for patients with a variety of primary disorders. Approximately 40 % of patients have isolated Pierre Robin, with 60 % having additional syndromic features. The most commonly associated syndrome is Stickler syndrome [3]. There are over 30 other syndromes in which Pierre Robin is a common finding. Therefore, a diagnosis of Pierre Robin should be considered only as a starting point in the diagnostic work-up.

Clinical Features

The primary features of Pierre Robin sequence are micrognathia, wide U-shaped cleft palate, and respiratory compromise secondary to glossoptosis. These features are typically evident soon after birth and are sometimes identified on prenatal ultrasound.

(a) *Respiratory distress*: Respiratory distress often occurs immediately after birth and may be exacerbated by feeding. Glossoptosis, pharyngeal hypotonia, and tracheomalacia are common causes of respiratory distress in Pierre Robin sequence [4, 5]. Endotracheal or nasotracheal intubation and eventual placement of a tracheostomy may be necessary in severe cases. As a first step, many children undergo glossopexy (tongue–lip adhesion) and/or mandibular distraction to relieve upper airway obstruction.

(b) *Feeding difficulties*: Feeding difficulties related to the micrognathia, cleft palate, and respiratory distress often necessitate placement of nasogastric tube for feeding. Failure to thrive can be seen and has been attributed to expenditure of excess energy for respiration and difficulty feeding.

(c) *Developmental delay*: Delay of milestones and learning difficulties in Pierre Robin sequence can be acquired as a result of neonatal hypoxia or it may be intrinsic to an underlying genetic syndrome.

(d) *Middle ear disease*: Many children with Pierre Robin sequence have recurrent otitis media as the presence of a cleft palate alone increases their risk of having middle ear disease. In addition, in many of the associated syndromes hearing loss may also be present.

Heredity and Etiology

Pierre Robin sequence can be a result of micrognathia, which may be due to a variety of causes. Fusion of the palate occurs between the 9th and 11th week of embryogenesis. Prior to this, at 8 weeks gestation, the tongue rests against the skull base. As the mandible grows and descends, the tongue is pulled down and away from the palatal shelves. In Pierre Robin sequence, a variety of primary abnormalities prevent this from occurring and the tongue remains between the palatal shelves, preventing proper orientation and fusion of the palate. If descent of the tongue occurs late, a cleft may persist. Lateral head growth causes mechanical separation of the palatal shelves until after programmed cell growth has ended. Animal studies have demonstrated that mandibular constraint results in cleft palate [6–8]. After birth, the micrognathia and sometimes retrognathia persist with glossoptosis as a consequence. Since infants are obligate nose breathers, a posteriorly displaced tongue can cause airway obstruction [5].

The inheritance pattern of Pierre Robin sequence is entirely dependent on its primary etiology. In some cases such as Stickler syndrome, there is autosomal dominant inheritance, resulting in a 50 % recurrence risk. Alternatively, in cases resulting from deformation of the fetus such as multiple gestation or uterine anomalies, the risk of recurrence is extremely low. As a result of this wide variability, identification of an underlying cause for Pierre Robin sequence is critical before providing recurrence risk counseling.

There are several primary abnormalities that result in a common final phenotype of Pierre Robin sequence [6]. These include disorders of collagen (e.g., Stickler syndrome, cerebrocostomandibular syndrome); deformation (e.g., oligohydramnios, multiple gestations, uterine anomalies); chromosomal abnormalities (e.g., Trisomy 13, Trisomy 18; 22q11.2 deletion syndrome); and facial hypotonia causing improper movement of the mandible (e.g., myotonic dystrophy).

Diagnosis

Pierre Robin sequence is a clinical diagnosis based on physical findings (Fig. 1.1). Careful examination of a child with Pierre Robin sequence is essential in determining which associated genetic conditions should be excluded. Additional work-up should include a careful neurologic examination (to rule out primary central nervous system or neuromuscular disorder), ophthalmologic examination (to rule out myopia associated with Stickler syndrome), cardiac evaluation (to rule out congenital heart disease), and a chest X-ray (to evaluate for rib gaps as seen in cerebrocostomandibular syndrome or vertebral anomalies as seen in 22q11.2 DS), as abnormalities of these systems can greatly assist in diagnosis. For example, children with primary neuromuscular abnormalities can develop micrognathia secondary to poor fetal movement. Children with a cardiac defect should be evaluated for signs of 22q11.2 deletion. Cerebrocostomandibular

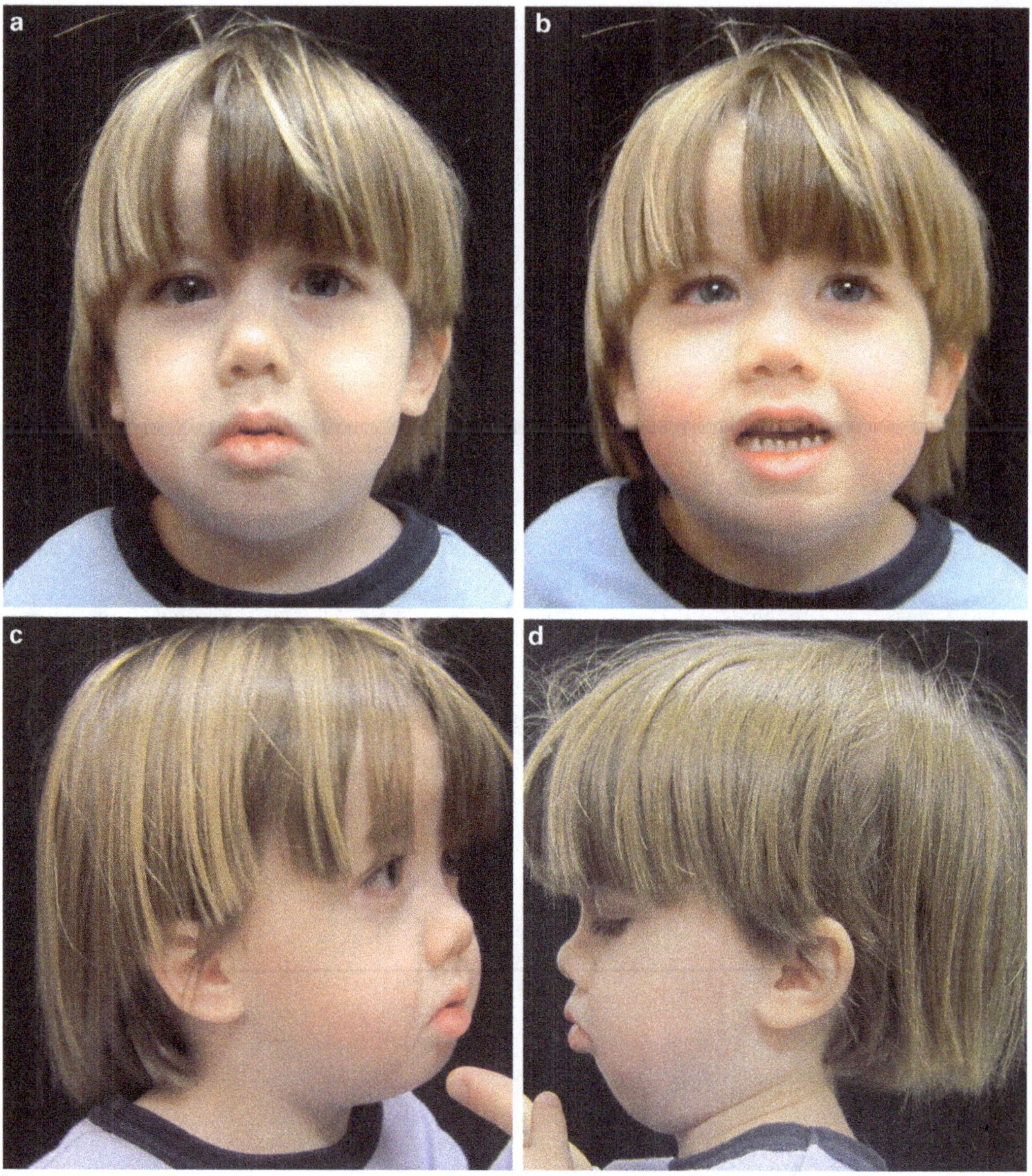

Fig. 1.1 Pierre Robin sequence in a child with Stickler Association

syndrome should be considered in children with abnormalities on chest X-ray (such as posterior rib gaps). Genomic microarray analysis should be considered in most cases, but sequencing of additional genes, such as COL2A1 (collagen, type II, alpha I gene) for Stickler syndrome, may be warranted.

Associations

CHARGE Association

Definition and Clinical Features

From the 1950s to 1970s, case reports began to emerge of children with combinations of coloboma, choanal atresia, and congenital

Table 1.1 Clinical features of children diagnosed with CHARGE syndrome

Acronym	Feature	Frequency (%)	Comments
C	C = coloboma	80–90	Colobomas of iris, retina, or optic disk. May be unilateral or bilateral
H	H = heart defects	60–85	Include patent ductus arteriosum (PDA), ventricular septal defect (VSD), atrial septal defect (ASD), endocardial cushion defect, coarctation of aorta, vascular ring, hypoplastic left heart, and tetralogy of Fallot
A	A = atresia choanae	55–85	May be unilateral or bilateral
R	R = retardation of growth	70–85	Usually normal birth weight with secondary failure to thrive, often falling below the third percentile
	R = retardation of development	60–100	Wide range of intellectual impairment, from normal to severe mental retardation
G	G = genital defects	53–100	Hypogonadism in 80–90 % of males and 15–20 % of females
E	E = ear anomalies and/or deafness	85–100	Characteristic appearance—short, wide, low-set, protruding, lop or cup shaped, with an unusual antihelix and often asymmetric. Mixed progressive hearing loss in 60–90 %. Abnormalities of semicircular canals often noted on computer tomography (CT)/magnetic resonance imaging (MRI)

heart disease. Pagon [9] reported an additional 21 cases and coined the moniker "CHARGE association" for the pattern of abnormalities most commonly seen in afflicted patients (Table 1.1) (Fig. 1.2).

Children with a diagnosis of CHARGE typically have at least four of the features, and coloboma or choanal atresia are considered requisite parts of the diagnosis. Other abnormalities seen in CHARGE include structural brain defects [10, 11], cleft lip or palate [12], cranial nerve abnormalities which may be asymmetric [13, 14], esophageal atresia and/or tracheoesophageal fistula, renal abnormalities including horseshoe kidney and ureteral abnormalities [14], and delayed tooth eruption [15].

Heredity and Etiology

CHARGE association results from multiple genetic etiologies (including genetic mutations of *CHD7*, a gene also known as "chromodomain helicase DNA-binding protein 7," which is thought to play a role in remodeling chromatin) and based on concordance studies in monozygotic twins and discordance in dizygotic twins is not caused by environmental factors [14, 16, 17]. For children with all major features of CHARGE, *CHD7* mutations will be detected in 90 %. For children with suspected CHARGE where some features are absent, a mutation in *CHD7* will be identified in fewer patients (60–70 %). Advanced paternal age at the time of conception compared with that of the general population may increase the risk of having a child with CHARGE association. Most cases occur sporadically, and the risk of recurrence in siblings of affected children is about 1 % [18]. There are case reports of children with normal *CHD7* sequencing who have mutations in *SEMA3E* (a member of the semaphorin family of genes that encodes a protein with an immunoglobulin-like domain, a PSI domain, and a Sema domain) [19, 20]. In addition, some children with mutations identified in *CHD7* and *SEM3AE* have also been found to have a deletion at 22q11.2. However, it is likely that additional mutations have not yet been discovered, which may account for the small number of patients with CHARGE who do not have an identified mutation.

Diagnosis

The clinical features of CHARGE are usually identified at birth with some abnormalities evident on prenatal ultrasound examination. In addition to a careful physical exam, a child with suspected CHARGE should undergo hearing and ophthalmologic examination to aid in diagnosis.

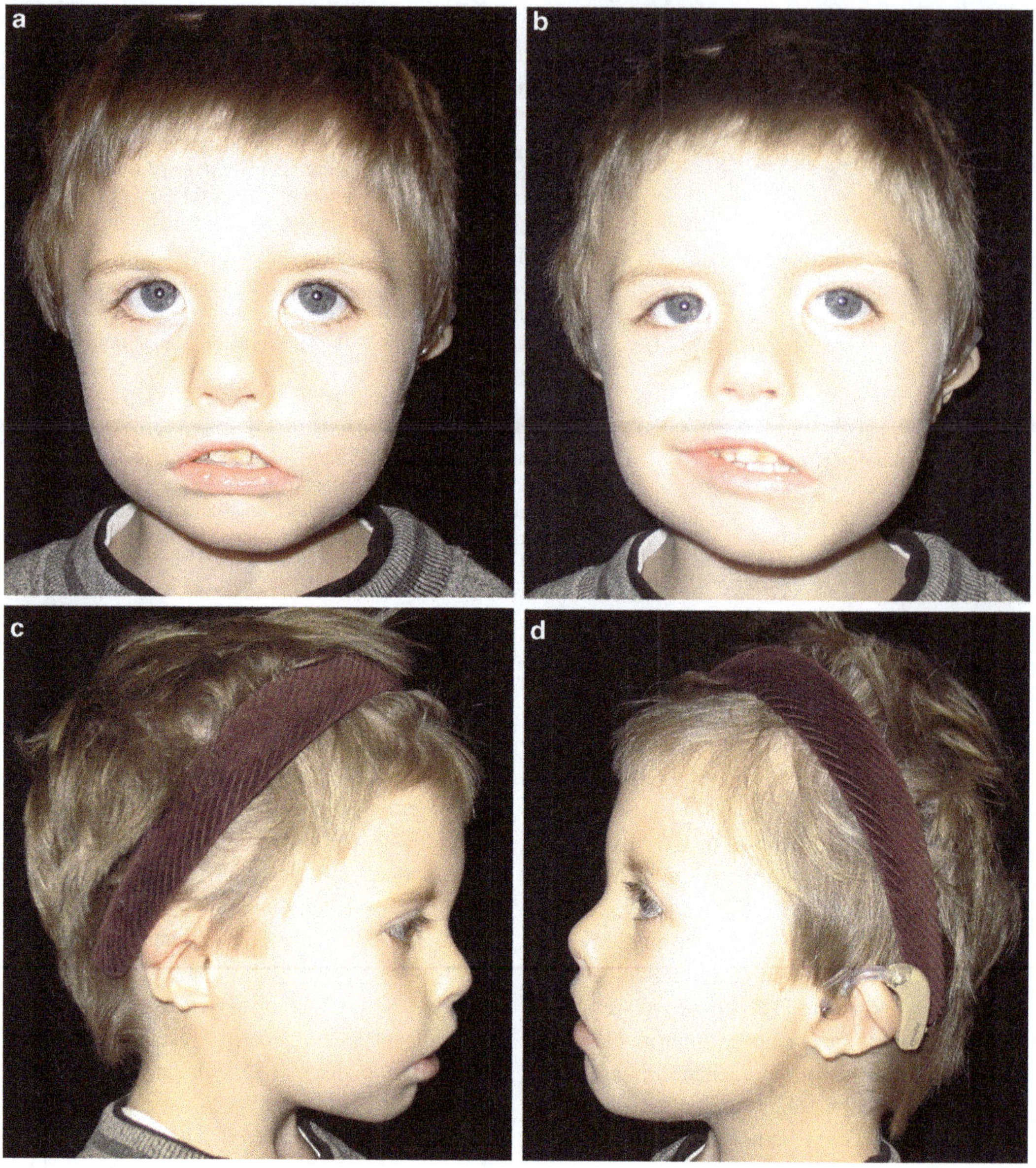

Fig. 1.2 Patient with CHARGE Association

Head imaging with CT or MRI can identify abnormalities of the semicircular canals as well as structural brain abnormalities. Molecular testing is clinically available and can assist in the diagnosis of CHARGE cases due to *CHD7* mutation. Because of the number of cytogenetic abnormalities that can result in a similar phenotype, genomic microarray analysis should be performed for all suspected cases who have normal *CHD7* sequencing. Children that are negative for *CHD7* mutation can be diagnosed clinically based on the above criteria.

Syndromes

22q11.2 Deletion Syndrome

Definition

The 22q11.2 deletion syndrome (22q11.2 DS) is the most common microdeletion syndrome, with an estimated incidence of 1/4,000 live births [11, 21–26]. Prior to the recognition of its genetic basis, children with different features of the disorder were described with a variety of terms: DiGeorge syndrome, velocardiofacial syndrome, conotruncal anomaly face syndrome, autosomal dominant Opitz/GBBB syndrome, and Cayler cardiofacial syndrome [27–34]. The prevalence of 22q11.2 deletion is even higher, having been identified in 1/68 children with congenital heart disease [35]. This deletion syndrome is the most common cause of syndromic palatal defects and a frequent cause of developmental delay [36].

Clinical Features

Children with 22q11.2 DS have recognizable facial features as well as somatic and functional abnormalities (Fig. 1.3). There are several features that occur frequently in children with 22q11.2 DS, and dozens of other features that have been reported in smaller number of children. The most common abnormalities [37] are listed in Table 1.2.

Each of these features occurs at a much greater rate than the general population.

Characteristic facial features in 22q11.2 DS include malar flatness, hooded eyelids, hypertelorism, downslanting or upslanting palpebral fissures, auricular anomalies including overfolded helices, attached earlobes, prominent nasal root with fullness to the nasal tip and hypoplastic alae nasi, nasal dimple or crease, small mouth, and asymmetric crying facies [38–43]. These facial features are variable in any individual child and are less consistently seen in non-Caucasian children [44].

Many other somatic birth defects and functional problems have been reported in children with 22q11.2 deletion, including but not limited to limb defects [45–49], neural tube defects [50], genitourinary anomalies [44], craniosynostosis [39], laryngeal abnormalities [51], autoimmune disorders [52–54], and hearing loss [55].

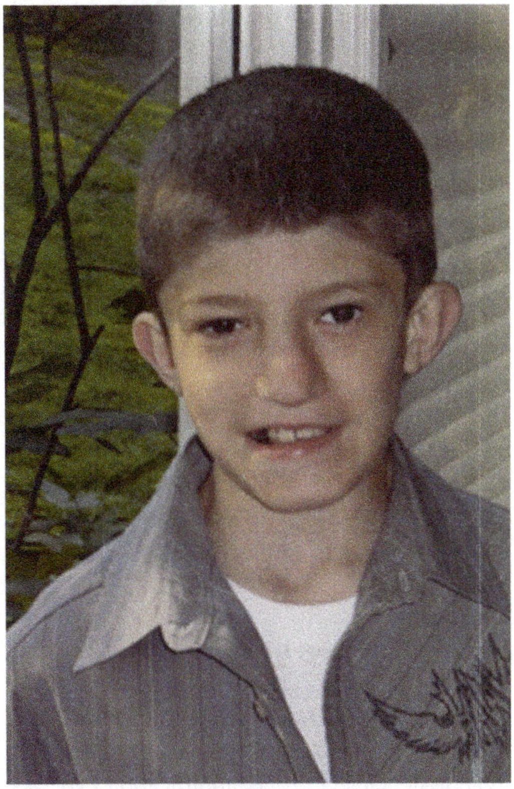

Fig. 1.3 Patient with 22q11.2 Deletion syndrome

Table 1.2 Clinical features of children diagnosed with 22 q11.2 deletion syndrome

Feature	Frequency (%)
Developmental delay	>90
Congenital heart defect	76
Palatal defects	76
Immunodeficiency	77
Hypocalcemia	49
Renal anomalies	36
Dysphagia	35
Schizophrenia	Approximately 25
Polydactyly	4
Congenital diaphragmatic hernia	1

Heredity and Etiology

The vast majority (85 %) of individuals have the same 2.54 Mb deletion, encompassing about 30 functional genes [37]. Ten percent of cases are familial with a parent usually demonstrating some signs of the disorder. A smaller subset of individuals has smaller deletions within this region [37, 56]. Congenital heart defects in

22q11.2 deletion have been linked with the TBX1 gene (T box transcription factor), as children with smaller deletions that include deletion of TBX1 have a high rate of congenital heart disease [37]. No other clear genotype–phenotype correlations have been made to date [57].

Most deletions are *de novo* and occur because the structure of the 22q11.2 region is vulnerable to mutations. There are segmental duplications that flank the typical breakpoints, which make it susceptible to rearrangements [58–62]. Like all contiguous gene deletion syndromes, the risk of a child inheriting the deletion from an affected parent is 50 %. However, because of phenotypic variability, the severity of features in a child born to an affected parent cannot be predicted based on the parent's own phenotype.

Diagnosis

Deletion of the 22q11.2 region can be identified using single-nucleotide polymorphism (SNP) or comparative genomic hybridization (CGH) genome-wide microarray or use of multiplex ligation-dependent probe amplification (MLPA). Although standard fluorescent in situ hybridization (FISH) can be used to detect a deletion of 22q11.2, this technique may miss patients with smaller atypical deletions in 22q11.2 [37, 63–65].

Pregnant women who have a family history of 22q11.2 DS may be offered genetic testing using chorionic villous sampling or amniocentesis. Fetuses with somatic defects noted on ultrasound can be tested utilizing amniocentesis. Sonographic abnormalities identified in pregnancies of fetuses with 22q11.2 DS include congenital heart defects, cleft palate, renal anomalies, polyhydramnios, polydactyly, congenital diaphragmatic hernia, clubfoot, and neural tube defects [44, 57].

Treacher Collins Syndrome

Definition

Treacher Collins syndrome, also known as mandibulofacial dysostosis, is an autosomal dominant disorder with characteristic facial anomalies resulting from malformations of structures arising from the first and second pharyngeal arch, groove, and pouch [66].

Clinical Features (Fig. 1.4)

(a) *Development*: Children with Treacher Collins usually display normal intelligence; however, occasional cases of developmental delay have been attributed to hearing loss [67].
(b) *Ears*: Malformations of the internal and external ear, include atresia of the external auditory canal, as well as, ossicle abnormalities of the middle ear, and pinnae. Hearing loss is common, secondary to noted defects.
(c) *Eyes*: Prominent downslanting of the palpebral fissures; coloboma or notching of the lateral portion of the lower eyelid with absence of eyelashes medial to the notch. Cataracts have also been reported [68].
(d) *Face*: Central face appears prominent because of deficiency of zygomatic arch and micrognathia. Micrognathia is the result of mandibular hypoplasia or the condyle, coronoid process, and the body of the mandible with abnormal ramus [66]. The condyle may have abnormalities of the cartilage and is covered with hyaline rather than fibrocartilage.
(e) *Palate*: Cleft palate—submucous cleft, often of Robin type (U-shaped cleft with micrognathia and glossoptosis). Cleft lip is rare.
(f) *Skull*: Skull anomalies including brachycephaly with bitemporal narrowing, absent or underdeveloped malar bones with nonfusion of the zygomatic arches, hypoplastic zygomatic process, lateral pterygoid plates and muscles, non-pneumatized mastoids, small or absent paranasal sinuses, and absence of infraorbital foramen.
(g) *Other characteristic features*: Brachycephaly, tongue-shaped extension of hair protruding in front of ear, preauricular ear tags, or fistulae externalizing between tragus and corner of mouth.

Heredity and Etiology

Treacher Collins is autosomal dominant with variable penetrance. Approximately 40 % of cases are familial. Mutations of *TCOF*-1, also known as *Treacle*, are identified in 70–93 %. Somatic mosaicism has been reported [69–72]. Treacle mutations lead to haploinsufficiency of a nucleolar phosphoprotein involved in ribosomal RNA production.

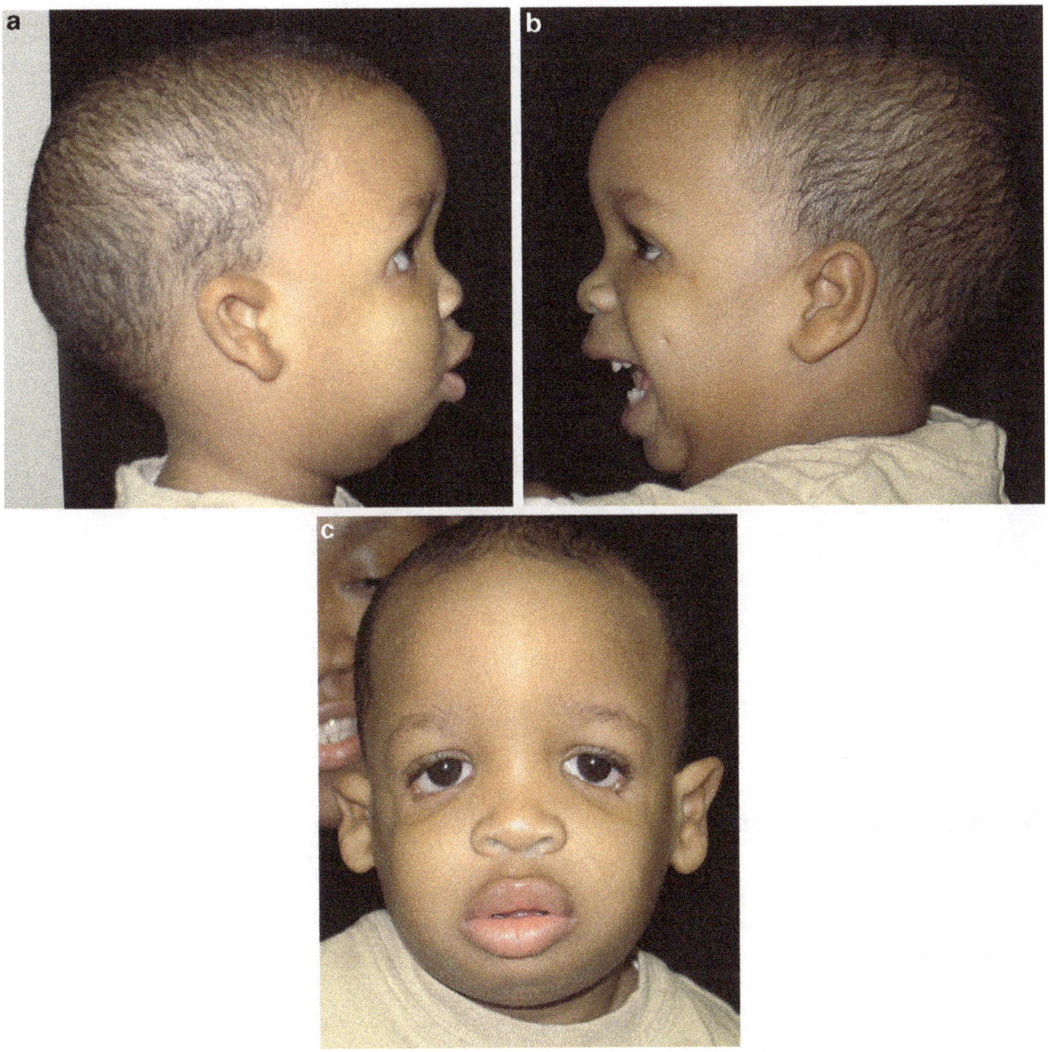

Fig. 1.4 Patient with Treacher Collins syndrome

Animal models of Treacher Collins have been produced by inducing haploinsufficiency of this gene. In mice, haploinsufficiency of Treacle is associated with apoptosis of neural crest cells and prefusion of the neural folds, although the mechanism of these events remains unclear. Occasional cases of Treacher Collins with normal *TCOF-1* have been associated with mutations of polymerase (RNA) 1 polypeptide C (*POLR1C*) [73]. Exposure to isotretinoin in utero can also reproduce craniofacial abnormalities similar to Treacher Collins.

Associated Malformations

Treacher Collins has clinical overlap with Nager syndrome, Miller syndrome, and Robin sequence.

Diagnosis

Sequencing and deletion analysis of *TCOF1* are diagnostic in 70–93 % of affected individuals [69–71]. Somatic mosaicism has been reported [72]. Prenatal sonogram successfully identified many cases [74–78].

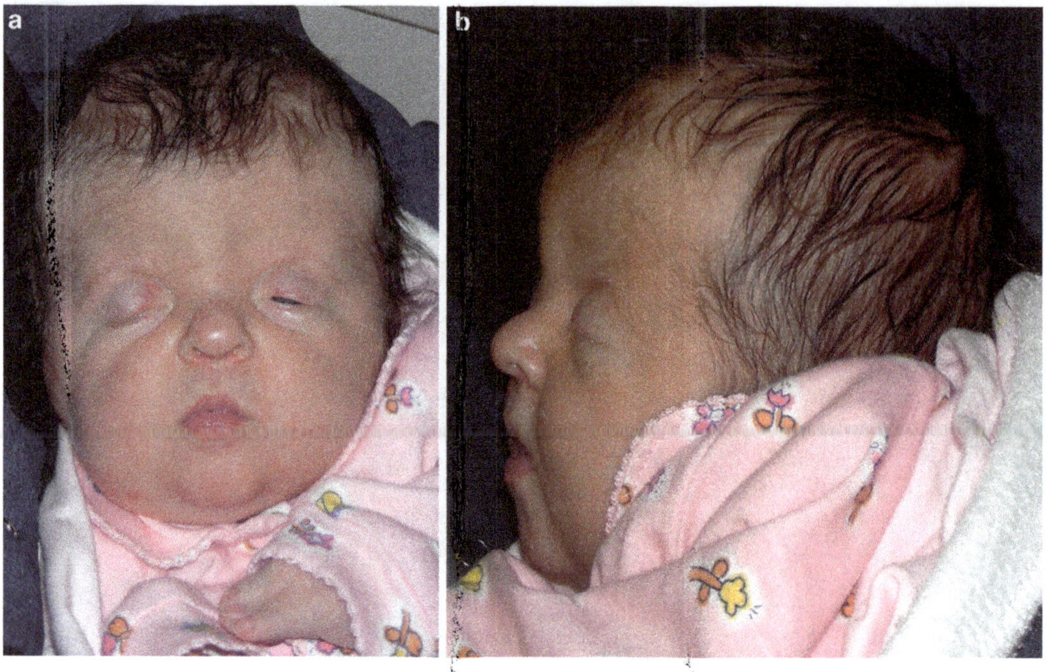

Fig. 1.5 Infant with Apert syndrome

Craniosynostosis Syndromes

Definition

Craniosynostosis, the premature fusion of cranial sutures, occurs in approximately 1/3,000 births. It is most often an isolated finding, affecting the sagittal or coronal sutures. Craniosynostosis can also occur as part of a syndrome, with additional findings such as limb defects and developmental delay. The most common craniosynostosis syndromes are Apert syndrome, Crouzon syndrome, Pfeiffer syndrome, Muenke syndrome, and Saethre–Chotzen syndrome, although more than 100 syndromes associated with craniosynostosis have been described. Figures 1.5, 1.6, and 1.7 demonstrate the typical facial features of children with Apert, Pfeiffer, and Crouzon syndrome respectively.

Clinical Features

Apert syndrome: Apert syndrome is easily distinguished from other craniosynostosis syndromes by the presence of bilateral severe syndactyly of the hands and feet. The thumb is typically spared, with most severe involvement of the second through fourth fingers. This gives the hand the appearance of a mitten. The feet typically involve all toes, with relative sparing of the hallux. The skull has a short anterior–posterior diameter which causes the child to have a high forehead due to bicoronal synostosis. There are often irregularities of the synostosis. Children with Apert syndrome have typical unusual facial features including supraorbital grooves, ocular hypertelorism and downslanting palpebral fissures, depressed nasal bridge with short, broad nose, and long upper lip with thin vermillion border [79]. Most affected individuals have cognitive impairment. Other clinical features in Apert include cardiac defects (10 %), genitorurinary abnormalities (10 %), cleft palate (43 %), choanal stenosis, agenesis of the corpus callosum, and ventriculomegaly [79–81].

Crouzon syndrome: Children with Crouzon syndrome also typically have bicoronal synostosis but lack involvement of the hands or the feet. Facial features include hypertelorism, proptosis, midfacial hypoplasia, and a beaked nose. Occasionally, radiographic abnormalities of the carpal bones may

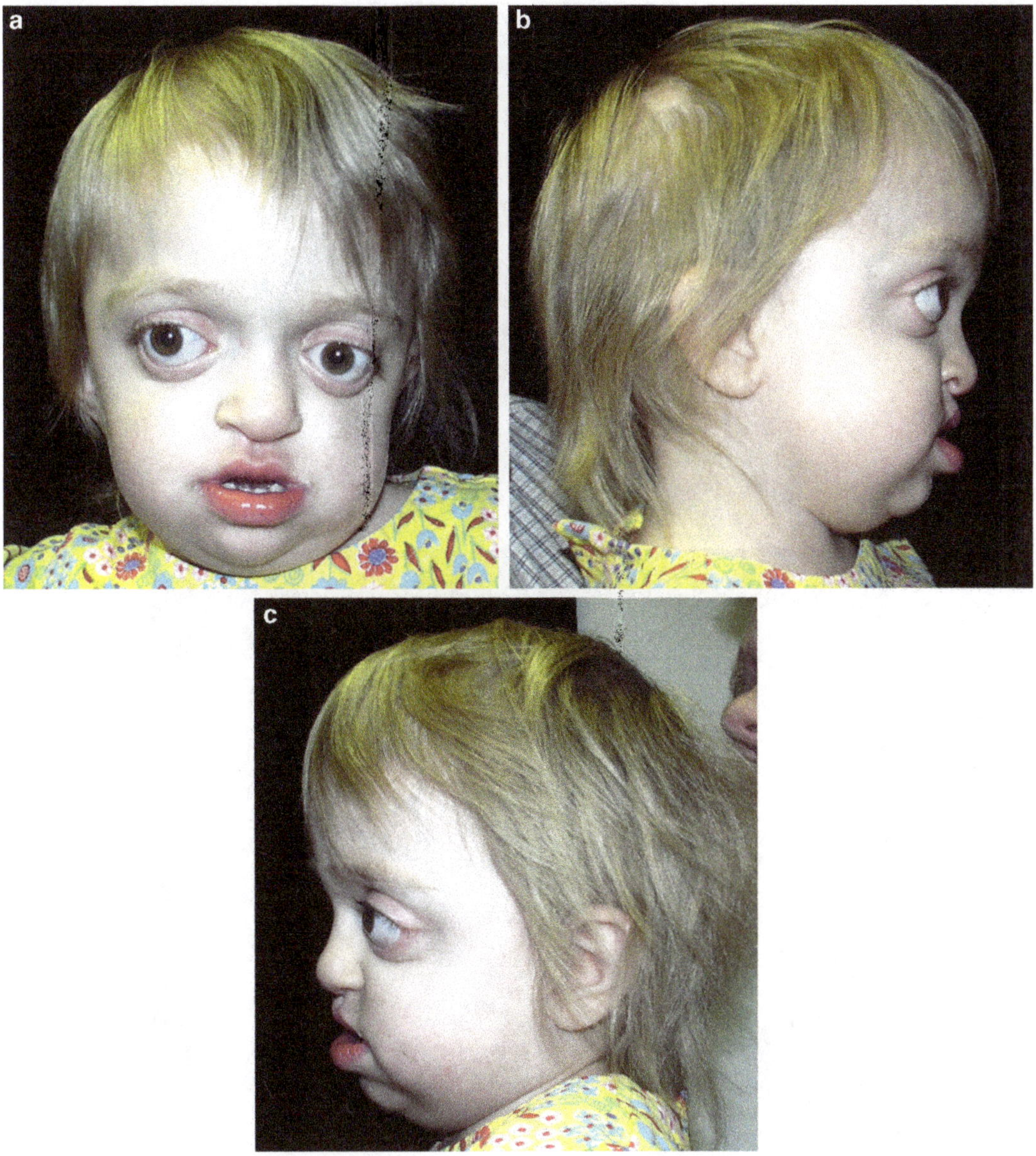

Fig. 1.6 Patient with Pfeiffer syndrome

be seen. Children with Crouzon do not typically have involvement of other organ systems, and cognitive development is normal [79].

Pfeiffer syndrome: Children with Pfeiffer syndrome can be distinguished from those with other craniosynostosis syndromes because they also have broad and medially deviated great toes and broad thumbs. The craniosynostosis in these children results in bicoronal synostosis, but they may also have deformities that result in a cloverleaf-shaped skull. The severity of the phenotype can vary in children with Pfeiffer syndrome, with some being severely affected. Children with Pfeiffer syndrome should also be evaluated for choanal stenosis and tracheal sleeve.

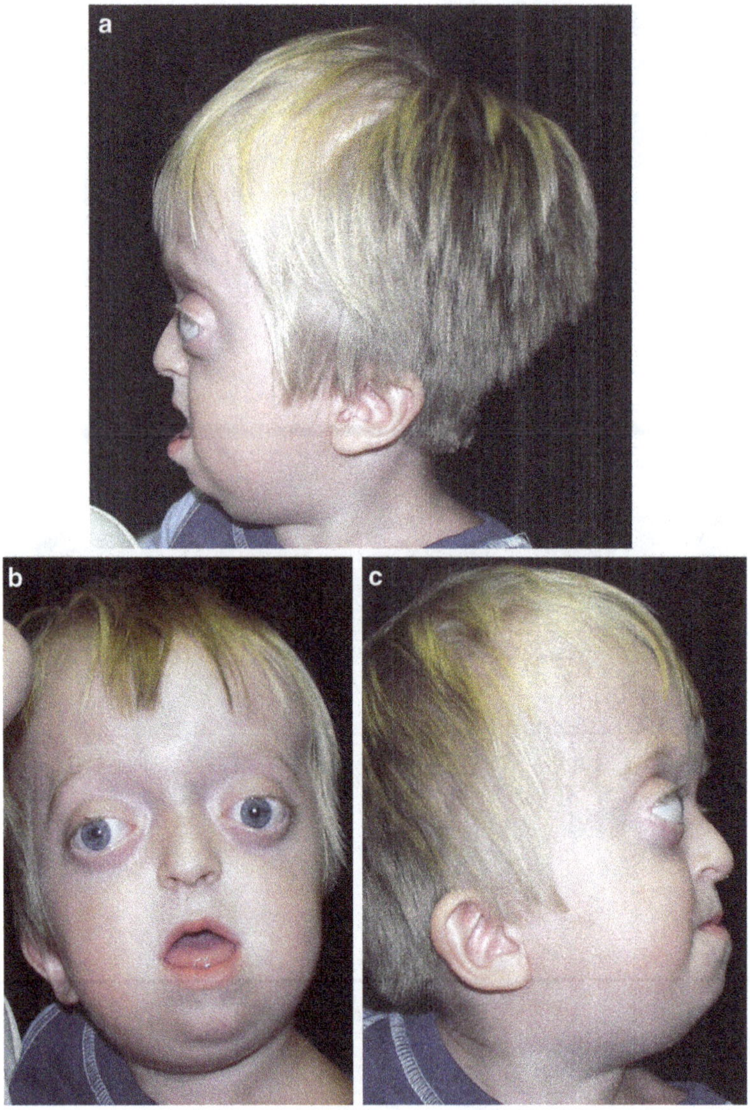

Fig. 1.7 Patient with Crouzon syndrome

Muenke syndrome: Muenke syndrome is characterized by bicoronal or unicoronal synostosis. Macrocephaly, hearing loss, and brachydactyly have also been reported. Abnormalities of the hands, such as thimble-shaped phalanges, may be seen radiographically. There are mild learning disabilities and variable hearing loss associated with this syndrome [79].

Saethre–Chotzen syndrome: Although Saethre–Chotzen is a craniosynostosis syndrome, the presence of craniosynostosis is not an obligate finding for diagnosis. There are a variety of minor clinical features that can be seen in family members, which may lead to genetic testing and diagnosis. There is variable presence and involvement of cranial sutures. The coronal sutures are typically involved in Saethre–Chotzen, but other sutures may be affected resulting in skull and facial asymmetry. Ocular abnormalities in Saethre–Chotzen include ptosis and tear duct stenosis. The ears have characteristic findings including prominent crus and helical roots. The hands are often short and have a single palmar crease and mild syndactyly. The feet have broad or bifid halluces and syndactyly of the toes, which deviate laterally, though not as severely as seen in those children who have Apert syndrome. The cognitive development of these children is normal in most individuals.

Heredity and Etiology

Most craniosynostosis syndromes, including those discussed here, are caused by mutations in *FGFR1*, *FGFR2*, *FGFR3* (fibroblast growth factor genes), and *TWIST* (a transcription gene affecting DNA binding and helix–loop–helix domains).

Apert syndrome: Apert syndrome is caused by one of two point mutations (S252W or P253R) in *FGFR2* leading to an amino acid change [82]. This leads to increased signaling activity due to reduced dissociation of the receptor/ligand complex. Apert syndrome is transmitted autosomal dominantly with complete penetrance, but most cases represent new mutations, and this is reflected in that the affected individuals are more severely affected. The incidence of Apert syndrome increases with advanced paternal age.

Crouzon syndrome: Crouzon syndrome has been associated with a variety of mutations in *FGFR2*. In addition, there is some overlap of mutations of genes that cause Crouzon syndrome and other craniosynostosis syndromes. These mutations are thought to be "gain-of-function mutations" because they confer new or enhanced activity on proteins such as the fibroblast growth factor receptor 2 protein as seen in Crouzon syndrome; however, about half of the cases of Crouzon are not a result of an identified mutation. Inheritance is autosomal dominant, and many cases are familial as there is no effect on reproductive fitness.

Pfeiffer syndrome: Like Crouzon, numerous mutations in *FGFR2* can lead to Pfeiffer syndrome. All mutations in familial cases of Pfeiffer are thought to be autosomal dominant. Mutations are generally de novo in severe cases where reproductive fitness is reduced. Occasional mild cases with mutation in *FGFR1* have been noted.

Muenke syndrome: Muenke syndrome is caused by a Pro250Arg mutation in *FGFR3*. This too is thought to be a "gain-of-function mutation" and is transmitted in an autosomal dominant pattern, and the syndrome may be unrecognized in mildly affected family members.

Saethre–Chotzen syndrome: Saethre–Chotzen is caused by mutations in *TWIST*, a developmentally regulated transcription factor [83–85]. A translocation at the *TWIST* locus has also been reported to result in Saethre–Chotzen [86]. Deletion of *TWIST* can also lead to Saethre–Chotzen. Inheritance of Saethre–Chotzen is autosomal dominant.

Diagnosis

The diagnostic evaluation of children with craniosynostosis should begin with a careful physical exam and attention to associated features as there is molecular overlap in some of the craniosynostosis-related syndromes. Clinical testing is available for *FGFR1*, *FGFR2*, *FGFR3*, and *TWIST*. Special considerations and individual testing recommendations are given below:

Apert syndrome: *FGFR2* sequencing only.

Crouzon syndrome: *FGFR2* sequencing should be done, but mutations are only identified in 60 % of cases, so a negative result does not rule out a diagnosis.

Pfeiffer syndrome: *FGFR2* sequencing is recommended. If negative, consider sequencing of *FGFR1*. Sequencing of *FGFR1* can also be considered as part of the original work-up in mild cases.

Muenke syndrome: *FGFR3* sequencing for Pro250Arg mutation.

Saethre–Chotzen syndrome: *TWIST* sequencing and microdeletion analysis. If these results are normal and the diagnosis is suspected, chromosome analysis for balanced translocations should be performed.

Oculo-Auriculo-Vertebral Spectrum (Hemifacial Microsomia, Goldenhar Syndrome)

Definition

Goldenhar syndrome, part of the oculo-auriculo-vertebral spectrum (OAVS), is characterized by variable degrees of underdevelopment of the ear, mouth, and mandible of one or both sides of the face as well as vertebral anomalies, epibulbar dermoids, cleft palate, and/or hearing loss. Hemifacial macrosomia, in which no epibulbar dermoids are noted, is also part of the OAVS. This group of disorders has also been termed "first and second branchial arch syndrome" based on the embryologic etiology [87–90]. Other disorders in the OAVS include craniofacial microsomia, Goldenhar–Gorlin syndrome, first arch syndrome, facio-auriculo-vertebral syndrome, and lateral facial dysplasia. The distinction of specific disorders along the OAVS has been an area of debate, but cases classified as Goldenhar are thought to represent 10–35 % of cases. The incidence of OAVS is estimated to be 1/5,600 [91]. The male:female ratio is approximately 3:2.

Clinical Features

There is considerable variability in the type and severity of abnormalities in OAVS. Facial features of hemifacial microsomia can be seen in Fig. 1.8, and features typical of Goldenhar can be seen in Fig. 1.9. The phenotypic appearance of the facial findings has been used for further classification within the spectrum, but many other organ systems can also be involved.

(a) *Facies*: Facial asymmetry is seen in the majority of cases, even in children who may have bilateral involvement. Mild cases are often not noticed in infancy but are usually obvious by the age of four [87]. The appearance of asymmetry is produced by a combination of abnormalities of the bony structures, musculature, and soft tissue. Kaban et al. [92] published a revised classification of this disorder based on facial bone abnormalities:
   - Type I, miniature mandible with normal morphology
   - Type IIA, mandibular ramus abnormal in size and shape
   - Type IIB, mandibular ramus abnormal in size, and shape and location requiring costochondral graft construction
   - Type III, absent ramus, condyle, and temporomandibular joint

   In all cases, the temporal bone, orbit, zygoma, nasal bones, and maxilla may be distorted. Those with types IIB and III have the most severe distortion, and affected children often have absent zygomatic arch and hypoplastic or inferiorly displaced orbit.

(b) *Eyes*: A variety of ocular abnormalities are evident. Epibulbar dermoids are the most common ocular abnormality, occurring in up to 35 % of individuals with OAVS [93, 94]. Epibulbar dermoids are white or yellow solid masses that appear on the globe or the orbit, most commonly on the inferotemporal quadrant at the limbus. Typically, children with epibulbar dermoids are classified as having Goldenhar syndrome. Bilateral lesions occur in 25 % of patients and often appear at the same location in each eye. Vision may be impaired as a result of obstruction of the papillary axis, astigmatism, or lipid infiltration of the cornea. Other structural ocular abnormalities may include unilateral colobomas of the upper lid (20 %), bilateral colobomas (3 %), blepharoptosis (narrowing of the palpebral fissure) (10 %), elevation of the orbit (7 %) [95], and, in severe cases, anophthalmia and microphthalmia [93, 94, 96–100]. Patients with epibulbar dermoids have a higher rate of other ocular abnormalities such as blepharoptosis, microphthalmia, and anophthalmia [93, 101, 102]. Ocular motility defects are seen in 25 % of cases, including Duane syndrome, esotropia, and exotropia.

(c) *Ears*: Ear anomalies are found in 65 % of cases and range from anotia to mild underdevelopment of the pinna [97]. There is often a mass of tissue located anteriorly and inferiorly

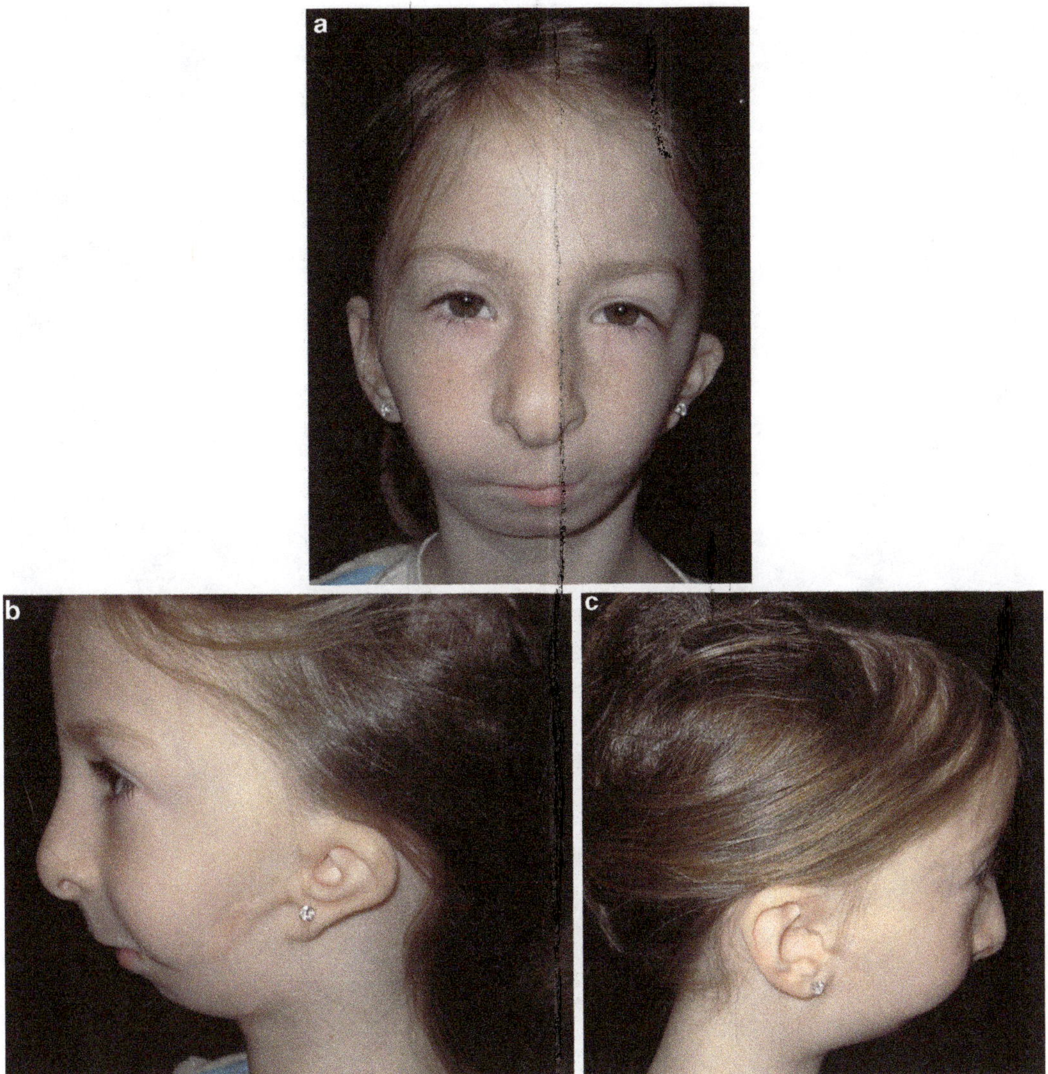

Fig. 1.8 Patient with Hemifacial microsomia

to the location where the ear should have been. Bilateral involvement may be evident. Preauricular skin and cartilage tags or sinuses are seen in at least 40 % of cases [87]. Ear tags are found anywhere between the tragus and the angle of the mouth. Isolated microtia is considered to be part of the OAVS [103], and some consider ear involvement to be a mandatory feature required for diagnosis. Hearing loss may be caused by a variety of structural abnormalities of the ear, including a variable degree of atresia of the auditory canal, ossicle malformations, or skull base abnormalities. Hearing loss is commonly conductive but may include a sensorineural component in 15 % of patients, caused by cranial nerve anomalies [87, 104].

(d) *Mouth*: An appearance of a large mouth may be evident in some individuals either as a result of true macrostomia or because a lateral facial cleft is present. Unilateral agenesis of the parotid gland has been reported in

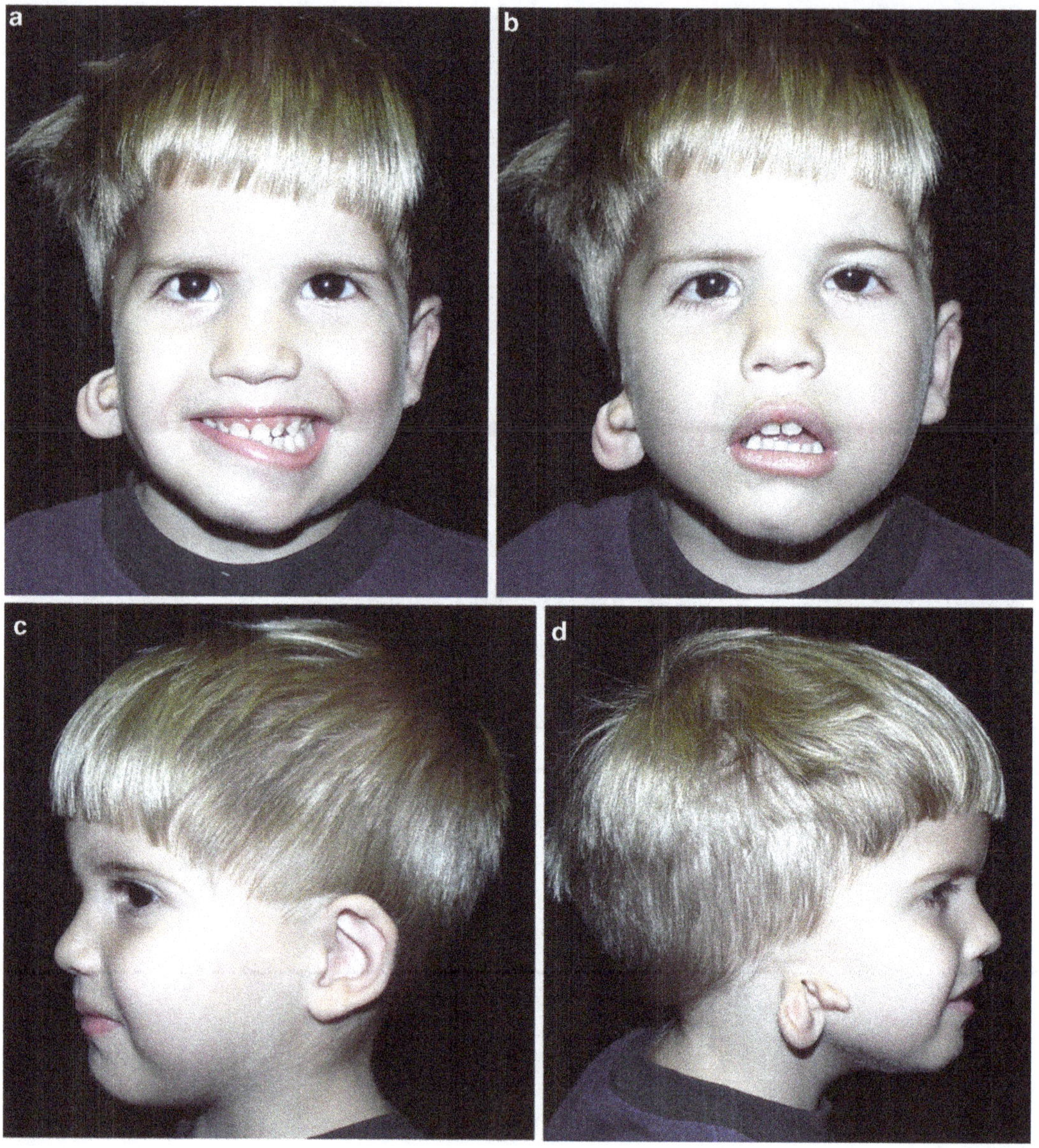

Fig. 1.9 Patient with Goldenhar syndrome

addition to displaced salivary glands and salivary fistulas. Palatal abnormalities may result from defects in the development of bone, musculature, and/or soft tissue. Unilateral or bilateral cleft lip and/or cleft palate occur in 7–15 % of patients. Cleft palate occurs twice as frequently as does cleft lip. The muscles of the tongue or the palate may be hypoplastic or function abnormally, and this may result in velopalatine insufficiency (35 %) because the lateral pharyngeal wall and palate move asymmetrically [105]. Structural palatal abnormalities and dysfunction may cause feeding difficulties in infants with OAVS.

(e) *Neurologic*: Developmental delay is seen in 5–15 % of patients [99]. Cranial nerve involvement is common, and the facial nerve is most often affected [106]. Abnormalities of cranial nerves I, II, III, IV, VI, VIII, IX, and X have also been reported [94, 96, 107, 108]. Though most patients with OAVS have structurally normal brains, a small proportion of cases have a wide variety of structural brain abnormalities, including frontal and occipital encephaloceles, hydrocephalus, lipoma of the corpus callosum, dermoid cyst, teratoma, Arnold–Chiari malformation, lissencephaly, arachnoid cyst, holoprosencephaly, porencephalic cyst, unilateral arhinencephaly, anomalies of the pons, pseudotumor cerebri, and hypoplasia of the corpus callosum [87, 109].

(f) *Trachea and lung*: Tracheoesophageal fistula is seen in 5 % of children with OAVS [110]. Incomplete lung lobulation or agenesis is sometimes noted and is usually ipsilateral to the facial anomalies [111].

(g) *Cardiac*: Cardiac defects occur in approximately 35 % of patients (ranging in incidence from 5 to 60 %). Ventricular septal defect or Tetralogy of Fallot with or without right aortic arch accounts for 65 % of defects, but many other structural cardiac defects have been reported. These include Transposition of the Great Vessels, tubular hypoplasia of the aortic arch, coarctation of the aorta, abnormal situs, cardiomegaly, isolation of the left innominate artery with bilateral patent ductus arteriosus, pulmonic stenosis, dextrocardia, double-outlet right ventricle, hypoplasia of the internal carotid artery, and external carotid artery [112].

(h) *Skeletal abnormalities*: In addition to skull and facial anomalies discussed above, there are a variety of other skeletal abnormalities and some are common, such as cervical spine malformations. Fusion of the cervical spine is seen in up to 60 %. Platybasia and occipitalization of the atlas are seen in 30 % [113]. Instability of C1–C2 has also been reported [80]. Structural abnormalities of the vertebrae (spina bifida, hemivertebrae, butterfly vertebrae, Klippel–Feil anomaly, scoliosis) and rib abnormalities are seen in a third of patients with OAVS [89]. A variety of radial limb defects are seen in 10 %, including radial or thumb hypoplasia or digitalized thumb [87, 114].

(i) *Other*: Other abnormalities include renal malformations, including absent kidney, double ureter, crossed renal ectopia, anomalous blood supply to the kidney, renal artery stenosis, hydronephrosis, and hydroureter [115]. Additionally, imperforate anus, rectovaginal fistula, situs inversus, tracheoesophageal fistula, duodenal atresia, and portal vein cavernoma have been described in these patients [116–120].

Heredity and Etiology

Abnormalities seen in OAVS originate between days 30 and 45 of gestation. The seemingly unconnected abnormalities in OAVS are thought to be the result of abnormal development of a "developmental field," a set of cells in the embryo that are susceptible to the same genetic, toxic, or vascular insult [121]. Animal and human studies have shown that vascular disruption during this time period is sufficient to result in an OAVS phenotype [88, 122–124]. Other insults to the developing embryo such as exposure to thalidomide [125], primidone [126], and retinoic acid [127] and maternal diabetes [128, 129] can result in damage to the first and second branchial arches and an OAVS-like appearance.

OAVS has been diagnosed in cases of children with a variety of cytogenetic abnormalities, including del 1p22.2-p31.1 [130], del(5p) [131, 132], del(6q), del(8q) [133], trisomy 10p [134], trisomy 18 [135], recombinant chromosome 18 [136], del(18q) [137], ring 21 chromosome, del (22qter) [138], dup(22q) [139], trisomy 22 [140], 22q11.2 DS [112, 141, 142], 45, X [143], 49, XXXXX [144], 49 XXXXY [145], 47, XXY [146], mosaic trisomy 7 [147], mosaic trisomy 9 [148, 149], and mosaic trisomy 22 [148].

Most cases are isolated, and empiric recurrence risk is 2–3 %. There is a higher rate in twins as compared with singleton pregnancies, but there is no difference in the concordance rate in monozygotic and dizygotic twins, suggesting that most cases are sporadic [150]. However, there have been occasional reports of recurrence in subsequent generations and occasional cases of affected siblings born to unaffected parents [87]. Eye and vertebral anomalies were rare in these familial cases. Using segregation analysis, Kaye et al. [151] suggested autosomal dominant inheritance with variable expressivity for these families. Genetic counseling for recurrence would be beneficial in familial cases and when cytogenetic abnormalities have been identified as noted above.

Diagnosis

Diagnosis is based on clinical features, as most cases are sporadic with no genetic abnormality identified. Genomic microarray analysis should be included as part of the work-up because of the high prevalence of abnormalities but is normal in most cases of OAVS.

References

1. Robin P. La chute de la base de la langue consideree comme une nouvelle cause de gene dans la respiration nase-pharyngienne. Bull Acad Med (Paris). 1923;89:37–41.
2. Robin P. Glossoptosis due to atresia and hypotrophy of the mandible. Am J Dis Child. 1934;48:541–7.
3. Izumi K, Konczal LL, Mitchell AL, Jones MC. Underlying genetic diagnosis of Pierre Robin Sequence: retrospective chart review at two children's hospitals and a systematic literature review. J Pediatr. 2012;160:645–50.
4. Sher AE, Shprintzen RJ, Thorpy MJ. Endoscopic observations of obstructive sleep apnea in children with anomalous upper airways: predictive and therapeutic value. Int J Pediatr Otorhinolaryngol. 1986;11:135–46.
5. Shprintzen RJ. Robin sequence. In: Cassidy SB, Allanson JE, editors. Management of genetic syndromes. 2nd ed. Hoboken, NJ: WileyLiss; 2005. p. 469–78.
6. Cohen MM. The Robin anomalad – its nonspecificity and associated syndromes. J Oral Surg. 1976; 34(7):587–93.
7. Poswillo D. The aetiology and surgery of cleft palate with micrognathia. Ann R Coll Surg Eng. 1968;43: 61–88.
8. Latham RA. The pathogenesis of cleft palate associated with the Pierre Robin syndrome. Br J Plast Surg. 1966;19:205–14.
9. Pagon RA, Graham JM, Zonana J, Yong SL. Coloboma, congenital heart disease, and choanal atresia with multiple anomalies: CHARGE association. J Pediatr. 1981;99(2):223–7.
10. Lin AE, Chin AJ, Devine W, Park SC, Zackai E. The pattern of cardiovascular malformation in the CHARGE association. Am J Med Genet. 1990;37:304–10.
11. Pinto G, Abadie V, Mesnage R, et al. CHARGE syndrome includes hypogonadotropic hypogonadism and abnormal olfactory bulb development. J Clin Endo Metab. 2005;90(10):5621–6.
12. Hennekam RCM, Krantz, ID, Allanson JE. Well-known miscellaneous syndromes. In: Gorlin's syndromes of the head and neck. 5th ed. New York: Oxford University Press; 2010. p. 1258–94.
13. Sanlaville D, Verloes A. CHARGE syndrome: an update. Eur J Hum Genet. 2007;15:389–99.
14. Oley CA, Baraitser M, Grant DB. A reappraisal of the CHARGE association. J Med Genet. 1988;25:147–56.
15. Stromland K, Sjogreen L, Johansson M, et al. CHARGE association in Sweden: malformations and functional deficits. Am J Med Genet A. 2005;133A(3):331–9.
16. Farquhar J, Carachi R, Raine PAM. Twins with oesophageal atresia and the CHARGE association. Eur J Pediatr Surg. 2002;12:56–8.
17. Levin DL, Muster AJ, Newfeld EA, Paul MH. Concordant aortic arch anomalies in monozygotic twins. J Pediatr. 1973;83:459–61.
18. Tellier AL, Cormier-Daire V, Abadle V, et al. CHARGE syndrome: report of 47 cases and review. Am J Med Genet. 1998;76:402–9.
19. Vissers LELM, van Ravenswaaij CMA, Admiraal R, et al. Mutations in a new member of the chromodomain gene family cause CHARGE syndrome. Nat Genet. 2004;36:955–7.
20. Lalani SR, Safiullah AM, Molinari LM, Fernbach SD, Martin DM, Belmont JW. *SEMA3E* mutation in a patient with CHARGE syndrome. J Med Genet. 2004;41:e94.
21. Wilson DI, Cross IE, Goodship JA, Brown J, Scambler JP, Bain HH, Taylor JFN, Walsh K, Bankier A, Burn J, Wolstenholme J. A prospective cytogenetic study of 36 cases of DiGeorge syndrome. Am J Hum Genet. 1992;51:957–63.
22. Devriendt K, Fryns JP, Mortier G, van Thienen MN. The annual incidence of DiGeorge/velocardiofacial syndrome. J Med Genet. 1998;35:789–90.
23. Goodship J, Cross I, LiLing J, Wren C. A population study of chromosome 22q11 deletions in infancy. Arch Dis Child. 2000;79:348–51.
24. Scambler PJ. The 22q11.2 deletion syndromes. Hum Mol Genet. 2000;10:2421–6.
25. Botto LD, May K, Fernhoff PM, Correa A. A population based study of the 22q11.2 deletion: phenotype, incidence and contribution to major birth defects in the population. Pediatrics. 2003;112: 101–7.
26. Oakarsdottir S, Vujic M, Fasth A. Incidence and prevalence of the 22q11 deletion syndrome: a population-based study in Western Sweden. Arch Dis Child. 2004;89:148–51.

27. De la Chapelle A, Herva R, Koivisto M, Aula P. A deletion in chromosome 22 can cause DiGeorge syndrome. Hum Genet. 1981;57:253–6.
28. Kelley RI, Zackai EH, Emanuel BS, Kistenmacher M, Greenberg F, Punnett HH. The association of the DiGeorge anomalad with partial monosomy of chromosome 22. J Pediatr. 2005;197:229–33.
29. Driscoll DA, Budarf ML, Emanuel BS. A genetic etiology for DiGeorge syndrome: consistent deletions and microdeletions of 22q11. Am J Hum Genet. 1992;50:924–33.
30. Driscoll DA, Salvin J, Sellinger B, McDonald-McGinn D, Zackai EH, Emanuel BS. Prevalence of 22q11 microdeletions in DGS and VCFS: implications for genetic counseling and prenatal diagnosis. J Med Genet. 1993;30:813–7.
31. Burn J, Takao A, Wilson D, Cross I, Momma K, Wadey R, Scambler P, Goodship J. Conotruncal anomaly face syndrome is associated with a deletion within chromosome 22. J Med Genet. 1993;30: 822–4.
32. Matsouka R, Takao A, Kimura M, Imamura S-I, Kondo C, Joh-o K, Ikeda K, Nishibatake M, Ando M, Momma K. Confirmation that the conotruncal anomly face syndrome is associated with a deletion within 22q11.2. Am J Med Genet. 1994;53:285–9.
33. Giannoti A, Diglio MC, Marino B, Mingarelli R, Dallapiccola B. Cayler cardiofacial syndrome and del 22q11: Part of the CATCH22 pehnotype. Am J Med Genet. 1994;30:807–12.
34. Bawle EV, Conard J, Van Dyke DI, Czarnecki P, Driscoll DA. Letter to the Editor: Seven new cases of Cayler cardiofacial syndrome with chromosome 22q11.2 deletion, including a new familial case. Am J Med Genet. 1998;79:406–10.
35. Wilson DI, Cross IE, Wren C. Minimum prevalence of chromosome 22q11 deletions. Am J Hum Genet Suppl. 1994;55:A169.
36. Rausch A, Hoyer J, Guth S, Sweier C, Kraus C, Becker C, Zenker M, Huffmeier U, Thiel C, Ruschendorf F, Nurnberg P, Reis A, Trautmann U. Diagnostic yield of various genetic approaches in patients with unexplained developmental delay or mental retardation. Am J Med Genet A. 2006;140:2063–74.
37. McDonald-McGinn DM, Kohut T, Zackai EH. Deletion 22q11.2 (Velocardiofacial syndrome/ DiGeorge syndrome). In: Cassidy SB, Allanson JE, editors. Management of genetic syndromes. 3rd ed. Hoboken, NJ: John Wiley & Sons; 2010. p. 263–84.
38. Gripp KW, McDonald-McGinn DM, Driscoll DA, Reed LA, Emanuel BS, Zackai EH. Nasal dimple as part of the 22q11.2 deletion syndrome. Am J Med Genet. 1997;69:290–2.
39. McDonald-McGinn DM, Kirschner R, Goldmuntz E, Sullivan K, Eicher P, Gerdes M, Moss E, Solot C, Wang P, Jacobs I, Handler S, Knightly C, Heher K, Wilson M, Mig JE, Grace K, Driscoll D, Pasquariello P, Randall P, LaRossa D, Emanuel BS, Zackai EH. The Philadelphia story: the 22q11.2 deletion: report on 250 patients. Genet Couns. 1999;10:11–24.
40. Swillen A, Devriendt K, Vantrappen G, et al. Familial deletions of 22q11.2: the Leuven experience. Am J Med Genet. 1997;80:531–2.
41. Bassett A, Hodgkinson K, Chow E, Correia S, Scutt L, Weksberg R. 22q11 deletion syndrome in adults with schizophrenia. Am J Med Genet. 1998;81(4):328–37.
42. Murphy KC, Jones LA, Own MJ. High rates of schizophrenia in adults with velo-cardio-facial syndrome. Arch Gen Psychiatr. 1999;56(10):940–5.
43. Beauchesne LM, Warnes CA, Connolly HM, Ammash NM, Grogan M, Jala SM, Michels VV. J Am Coll Cardiol. 2005;45:595–8.
44. McDonald-McGinn DM, Minugh-Purvis N, Kirschner R, Jawad A, Tonnesen MK, Catazaro JR, Driscoll D, LaRossa D, Emanuel B, Zackai EH. The 22q11.2 deletion in African-American patients? An underdiagnosed population. Am J Med Genet. 2005;134:242–6.
45. Cormier-Daire V, Iserin L, Theophile D, Sidi D, Vervel C, Padovani JP, Vekemans M, Munnich A, Lyonnet S. Upper limb malformations in DiGeorge syndrome. Am J Med Genet. 1995;56:39–41.
46. Diglio MC, Giannotti A, Marino B, Guadagni AM, Orzalesi M, Dallapiccola B. Radial aplasia and chromosome 22q11. deletion. J Med Genet. 1997;34:942–4.
47. Devriendt K, de Smet L, de Boeck K, Fryns JP. DiGeorge syndrome and unilateral symbrachydactyly. Genet Couns. 1997;8:345–7.
48. Ming JE, McDonald-McGinn DM, Megerian TE, Driscoll DA, Elias ER, Russell BM, Irons M, Emanuel BS, Markowitz RI, Zackai EZ. Skeletal anomalies and deformities in patients with deletions of 22q11. Am J Med Genet. 1997;72(2):210–5.
49. Prasad C, Quackenbush EJ, Whitemena D, Korf B. Limb anomalies in DiGeorge and CHARGE syndromes. Am J Med Genet. 1997;68:179–81.
50. Nickel RE, Magenis RE. Neural tube defects and deletions of 22q11.2. Am J Med Genet. 1996;66(1):25–7.
51. McDonald-McGinn DM, Driscoll DA, Bason L, Christensen K, Lynch D, Sullivan K, Canning D, Zavod W, Quinn N, Rome J, Paris Y, Weinberg P, Clark BJ, Emanuel BS, Zackai EH. Autosomal dominant "Opitz" GBBB syndrome due to a 22q11.2 deletion. Am J Med Genet. 1995;59:103–13.
52. Keenan GF, Sullivan KE, McDonald-McGinn DM, Zackai EH. Letter to the Editor: Arthritis associated with 22q11.2: more common than previously suspected. Am J Med Genet. 1997;71:488.
53. Sullivan KE, McDonald-McGinn DM, Driscoll DA, Zmijewski CM, Ellabban AS, Reed L, Emanuel BS, Zackai EH, Athreya BH, Keenan G. JRA-like polyarthritis in chromosome 22q11.2 deletion syndrome (DiGeorge anomalad/velocardiofacial syndrome/ conotruncal anomaly face syndrome). Arthritis Rheum. 1997;40:430–6.
54. Kawame H, Adachi M, Tachibana K, Kurosawa K, Ito F, Gleason MM, Weinzimer S, Levitt-Katz L, Sullivan K, McDonald-McGinn DM. Graves' disease in patients with 22q11.2 deletion. J Pediatr. 2001;139:892–5.

55. Ryan AK, Goodship JA, Wilson DI, Philip N, Levy A, et al. Spectrum of clinical features associated with interstitial chromosome 22q11.2 deletions: a European collaborative study. J Med Genet. 1997;34:798–804.
56. Gong W, Emanuel BS, Collins J, Kim DH, Wang Z, Chen F, Zhang G, Roe B, Budarf ML. A transcription map of the DiGeroge and velo-cardio-facial syndrome minimal critical region on 22q11. Hum Mol Genet. 1996;58:1377–81.
57. McDonald-McGinn DM, Catania C, Saitta S, Kaplan P, Coppinger J, Shaffer L, Emanuel BS, Zackai EH. Atypical 22111.2 deletions. Proc Greenwood Genet Cent. 2008;27:106–7.
58. Emanuel BS, Budard ML, Shaikh T, Driscoll D. Blocks of duplicated sequence define the endpoints of DGS/VCFS 22q11.2 deletions. Am J Hum Genet. 1998;63:A11.
59. Edelman L, Pandita RK, Morrow BE. Low-copy repeats mediate the common 3-Mb deletion in patients with velo-cardio-facial syndrome. Am J Hum Genet. 1999;64:1076–86.
60. Shaikh TH, Kurahashi H, Saitta SC, Hu P, Rose BA, Driscoll DA, McDonald-McGinn DM, Zackai EH, Budarf ML, Emanuel BS. Chromosome 22-specific low copy repeats and the 22q11.2 deletion syndrome: genomic organization and deletion endpoint analysis. Hum Mol Genet. 2000;9:489–501.
61. Baumer A, Riegel M, Schinzel A. Non-random asynchronous replicate ion at 22q11.2 favours unequal meiotic crossovers leading to the human 22q11.2 deletion. J Med Genet. 2004;41:413–20.
62. Saitta SC, Harris SE, McDonald-McGinn DM, Emanuel BS, Tonnesen MK, Zackai EH, Seitz SC, Driscoll DA. Independent *de novo* 22q11.2 deletions in first cousins with DiGeorge/velocardiofacial syndrome. Am J Med Genet. 2004;124:313–7.
63. Kariyazono H, Ohno T, Ihara K, Igarashi H, Joh-o K, Ishikawa S, Hara T. Rapid detection of the 22111.2 deletion with quantitative real-time PCR. Mol Cell Probes. 2001;15:71–5.
64. Mantripragada KK, Tapia-Paez I, Blennow E, Nilsson P, Wedell A, Dumanski JP. DNA copy-number analysis of the 22q11 deletion-syndrome region using array-CGH with genomic and PCR-based targets. Int J Mol Med. 2004;13:273–9.
65. Fernandez L, Lapunzina P, Pajares IL, Criado GR, Garcia-Guereta I, Perez J, Quero J, Delicado A. Higher frequency of uncommon 1.5–2 Mb deletions found in familial cases of 22q11.2 deletion syndrome. Am J Med Genet. 2005;136:71–5.
66. Hennekam RCM, Krantz, ID, Allanson JE. Orofacial clefting syndromes: general aspects. In: Gorlin's syndromes of the head and neck. 5th ed. New York: Oxford University Press; 2010. p. 943–72.
67. Stovin JJ, Lyon JA, Clemens RL. Mandibulofacial dysostosis. Radiology. 1960;74:225–31.
68. Biebersheimer JB, Fredrick DR. Delayed-onset infantile cataracts in a case of Treacher Collins syndrome. Arch Ophthalmol. 2004;122:1721–2.
69. Dixon J, Ellis I, Bottani A, Temple K, Dixon MJ. Identification of mutations in TCOF1: Use of molecular analysis in the pre- and postnatal diagnosis of Treacher Collins syndrome. Am J Med Genet. 2004;127A:244–8.
70. Splendore A, Silva EO, Alonso LG, et al. High mutation detection rate in *TCOF1* among Treacher Collins syndrome patients reveals clustering of mutations and 16 novel pathogenic changes. Hum Mutat. 2000;16:315–22.
71. Teber OA, Gillessen-Kaesbach G, Fischer S, et al. Genotyping in 46 patients with tentative diagnosis of Treacher Collins syndrome revealed unexpected phenotypic variation. Eur J Hum Genet. 2004;12:879–80.
72. Shoo BA. Mosaicism of a *TCOF1* mutation in an individual clinically unaffected with Treacher Collins syndrome. Am J Med Genet. 2004;126A:84–8.
73. Dauwerse JG, Dixon J, Seland S, et al. Mutations in gene encoding subunits of RNA polymerases I and III cause Treacher Collins syndrome. Nat Genet. 2011;43:20–2.
74. Behrents RG, McNamara JA, Avery JK. Prenatal mandibulofacial dysostosis (Treacher Collins in man). Cleft Palat J. 1977;14:13–34.
75. Crane JP, Beaver HA. Midtrimester sonographic diagnosis of mandibular dysostosis. Am J Med Genet. 1986;25:251–5.
76. Hsu TY, Hus JJ, Chang SY, Chang MS. Prenatal three-dimensional sonographic images associated with Treacher Collins syndrome. Ultrasound Obstet Gynecol. 2002;19:413–22.
77. Meizner I, Carmi R, Katz M. Prenatal ultrasonic diagnosis of mandibulofacial dysostosis (Treacher Collins syndrome). J Clin Ultrasound. 1991;19:124–7.
78. Tanaka Y, Kanenishi K, Tanaka H, Yanagihara T, Hata T. Antenatal three-dimensional sonographic features of Treacher Collins syndrome. Ultrasound Obstet Gynecol. 2002;19:414–5.
79. Gripp KW, Zackai EH. Craniosynostosis syndromes. In: Cassidy SB, Allanson JE, editors. Management of genetic syndromes. 2nd ed. Hoboken, NJ: WileyLiss; 2005. p. 163–70.
80. Slaney SF, Oldridge M, Hurst JA, et al. Differential effects of *FGFR2* mutations on syndactyly and cleft palate in Apert syndrome. Am J Hum Genet. 1996;58(5):923–32.
81. Cohen Jr MM. Apert syndrome In: Cohen MM Jr, MacLean RE, editors. Craniosynostosis, diagnosis, evaluation and management. New York: Oxford University Press; 2000.
82. Wilkie AOM. Craniosynostosis: genes and mechanisms. Hum Mol Genet. 1997;6(10):1647–56.
83. El Ghouzzi V, Le Merrer M, Perrin-Schmitt F, et al. Mutations of the *TWIST* gene in the Saethre-Chotzen syndrome. Nat Genet. 1997;15:42–6.
84. Howard TD, Paznekas WA, Green ED, et al. Mutations in *TWIST*, a basic helix-loop-helix transcription factor, in Saethre-Chotzen syndrome. Nat Genet. 1997;15:35–41.

85. Johnson D, Horsley SW, Maloney DM, et al. A comprehensive screen for *TWIST* mutations in patients with craniosynostosis identifies a new microdeletion syndrome of chromosome band 7p21.1. Am J Hum Genet. 1998;63(5):1282–93.
86. Reid CS, McMorrow LE, McDonald-McGinn DM, et al. Saethre-Chotzen syndrome with familial translocation at chromosome 7p22. Am J Med Genet. 1993;47(5):637–9.
87. Hennekam RCM, Krantz, ID, Allanson JE. Branchial arch and oral-acral disorders. In: Gorlin's syndromes of the head and neck. 5th ed. New York: Oxford University Press; 2010. p. 879–942.
88. Gorlin RJ, Jue KL, Jacobsen U, Goldschmidt E. Oculoauriculovertebral dysplasia. J Pediatr. 1963;63:991–9.
89. Gibson JNA, Sillence DO, Taylor TKF. Abnormalities of the spine in Goldenhar's syndrome. J Pediatr Orthop. 1996;16:344–9.
90. Jongbloet PH. Goldenhar syndrome and overlapping dysplasias in vitro fertilization and ovopathy. J Med Genet. 1987;24:616–20.
91. Grabb WC. The first and second branchial arch syndrome. Plast Reconstr Surg. 1965;36:485–508.
92. Kaban LB, Moses MH, Mulliken JB. Surgical correction of hemifacial microsomia. Plast Reconstr Surg. 1988;82:9–19.
93. Baum JL, Feingold M. Ocular aspects of Goldenhar's syndrome. Am J Ophthalmol. 1973;75:250–7.
94. Margolis S, Aleksic S, Charles N, McCarthy J, Greco A, Budzilovich G. Retinal and optic nerve findings in Goldenhar-Gorlin syndrome. Ophthalmology. 1984;91:1327–33.
95. Padwa BL, Bruneteau RJ, Mullikan JB. Association between "Plagiocephaly" and hemifacial microsomia. Am J Med Genet. 1993;47:1202–7.
96. Aleksic S, Budzilovich G, Reuben R, et al. Unilateral arhinencephaly in Goldenhar-Gorlin syndrome. Dev Med Child Neurol. 1975;17:498–504.
97. Coccaro PJ, Becker MH, Converse JM. Clinical and radiographic variations in hemifacial microsomia. Birth Defects. 1975;11(2):314–24.
98. Cohen Jr MM. Variability versus "incidental findings" in the first and second branchial arch syndrome: unilateral variants with anophthamia. Birth Defects. 1971;7(7):103–8.
99. Shokeir MHK. The Goldenhar syndrome: a natural history. Birth Defects. 1977;13(3C):67–83.
100. Wilson GN. Cranial defects in Goldenhar's syndrome. Am J Med Genet. 1983;14:435–43.
101. Mansour AM, Wang F, Henkind P, Goldberg R, Shprintzen R. Ocular findings in the facio-auriculovertebral sequence (Goldenhar-Gorlin syndrome). Am J Ophthalmol. 1985;100:555–9.
102. Rollnick BR, Kaye CE, Nagatoshi K. Oculo-auriculo-vertebral dysplasia and variants: phenotypic characteristics of 194 patients. Am J Med Genet. 1987;26:361–75.
103. Bennun RD, Mulliken JB, Kaban LB, Murray JE. Microtia: a microform of hemifacial microsomia. Plast Reconstr Surg. 1985;76:859–63.
104. Scholtz AW, Fish 3rd JH, Kammen-Jolly K, et al. Goldenhar's syndrome: congenital hearing deficit of conductive or sensorineural origin? Temporal bone histopathologic study. Otol Neurotol. 2001;4:501–5.
105. Shprintzen RJ. Palatal and pharyngeal anomalies in craniofacial syndromes. Birth Defects. 1982;18(1):53–78.
106. Carvalho GJ, Song CS, Vargervik K, Lalwani AK. Auditory and facial nerve dysfunction in patients with hemifacial microsomia. Arch Otolaryngol Head Neck Surg. 1999;125(2):209–12.
107. Aleksic S, Budzilovich G, Choy A, et al. Congenital opthalmoplegia in oculoauriculovertebral dysplasia-hemifacial microsomia (Goldenhar-Gorlin syndrome). A clinicopathologic study and review of the literature. Neurology. 1976;26(7):638–44.
108. Aleksic S, Budzilovich G, Greco MA, et al. Intracranial lipomas, hydrocephalus and other CNS anomalies in oculo-auriculo-vertebral dysplasia (Goldenhar-Gorlin syndrome). Childs Brain. 1984;11:285–97.
109. Schrander-Stumpel CT, de Die-Smulders CE, Hennekam RC, et al. Oculoauriculovertebral spectrum and cerebral anomalies. J Med Genet. 1992;29(5):326–32.
110. Sutphen R, Galan-Gomez E, Cortada X, Newkirk PN, Kousseff BG. Tracheoesophageal anomalies in oculoauriculovertebral (Goldenhar) spectrum. Clin Genet. 1995;48(2):66–71.
111. Milani D, Selicorni A. Right pulmonary agenesis with ipsilateral microtia: a new laterality association or part of the aculoauriculovertebral spectrum? Prenat Diag. 2002;22(11):1053–4.
112. Digilio MC, Calzolari F, Capolino R, et al. Congenital heart defects in patients with oculo-auriculo-vertebral spectrum (Goldenhar syndrome). Am J Med Genet A. 2008;146A(14):1815–9.
113. Gosain AK, McCarthy JG, Pinto RS. Cervicovertebral anomalies and basilar impression in Goldenhar syndrome. Plast Reconstr Surg. 1994;93(3):498–506.
114. Moeschler J, Clarren SK. Familial occurrence of hemifacial microsomia with radial limb defects. Am J Med Genet. 1982;12:371–5.
115. Ritchey ML, Norbeck J, Huang C, Keating MA, Bloom DA. Urologic manifestations of Goldenhar syndrome. Urology. 1994;43(1):88–91.
116. Gorgu M, Aslan G, Erdooan B, Karaca C, Akoz T. Goldenhar syndrome with situs inversus totalis. Int J Oral Maxillofacial Surg. 1998;27:404.
117. Hacihamdioglu B, Unay B, Hacihamdioglu DO, Vurucu S, Gul D, Akin R. Goldenhar syndrome with duodenal atresia: a new finding. Clin Dysmorphol. 2008;17(2):141–2.
118. Handa R, Upadhyay KK. Goldenhar Syndrome with H type tracheo esophageal fistula. Indian Pediatr. 2003;40(6):583–4.
119. McCarthy VP, Zimo DA, Lucas MA. Airway in the oculo-auriculo-vertebral spectrum: two cases and a review of the literature. Pediatr Pulmonol. 2001;32(3):250–6.

120. Stringer MD, Tovar JA, McKiernan PJ, Tanner S. Portal vein cavernoma associated with goldenhar syndrome. J Pediatr Gastroenterol Nutr. 2005;41(3): 368–70.
121. Cousley RRJ, Wilson DJ. Hemifacial microsomia: developmental consequence of perturbation of the auriculofacial cartilage model? Am J Med Genet. 1992;42:461–6.
122. Hennekam RCM, Hofstee N. Familial liability to intrauterine vascular impairments. Pediatrics. 1990;86:326–7.
123. Robinson LK, Hoyme HE, Edwards DK, Jones KL. The vascular pathogenesis of unilateral craniofacial defects. J Pediatr. 1987;111:236–9.
124. Soltan HC, Holmes LB. Familial occurrence of malformations possible attributable to vascular abnormalities. J Pediatr. 1986;109:112–4.
125. Rosenal TH. Aplasia-hypoplasia of the otic labyrinth after thalidomide. Acta Radiol. 1965;3:225–36.
126. Gustavson EE, Chen H. Goldenhar syndrome, anterior encephalocele and aqueductal stenosis following fetal primidone exposure. Teratology. 1985; 32:13–7.
127. Lammer EJ, Chen DT, Hoar RM, et al. Retinoic acid embryopathy. N Engl J Med. 1985;313(14):837–41.
128. Grix Jr A. Malformations in infants of diabetic mothers. Am J Med Genet. 1982;13:131–7.
129. Wang R, Martinez-Frias ML, Graham Jr JM. Infants of diabetic mothers are at increased risk for the oculo-auriculo-vertebral sequence: a case-based and case-control approach. J Pediatr. 2002;141(5): 611–7.
130. Callier P, Faivre L, Thauvin-Robinet C, et al. Array-CGH in a series of 30 patients with mental retardation, dysmorphic features, and congenital malformations detected an interstitial 1p22.2-p31.1 deletion in a patient with features overlapping the Goldenhar syndrome. Am J Med Genet. 2008;146A: 2109–15.
131. Josifova DJ, Patton MA, Marks K. Oculoauriculovertebral spectrum phenotype caused by an unbalanced t(5;8)(p15.31;p23.1) rearrangement. Clin Dysmorphol. 2004;13(3):151–3.
132. Neu KW, Friedman JM, Howard-Peebles PN. Hemifacial microsomia in cri du chat (5p-) syndrome. J Craniofac Genet Dev Biol. 1982;2(4): 295–8.
133. Townes PL, White MR. Inherited partial trisomy 8q(22 qter). Am J Dis Child. 1978;132:498–501.
134. Dabir TA, Morrison PJ. Trisomy 10p with clinical features of facio-auriculo-vertebral spectrum: a case report. Clin Dysmorphol. 2006;15(1):25–7.
135. Bersu ET, Ramirez-Castro JL. Anatomical analysis of the developmental effects of aneuploidy in man: Tre trisomy 18 syndrome: I. Anomalies of the head and neck. Am J Med Genet. 1988;1:173–93.
136. Sujansky E, Smith ACM. Recombinant chromosome 18 in two male sibs with first and second branchial arch syndrome. Am Soc Hum Genet 1981;92A.
137. Curran JP, alSalihi FL, Ilderdice PW. Partial deletion of the long arm of chromosome E-18. Pediatrics. 1970;46(5):721–9.
138. Herman GE, Greenberg F, Ledbetter DH. Multiple congenital anomaly/mental retardation (MCA/MR) syndrome with Goldenhar complex due to a terminal del(22q). Am J Med Genet. 1988;29(4):909–15.
139. Hathout EH, Elmendorf E, Bartley J. Hemifacial microsomia and abnormal chromosome 22. Am J Med Genet; 1998;76(1):71–3.
140. Kobrynski L, Chitayat D, Zahed L, et al. Trisomy 22 and facioauriculovertebral (Goldenhar) sequence. Am J Med Genet. 1993;46(1):68–71.
141. Derbent M, Yilmaz Z, Baltaci V, Saygili A, Varan B, Tokel K. Chromosome 22q11.2 deletion and phenotypic features in 30 patient with conotruncal heart defects. Am J Med Genet A. 2003;116A(2):129–35.
142. Xu J, Fan YS, Siu VM. A child with features of Goldenhar syndrome and a novel 1.12 Mb deletion in 22q11.2 by cytogenetics and oligonucleotide array CGH: is this a candidate region for the syndrome? Am J Med Genet A. 2008;146A(14): 1886–9.
143. Rao VA, Kaliaperumal S, Subramanyan T, Rao KR, Bhargavan R. Goldenhar's sequence with associated juvenile glaucoma in Turner's syndrome. Indian J Ophthalmol. 2005;53(4):267–8.
144. Schroeter C, Jahrig K, Weinke I. A new case of pentasomy X. Helv Paediatr Acta. 1980;35(3):233–41.
145. Kushnick T, Colondrillo M. 49, XXXXY patient with hemifacial microsomia. Clin Genet. 1975;7:442–8.
146. Poonawalla HH, Kaye CI, Rosenthal IM, Pruzansky S. Hemifacial microsomia in a patient with Klinefelter syndrome. Cleft Palate J. 1980;17(3): 194–6.
147. Hodes ME, Gleiser S, DeRosa GP, et al. Trisomy 7 mosaicism and manifestations of Goldenhar syndrome with unilateral radial hypoplasia. J Craniofac Genet Dev Biol. 1981;1(1):49–55.
148. DeRavel TJ, Lequis E, Brems H, Van Hoestenberghe R, Gillis PH, Fryns JP. Hemifacial microsomia in two patients further supporting chromosomal mosaicism as a causative factor. Clin Dysmorphol. 2001;10(4):263–7.
149. Wilson GN, Barr Jr M. Trisomy 9 mosaicism: another etiology for the manifestations of Goldenhar syndrome. J Craniofac Genet Dev Biol. 1983;3: 313–6.
150. Burck U. Genetic aspects of hemifacial microsomia. Hum Genet. 1983;64:291–6.
151. Kaye CI, et al. Oculo-auriculo-vertebral anomaly: segregation analysis. Am J Med Genet. 1992;43(6): 913–7.

Congenital Malformations of the Ear

2

Nael M. Shoman, Ravi N. Samy, and Daniel I. Choo

Abstract

Malformations affecting the ear encompass a wide spectrum of clinical entities. Interestingly, 50 % of all congenital malformations of the head and neck involve the ear. These malformations may present themselves as cosmetic and/or functional defects and can occur in isolation or as part of a constellation of features that define various associations and syndromes. They can affect the outer, middle, and/or inner ear, frequently in combination. The embryologic development of the outer and middle ear differs from that of the inner ear; this is reflected in the clinical presentation of ear malformations and forms the basis for many of the classification systems employed in clinical practice. This chapter reviews the embryology of the ear as well as the diagnosis and management of the most common malformations.

Keywords

Auricular atresia • Microtia • Congenital cholesteatoma • Common cavity malformations • Cochlear malformations

Embryology of the Ear and Associated Congenital Malformations

Malformations affecting the ear encompass a wide spectrum of clinical entities. Interestingly, 50 % of all congenital malformations of the head and neck involve the ear. These malformations may present themselves as cosmetic and/or functional defects and can occur in isolation or as part of a constellation of features that define various associations and syndromes. They can affect the outer, middle, and/or inner ear, frequently in combination. The embryologic development of

N.M. Shoman, M.D., F.R.C.S.(C) (✉)
Division of Otolaryngology – Head and Neck Surgery, Department of Surgery, St. Paul's Hospital, B 2.85, 1702 – 20th Street West, Saskatoon, SK, Canada, S7M 0Z9
e-mail: shoman@me.com

R.N. Samy, M.D.
Department of Otolaryngology Head and Neck Surgery, University Hospital/University of Cincinnati, 231 Albert Sabin Way, Cincinnati, OH 45267, USA

D.I. Choo, M.D.
Division of Pediatric Otolaryngology, Department of Otolaryngology Head and Neck Surgery, Cincinnati Children's Hospital Medical Center, 3333 Burnet Avenue, Cincinnati, OH 45229, USA

L.M. Elden and K.B. Zur (eds.), *Congenital Malformations of the Head and Neck*,
DOI 10.1007/978-1-4419-1714-0_2,

the outer and middle ear differs from that of the inner ear; this is reflected in the clinical presentation of ear malformations and forms the basis for many of the classification systems employed in clinical practice. This chapter reviews the embryology of the ear as well as the diagnosis and management of the most common malformations.

Outer Ear

Embryology

The first signs of auricular development are apparent at 4 weeks gestation as tissue condensations of the mandibular and hyoid arches. These condensations appear at the distal portion of the first pharyngeal groove; within 2 weeks, they give rise to six small buds of mesenchyme, known traditionally as the hillocks of His. The mandibular arch gives rise to hillocks 1–3, and the hyoid arch gives rise to hillocks 4–6 [1–3] (Fig. 2.1). The specific contribution of each arch to the formation of the auricle varies amongst published studies. However, a reasonable developmental scheme proposes that hillock 1 gives rise to the tragus, hillocks 2 and 3 the helix, and hillocks 4 and 5 the antihelix and hillock 6 eventually differentiates into the lobule. Other theories suggest that the hyoid arch contributes approximately 85 % of the auricle, with most of the central ear formed from hillocks 4 and 5, while the tragus is formed from hillocks 1–3 [4]. Regardless of the proposed auricular developmental model, the lobule is the last component of the external ear to develop. The concha is derived from the ectoderm forming the external auditory canal (EAC) [5, 6]. Initially, the auricle begins development in the anterior neck region. As the mandible develops during weeks 8–12, the auricle migrates dorsally and cephalad and lies in its relative adult location by week 20 [7].

The EAC develops from the dorsal portion of the first pharyngeal groove, which progressively deepens during the second month (Fig. 2.2). The ectoderm of the groove eventually abuts the endoderm of the tubotympanic recess, which is derived from the first pharyngeal pouch. This contact is brief and at the sixth month is broken by a mesodermal ingrowth. At 8 weeks, the inferior portion of the first pharyngeal groove deepens again. This forms the primary EAC, which corresponds to the cartilaginous canal in the adult. At 9 weeks, a cord of epithelial cells at the bottom of the primary EAC grows medially into the surrounding mesenchyme to terminate in a solid epithelial plate, which is known as the meatal plug. It is not until after the fifth month that the plug splits open, initially at its medial terminus, forming the bony EAC by the seventh month. The cells remaining at the periphery form the epithelial lining of the bony EAC, whereas those remaining medially form the superficial layer of the tympanic membrane (TM). These developmental changes in the EAC occur at a time when the outer, middle, and inner ear are already well developed.

The TM is trilaminar. The primordium of the TM is the pharyngeal membrane, which separates the first pharyngeal groove from the first pharyngeal pouch. At 9 weeks, the mesenchyme adjacent to the meatal plug gives rise to the lamina propria of the TM. This mesenchyme is surrounded by the four ossification centers of the tympanic ring. By the tenth week, the tympanic ring elements fuse except for a small region superiorly where a defect remains; this becomes the notch of Rivinus. These elements then expand, accompanied by the growth of the solid epithelial cord of cells of the meatal plug. Thus, the TM develops from three sources that correspond to its trilaminar structure. Its lateral surface arises from ectoderm of the first pharyngeal groove; its medial surface from endoderm of the tubotympanic recess, a derivative of the first pharyngeal pouch; and its middle layer, a fibrous stratum of connective tissue, from mesenchyme of the first and second pharyngeal arches.

Preauricular Sinus

Definition

A preauricular sinus is a congenital malformation that manifests as an external small opening in the preauricular region. It has been variably termed preauricular pit, preauricular fistula, preauricular tract, and preauricular cyst.

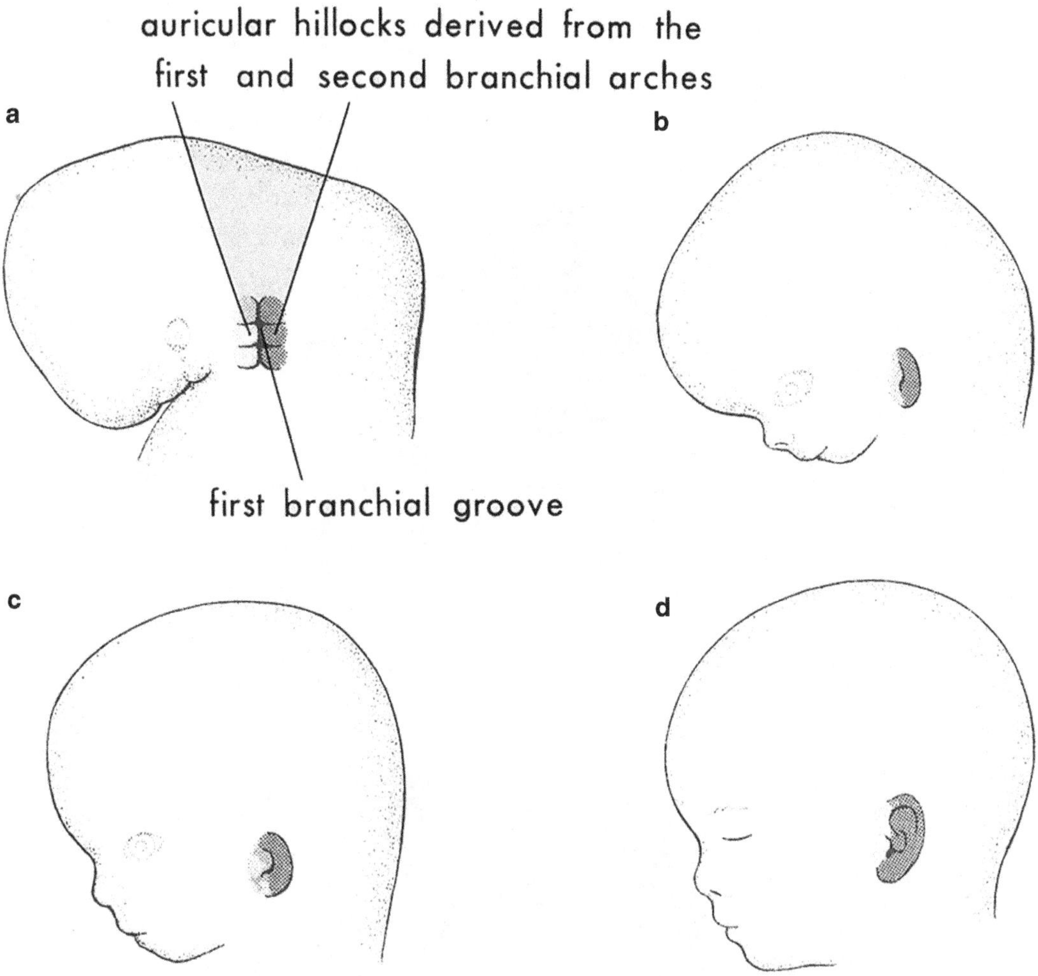

Fig. 2.1 Schematic demonstrating the hillocks of His that develops into the mature auricle (reprinted with permission from Moore KL, Persaud TVN. The Developing Human: Clinically Oriented Embryology. 5th ed. Philadelphia: W.B. Saunders; 1993:438)

Incidence

Preauricular sinuses have an estimated incidence of 0.1–0.9 % in the United States, 0.47 % in Hungary, 0.9 % in England, 2.5 % in Taiwan, and as high as 4–10 % in some parts of Africa [8–13].

Etiology

The most accepted theory attributes the development of a preauricular sinus to incomplete or defective fusion of the six hillocks of His [10].

Associated Malformations

The preauricular sinus has been described as part of a number of syndromes, most commonly branchio-oto-renal (BOR) syndrome [14, 15]. Others include brancho-oto-costal syndrome [16], cat eye syndrome [17], Waardenburg's syndrome [18], and trisomy 22 [19, 20].

Some studies have found an association between hearing loss (conductive and sensorineural) in newborn infants with isolated preauricular tags and pits. This incidence has been

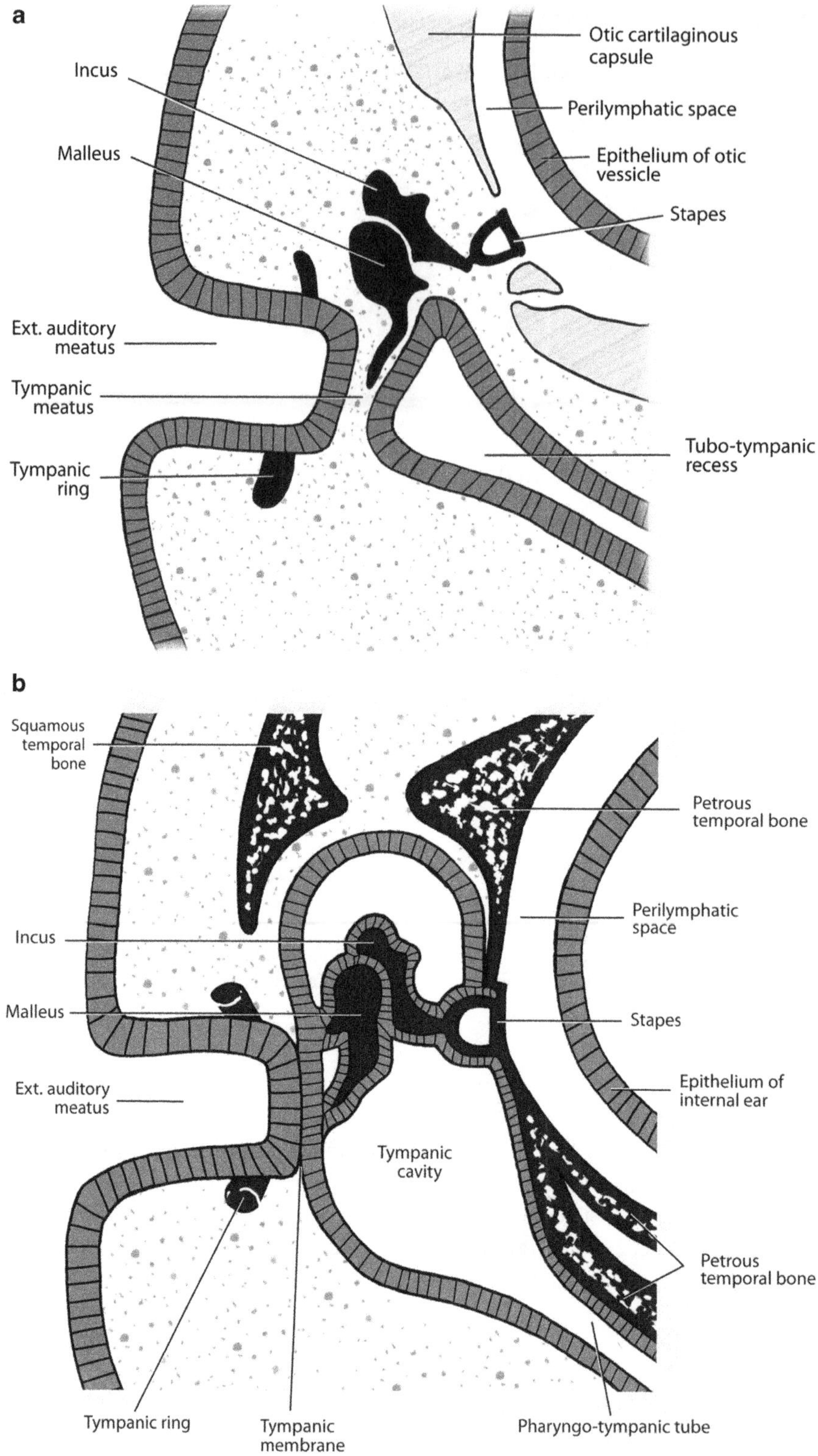

Fig. 2.2 Embryology of ear canal

reported as high as 15–30 % [21]. Interestingly, the hearing loss may evolve after a few years. However, many studies have found no statistically significant associated hearing loss with isolated preauricular sinuses and tags compared to control groups [10, 22]. The incidence of external or middle ear anomalies does not appear to be higher in patients with an isolated preauricular sinus. Conversely, individuals with congenital branchial cleft anomalies may have a higher incidence of concomitant preauricular sinus, reported as high as 60 % in the literature [23]. It is well known that patients with syndromic preauricular sinuses may have associated hearing loss as part of the clinical spectrum [24, 25].

Studies have shown an association between preauricular sinus and renal structural abnormalities. The percentage of children with isolated preauricular sinus and associated major renal structural abnormalities is reported to be 2.2–4.3 % [14, 26]. A prospective study of over 32,000 live births suggested a slightly increased risk (odds ratio 1.3) of renal anomalies in children with ear anomalies [21].

Clinical Features

Over 50 % of cases overall are unilateral [27], although some studies have found the incidence of bilateral lesions to be 25–50 % of cases [9]. They occur more commonly on the right side [8, 10]. They are frequently noted during routine physical examination as a small pit adjacent to the external ear, usually located at the anterior margin of the ascending limb of the helix, although the opening has also been reported along the posterosuperior margin of the helix, the tragus, or the lobule [8, 28]. The extent of the depth of the pit may vary, and can be shallow, limited to the visible portion of the pit, or may form a sinus tract that can extend to a variable depth or branch or follow a tortuous course. A preauricular sinus may also result in the formation of a subcutaneous cyst. These cysts are intimately related to the tragal cartilage and the anterior crus of the helix, whereby they are always adherent to the perichondrium of the auricular cartilage [29]. Unlike the tract of first branchial arch anomalies, a preauricular sinus tract is lateral and superior to the facial nerve and parotid gland.

Patients may present with discharge from the sinus either as a result of desquamating epithelial debris or infection. The latter may manifest with erythema, swelling, pain, and discharge. The most common culture pathogens implicated in infection are Staphylococcal species and, less commonly, Proteus, Streptococcus, and Peptococcus species [9].

Classification

A preauricular sinus can be inherited or can occur sporadically. Most cases are sporadic. Bilateral cases are more likely to be inherited [9]. When inherited, the pattern is of incomplete autosomal dominance with reduced (around 85 %) penetrance [27, 30]. Research studies have mapped a possible locus for congenital preauricular fistula to chromosome 8q11.1–q13.3 [31].

Diagnosis

Most patients are asymptomatic, and a sinus pit in a typical site is highly suggestive of the diagnosis (Fig. 2.3). A thorough history and head and neck examination are mandatory in all cases, seeking evidence of associated anomalies that may lead to the diagnosis of a syndromic etiology. Assessment of bilateral involvement, facial nerve function, and external ear development is important.

Management

Assessment of a child with a preauricular sinus, pit, or tag entails a thorough head and neck examination as well as systems review to elicit any obvious syndromal association. Assessment of the auricle as well as otomicroscopic examination of the external auditory canal and tympanic membrane are carried out to assess for any concomitant outer ear malformations.

The necessity of performing a renal ultrasound in patients with an isolated preauricular sinus has been controversial. Some authors have recommended that renal ultrasounds be performed on all patients with isolated preauricular sinuses [14], although this view is not shared by others [28]. Compelling arguments for attaining a

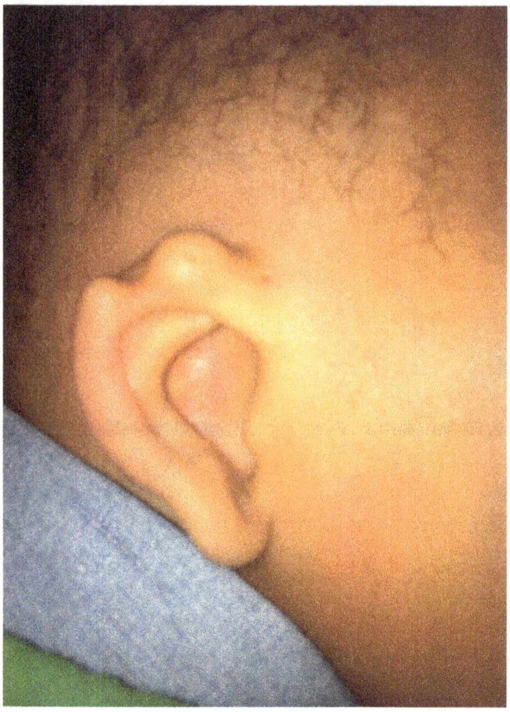

Fig. 2.3 Child with two ear pits (the more common preauricular pit and a less common helical pit adjacent to the notch in the helix)

renal ultrasound include the low cost and risk associated with the test as well as the significant clinical implications of a detected renal anomaly. Wang et al. [21], based on a retrospective review of 42 children with external ear anomalies who had undergone renal ultrasound in two genetics medical centers between 1981 and 2000, suggested that renal ultrasound should only be performed on patients with a preauricular sinus and one or more of the following:

1. Another malformation or dysmorphic feature
2. A family history of deafness
3. An auricular and/or renal malformation
4. A maternal history of gestational diabetes

Routine audiometric testing in patients with an isolated preauricular sinus has also been controversial. Most of the conducted studies constituted small patient cohorts. Moreover, confounding factors, including otitis media with effusion in the young age group, make data interpretation difficult. There has been no definitive evidence that hearing assessment should be carried out in the routine evaluation of the newborn with an isolated preauricular sinus, at least no more so in these children than in those without preauricular pits.

Management of an acutely infected preauricular sinus entails administration of appropriate antibiotics active against the causative pathogen. In the case when an abscess is present, incision and drainage are commonly undertaken. This can however result in scarring that may make subsequent definitive surgical excision of the sinus more challenging. Coatesworth et al. [32] have described a technique for drainage of a preauricular abscess using a lacrimal probe, in an attempt to minimize trauma to the underlying sinus, potentially reducing the impact of fibrosis on subsequent surgical excision if needed.

Management of recurrent or persistent preauricular sinus infections usually requires surgical excision of the sinus and its tract, preferably at a time of quiescence. Various surgical techniques have been described, with the primary surgical goal of obtaining complete excision to reduce the risk of recurrence. In reviewing the literature, recurrence rates have been reported between 0 and 42 % [33, 34]. The classic approach to surgical excision involves an elliptical skin incision with removal of the skin and sinus opening and medial dissection of the sinus tract. Wide local excision in the form of a radical supra-auricular approach has also been described [34]. This approach involves a postauricular extension of the elliptical incision around the sinus opening, with subsequent medical dissection to the temporalis fascia and continued over the cartilage of the anterior helix. Tissue superficial to the temporalis fascia is removed together with the preauricular sinus as well as a portion of the cartilage or perichondrium of the helix at the base of the sinus. Studies have shown that the supra-auricular approach has a lower recurrence rate compared with simple sinus and tract excision (3.7–5 % vs. 32–42 %, respectively) [35, 36].

Currie et al. [33] carried out a retrospective review over a period of 8 years to assess risk factors that influenced recurrence rates following surgical excision of preauricular sinuses. Factors found to reduce the risk of recurrence were the use of the supra-auricular approach with clearance down to the temporalis fascia, avoidance of sinus rupture, and closure of wound dead space. To facilitate complete surgical excision, many techniques have been employed to aid in the visualization of the sinus tract and its branches. These include preoperative sonographic imaging, preoperative sinograms, intraoperative methylene blue injection, and the use of a lacrimal probe [37, 38]. These have proven to be of variable benefit, and their use is mostly dictated by surgeon preference.

Aural Atresia

Definition

Congenital aural atresia (CAA) refers to a spectrum that involves varying degrees of failure of development of the EAC.

Incidence

The prevalence rates reported for CAA have been variable, reasons for which include variable registration systems and lack of a standardized definition and diagnosis [39]. Furthermore, CAA is often associated with microtia; accurately capturing CAA data from this overlapping dataset has been difficult. According to the Swedish Board of Welfare statistics, the frequency of isolated EAC malformations in 1980 was reported as 0.92 per 10,000 live births.

Etiology

Failure of canalization of the EAC canal during the seventh gestational month results in membranous and/or bony CAA. The etiology of CAA, as with microtia, is multifactorial. A number of factors have been implicated in the pathogenesis, including teratogens, vascular insults, and genetic aberrations [40, 41].

Associated Malformations

Microtia is commonly associated with CAA, and the degree of auricular malformation usually correlates with the degree of CAA as well as the middle ear deformity. However, even though segments of the auricle, EAC, and ossicular chain originate from the same pharyngeal arches, they are from different segments of neural crest cells and evolve at different times in embryonic development. As such, a severe microtia with accompanying CAA is not always accompanied by a disruption in the development of the ossicular chain or middle ear cavity. Likewise, cases of a normal auricle with CAA or, albeit rarely, of microtia with normal EAC and middle ear cavity have been reported [42]. Given the separate embryologic origin of the inner ear, the incidence of inner ear abnormalities is relatively low in patients who have CAA (about 8 %) [43]. CAA has been reported in patients with chromosomal anomalies, especially terminal deletions at chromosome 18q23. A study by Veltman et al. found that atresia occurs in approximately 66 % of all patients who have a terminal deletion of 18q [44].

Clinical Features

CAA is more commonly unilateral (70–90 %) [45]. When bilateral, the deformity on either side can vary in complexity. For unknown reasons, males are affected more commonly than females, at a 2.5:1 ratio. In addition, the right ear is more commonly involved (~60 %) [46]. CAA is more often bony than membranous, and it can be complete or incomplete. The latter may result in a stenotic cartilaginous canal laterally, with a medial osseous canal of normal caliber and a normal TM.

Classification

Several classifications have been proposed based on various parameters including clinical, radiological, surgical, and histopathological findings. A commonly used classification of CAA is that described by Weerda [47], which categorizes these malformations into three types (Table 2.1).

Altmann was the first to describe a histopathological classification correlating the severity of CAA [48] (Table 2.2). He divided three categories: mildly, moderately, and severely malformed types. Many authors have since modified this classification system, further subclassifying type II based on the surgical findings and functional outcome [49] (Table 2.3).

Schuknecht described a classification system (types A–D) based on a combination of high-resolution computed tomography (CT) scan and surgical findings (Table 2.4) (Fig. 2.4a–d).

Table 2.1 Weerda classification of congenital aural atresia

Type A	Marked narrowing of the EAC with an intact skin layer
Type B	Partial development of the EAC with an atresia plate at the medial part
Type C	Complete bony EAC atresia

Table 2.2 Altmann classification of congenital aural atresia

Group 1 (mild)	Some part of the EAC, although hypoplastic, is present. The tympanic membrane is hypoplastic, and the eardrum is small. The tympanic cavity is either normal in size or hypoplastic
Group 2 (moderate)	The EAC is completely absent, the tympanic cavity is small and its contents deformed, and the "atresia plate" is partially or completely osseous
Group 3 (severe)	The EAC is absent, and the tympanic cavity is markedly hypoplastic or missing

Table 2.3 Modified Altmann classification of CAA

Type I: Mild	Tympanic membrane is smaller in area than normal; various kinds of ossicular malformations may be present
Type II: Moderate	Moderate: atretic plate; tympanic cavity is within normal limits
IIa	Tympanic bone hypoplastic; course of the facial nerve usually normal
IIb	Tympanic bone absent; abnormal course of the facial nerve
Type III: Severe	No canal, and a severely hypoplastic tympanic cavity

Adapted from Declau F, Offeciers F, Van de Heyning P. *Classification of the non-syndromal type of meatal atresia*, in *Proceedings of the XVth World Congress of Otorhinolaryngology Head and Neck Surgery: Panel Discussions*, Devranoglu I, Editor. 1999: Istanbul, Turkey. p. 135–7

Table 2.4 Schuknecht classification of CAA

Type A: Meatal atresia	Limited to a stenotic fibrocartilaginous portion of the EAC
Type B: Partial atresia	Narrowing and sometimes tortuousities of both the fibrocartilaginous and bony parts of the EAC. The TM size is often reduced and replaced at least in part by a bony septum, and there is usually middle ear deformities including ossicular malformations
Type C: Total atresia	Totally atretic canal, but well-developed pneumatization of the tympanic cavity. Characteristically, the TM is missing, the head of the malleus is slightly deformed with fixation to the atresia plate, and the head of the malleus and body of the incus are fused. The facial nerve occasionally takes a more anterior course, in which case it may partially overlap the oval window
Type D: Hypopneumatic total atresia	Displays the same dysmorphic features found in type C as well as reduced pneumatization of the temporal bone. There is usually an abnormal course of the facial nerve as well as abnormalities of the bony labyrinth

Diagnosis

CAA is typically evident on initial neonatal examination. The presence of microtia may draw attention to a possible associated CAA. In many countries and in all states within the United States, universal newborn hearing screening is mandatory. This has enhanced the early identification of children with more subtle presentations of CAA (e.g., unilateral CAA) who might not have been diagnosed until later in life.

In the absence of other major congenital malformations, it is most important to evaluate the status of the child's hearing. Even if the contralateral ear is normal on newborn screening, a diagnostic auditory brainstem response (ABR) test is typically recommended in order to assure that the child has at least one normal hearing ear for access to sound and speech. Aside from audiometric assessment, any patient with CAA in whom surgical repair is contemplated should undergo high-resolution CT scanning of the temporal bones (Fig. 2.5).

Management

In cases of unilateral CAA, hearing is typically normal in the contralateral ear [50]. Some syndromes, such as Goldenhar syndrome or hemifacial microsomia, present an important exception to this, because the uninvolved ear may demonstrate a conductive, sensorineural, or mixed hearing loss. CAA typically results in conductive hearing loss (CHL) in 80–90 % of the cases with

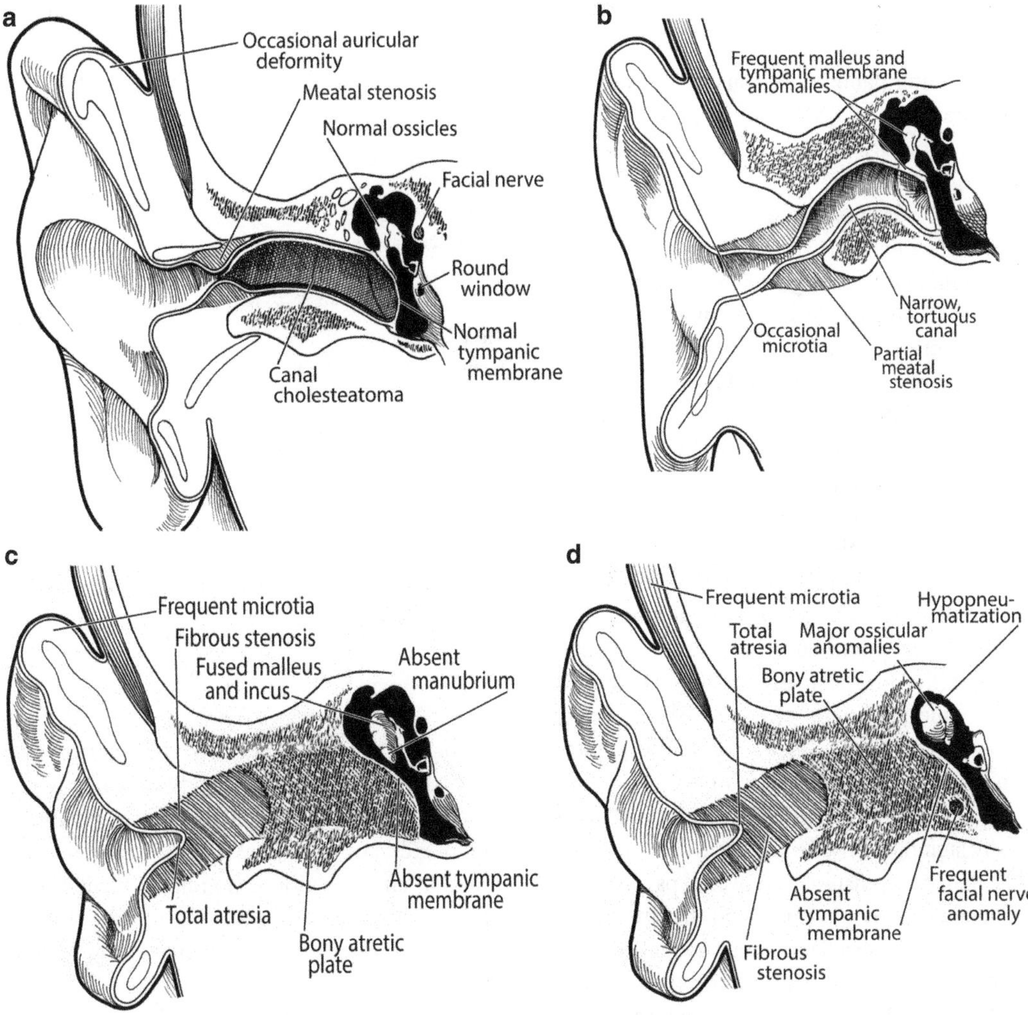

Fig. 2.4 (**a–d**) Schematics of types of ear canal stenosis/atresia (based on Schuknecht classification system)

Fig. 2.5 Axial computed tomography of left temporal bone demonstrating auricular atresia with absence of an ear canal (*white arrow*) and malformed middle ear space (*black arrow*)

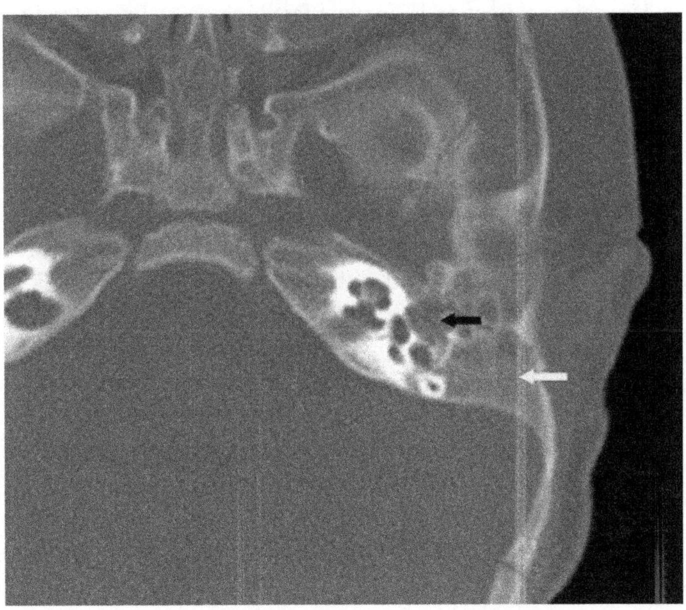

the remaining patients demonstrating a sensorineural hearing loss (SNHL) component [5]. The CHL is typically in the moderate hearing loss range of 40–60 dB.

Current literature suggests that there are many benefits to binaural stimulation, and children with a unilateral hearing loss are at a greater risk of delayed language development, attention-deficit disorders, and poor school performance. As such, patients with unilateral CAA are currently managed with various rehabilitative options, including a hearing aid, assistive listening devices, as well as surgical correction of the atresia. In patients with complete CAA who opt to use a hearing amplification device, a bone-conduction hearing aid must be used, while in cases of incomplete CAA, an air-conduction hearing aid is also an option, but can be problematic due to difficulties in effectively fitting a stenotic ear canal. In the classroom setting, an FM system can also be an extremely effective option for children with CAA and unilateral hearing loss.

In bilateral CAA, the degree of hearing loss is usually significant enough to cause delay in speech and language acquisition and overall psychological development. It is recommended that the medical and audiologic evaluation and management of infants with CAA should follow the American Academy of Pediatrics 1–3–6 newborn hearing loss guidelines: screen by 1 month, diagnose by 3 months, and begin intervention by 6 months of age.

If surgical correction is contemplated, preoperative CT scanning provides valuable information to help in the decision-making process. In 1992, Jahrsdoerfer et al. [51] proposed a CT grading system for CAA that was shown to correlate with postoperative hearing outcomes (Table 2.5). With respect to surgical management of unilateral CAA, the risks of atresia repair should be carefully discussed with the family and weighed against the alternatives of a bone- or air-conduction hearing aid or implantation of a bone-anchored hearing aid. CAA repair carries the risks of canal restenosis, facial nerve injury, sensorineural hearing loss, and postoperative chronic otorrhea. The degree of audiometric improvement is also somewhat unpredictable following atresia surgery. Delaying surgery until after adolescence, when patients can share in their own decision-making process, is advocated by some otologic surgeons. The goal of surgery in patients with bilateral CAA is to restore sufficient hearing such that amplification is no longer needed. This typically translates to a hearing threshold of 25 dB or better. The choice of which ear to operate on is based on imaging evaluation rather than audiometric assessment. Using the Jahrsdoerfer CT grading system, in cases of unilateral CAA, a good surgical candidate scores 8 or more points. In bilateral CAA, the better ear (higher score) is chosen for repair first. With proper patient selection in cases of aural atresia, it is possible to achieve a hearing level of 25 dB or better in 50–70 % of patients. If microtia is present, its repair is first carried out as the child approaches school age (typically 5 years of age). CAA repair follows thereafter at about 6–7 years of age.

Table 2.5 Jahrsdoerfer grading system of candidacy for CAA repair

Parameter	Points
Stapes present	2
Oval window open	1
Middle ear space	1
Facial nerve normal	1
Malleus–incus complex present	1
Mastoid well pneumatized	1
Incus–stapes connection	1
Round window normal	1
Appearance of external ear	1

Rating	Type of candidate
10	Excellent
9	Very good
8	Good
7	Fair
6	Marginal
≤5	Poor

The risk of cholesteatoma development with CAA is about 4–7 % [40]. A CT scan of the temporal bones should routinely be obtained around 4 years of age. It is not recommended that a CT scan be obtained at an earlier age, as it would have to be repeated closer to the time of surgery given the ongoing growth and maturity of the temporal bone. Furthermore, the risk of cholesteatoma development under 3 years of age is minimal.

This approach further minimizes unnecessary radiation exposure in the pediatric population. If cholesteatoma does exist, surgery is planned, in the form of either canal and middle ear surgery if the CT scan is favorable or canaloplasty alone.

Microtia

Definition

Microtia describes a spectrum of malformations that span a wide range of clinical presentations that can affect the size, orientation, position, and morphology of the auricle. Complete absence of the auricle can also occur (anotia).

Incidence

In Europe, a prevalence of 1.07 in 10,000 births for microtia and anotia was found in the period of 1980–2003 [39]. Jahrsdoerfer reported a prevalence of 1 in 5,800 births based on the Health Department statistics of the City of New York for a 10-year period (1952–1962) [52].

Etiology

The etiology of microtia is often multifactorial. Only 15 % of patients have a positive family history. In a minority of patients, a genetic or an environmental cause can be found; in these cases, microtia is usually part of a specific pattern of multiple congenital anomalies.

Associated Malformations

Microtia is commonly associated with CAA, and the degree of auricular deformity correlates with the degree of middle ear deformity and conductive hearing loss. Microtia occurs in association with several single-gene disorders, such as Treacher Collins syndrome, as well as chromosomal syndromes, such as trisomy 18. It is frequently associated with the oculoauriculovertebral dysplasia spectrum of congenital anomalies, including Goldenhar–Gorlin syndrome [53]. Furthermore, microtia is a component of isotretinoin and thalidomide teratogenicity and can be part of fetal alcohol syndrome and maternal diabetes embryopathy [33]. Women with four or more pregnancies are at increased risk for having a child with microtia, especially its most severe form (anotia) [54].

Table 2.6 De la Cruz classification of congenital aural atresia

Minor malformations	Major malformations
Normal mastoid pneumatization	Poor pneumatization
Normal oval window/footplate	Abnormal or absent oval window/footplate
Reasonable facial nerve–footplate relationship	Abnormal course of the facial nerve
Normal inner ear	Abnormalities of the inner ear

Clinical Features

As with CAA, microtia occurs more often on the right and in males. The occurrence of microtia is more common in Japanese, Hispanic, and Native American populations, but less common in the black and Caucasian populations [1, 6, 55].

Classification

Many classification systems have been proposed and modified over the years. In essence, all of the classification systems classify a normal or near-normal auricle as Grade I, with increasing grades signifying increasing deformity. Commonly used classification systems include the De la Cruz and Weerda classification systems. The De la Cruz classification divides malformations into minor and major categories (Table 2.6). In 1988, Weerda compiled all the classification systems into one scheme that is useful for clinical grading as well as basic management principles (Table 2.7) (Fig. 2.6a–c).

Anotia

Complete absence of any recognizable external ear structures. Management is similar to that of third-degree dysplasia.

Diagnosis

Microtia is evident on initial neonatal assessment. A thorough physical examination is important to accurately describe the auricular deformity, determine the status of the EAC, and assess for any associated malformations (preauricular pits/sinuses, cervical cysts, or sinuses),

Table 2.7 Weerda's combined classification of auricular defects, including surgical recommendations

First-degree dysplasia. Average definition: Most structures of a normal auricle are recognizable (minor deformities)

Surgical definition: Reconstruction does not require the use of additional skin or cartilage

a. Microtia
b. Protruding ear (synonyms: prominent ear, bat ear)
c. Cryptotia (synonyms: pocket ear, group IV B (Tanzer))
d. Absence of upper helix
e. Small deformities: Absence of the tragus, satyr ear, Darwinian tubercle, additional folds (Stahl ear)
f. Colobomata (synonyms: clefts, transverse coloboma)
g. Lobule deformities (pixed lobule, macrolobule, absence of lobule, lobule colobamata (bifid lobule))
h. Cup ear deformities

Type I: Cupped upper portion of the helix, hypertrophic concha, reduced height (synonyms: lidding helix, constricted helix, group IV A (Tanzer), lop ear)

Type II: More severe lopping of the upper pole of the ear; rib cartilage is used as support when a short ear must be expanded or the auricular cartilage is limp

Second-degree dysplasia

Average definition: Some structures of a normal auricle are recognizable

Surgical definition: Partial reconstruction requires the use of some additional skin and cartilage. Synonym: Second-degree microtia (Marx)

a. Cup ear deformity, type III: The severe *CUP* ear deformity is malformed in all dimensions (synonyms: cockleshell ear, constricted helix, group IV (Tanzer), snail-shell ear)
b. Mini-ear

Third-degree dysplasia

Average definition: None of the structures of a normal ear is recognizable

Surgical definition: Total reconstruction requires the use of skin and large amounts of cartilage. Synonyms: complete hypoplasia group II, peanut ear, third-degree microtia (Marx); normally concomitant congenital atresia is found

a. Unilateral: One ear is normal; no middle ear reconstruction is performed on any child; auricle reconstruction is begun at age 5 or 6 years
b. Bilateral: Bone-conduction hearing aid before the first birthday; middle ear surgery at age 4 years without transposition of the vestige; bilateral reconstruction of the auricle at age 5 or 6 years

Anotia—Complete absence of any recognizable external ear structures. Management is similar to that of third-degree dysplasia

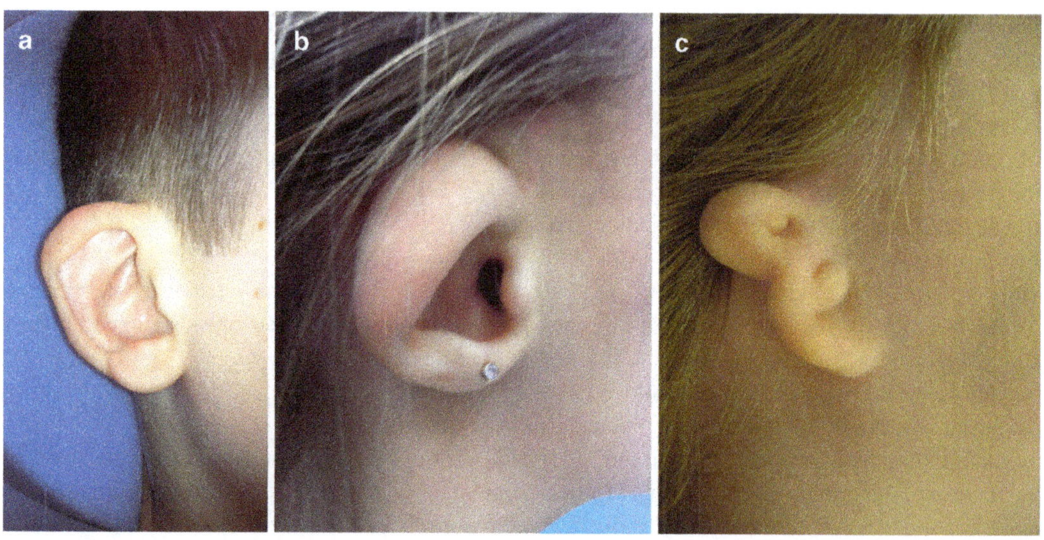

Fig. 2.6 (**a**) Photograph of child with first-degree dysplasia of pinna, demonstrating cupped ear, absent antihelical fold, and Darwinian tubercle. (**b**) Photograph of child with second-degree dysplasia demonstrating underdeveloped upper half of pinna. (**c**) Photograph of child demonstrating third-degree dysplasia. Note that the normal structures of the ear are not recognizable

craniofacial malformations (ocular, zygomatic, mandibular, palatal abnormalities), as well as other organ systems. This information will be helpful in determining a possible syndromic etiology. Microtia, as with CAA, is recognized by the American Academy of Pediatrics as a high-risk factor for congenital hearing loss. It is paramount that the hearing status of a neonate with a diagnosis of microtia be promptly determined. With bilateral microtia, early referral for audiologic evaluation is critical so that proper bone-conduction hearing aid use can be implemented. With unilateral microtia, a diagnostic ABR test is typically recommended to ensure that the child has at least one normal hearing ear. If there is associated CAA and surgical correction is contemplated, a preoperative CT scan is recommended.

Management

Management of microtia is commonly a multidisciplinary approach. If other congenital anomalies are present, either in association with a syndrome or as isolated findings, consultation from the appropriate services is indicated. From an otologic perspective, one must initially determine what type of auditory habilitation is required and feasible. Patients with microtia associated with CAA follow the algorithm previously discussed under CAA, as auditory habilitation of the associated CHL takes precedence in these cases. If surgery is contemplated, microtia repair is undertaken at approximately 5–6 years of age, with atresia repair following at approximately 6–7 years.

Using the Weerda classification, first-degree dysplasia encompasses many common and frequently isolated auricular malformations, including macrotia, protruding ears, and cup ear deformity. Reconstruction normally does not require the use of additional skin or cartilage. Instead, many otoplastic techniques have been described that attempt to achieve some auricular reduction. These techniques for the most part involve manipulation of the cartilage framework by using sutures or by cutting, abrading, or scoring. Examples of the former include the Mustarde and the Furnas techniques. Examples of the cartilage-cutting techniques include the Converse, Farrior, and Pitanguy techniques. These techniques make use of the observation that cut cartilage bends away from its cut side. Cartilage cutting is useful for manipulating cartilage that is stiff and thick but can cause scarring, irregularities along the cut edges, and a diminished auricle size. They are also generally more difficult to undertake and require an experienced surgeon for their maximal benefit and utilization.

Second-degree dysplasia, or atypical microtia, has most of the auricular structural components recognizable; there is however distinct tissue deficiency that necessitates the transposition of skin and cartilage. The main deficiency often lies in the vertical height of the affected ear. Augmenting this deficiency can be achieved by various techniques depending on the difference in height between the two ears. If the height difference is more than 20 mm, a cartilage graft is considered. Donor sites include the contralateral conchal bowl or a rib graft for large deficiencies. A staged skin graft in these instances is often required and may be advanced from a postauricular donor site.

Reconstruction for third-degree dysplasia (classic microtia) or anotia requires the use of skin and large amounts of cartilage. This is best initiated at the age of about 6 years, especially for unilateral cases, and the best donor tissue is autogenous costal cartilage. By this age, sufficient cartilage is present for the auricular reconstruction, and the patient is more able to cooperate with the necessary postoperative care. The reconstruction is multistaged and incorporates CAA repair.

Middle Ear

Embryology

The tympanomastoid compartment first appears at the 3-week stage as an outpouching of the first pharyngeal pouch (the tubotympanic recess) (Fig. 2.7). This is a stalklike diverticulum, which expands in a lateral direction until it comes in contact with the epithelial lining of the first pharyngeal cleft. The distal part of this diverticulum widens into a saclike structure, which is the primitive tympanic cavity. Expansion of the pouch begins at the inferior aspect of the definitive tympanic cavity and progresses by invasion of the adjacent mesenchyme. By 7 weeks, concomitant growth of the second branchial arch constricts the importation of the tubotympanic recess. The primary tympanic cavity lies lateral to this constriction, while the proximal part of the tubotympanic recess medial to this constriction remains narrow and develops into the Eustachian tube. The distal end of the first pharyngeal pouch buds into four sacci (anticus, posticus, superior, and medius), which expand to progressively pneumatize the middle ear and the epitympanum. Expansion of the sacci envelops the developing ossicles, which remain embedded in mesenchyme until the eighth month, when the surrounding tissue dissolves. The interface between two sacci gives rise to mesentery-like mucosal folds, which transmit blood vessels. Mesenchymal resolution may continue as late as 1 year postnatally (or even later in some rare cases). Persistence of this embryonic connective tissue in the adult may be evident as connective tissue strands draped over the oval and round windows.

By birth, the antrum approximates that of the adult. Mastoid pneumatization is evident as early as 33 weeks gestation and proceeds along well-established tracts. There is considerable variability amongst individuals in the degree and pattern of temporal bone pneumatization, and multiple factors are thought to play a role in this, including heredity, environmental, nutritional, infectious, and anatomic factors relating to the adequacy of ventilation by the Eustachian tube. Overall, the mastoid continues to grow for up to 19 years after birth.

The ossicular chain largely has its origins traced back to the pharyngeal arch apparatus, and studies have established that it is the phylogenetic equivalent of the jaw joint in all nonmammalian jawed vertebrates [56]. In these animals, the jaw joint is established between mesenchymal components of the first and second pharyngeal arches, namely, the quadrate and articular portions. In the typical living reptile, sound is transmitted through the *columella auris* from a primitive tympanic membrane to the inner ear [57]. During evolution, the jaw joint was modified, and the articulo-quadrate joint evolved to constitute the mammalian middle ear [58]. The articular became the malleus and the quadrate the incus. These ossicles, through their respective contacts with the tympanic membrane and stapes (the phylogenetic homolog of the columella auris), were incorporated into the sound-transmitting apparatus [59, 60].

The first evidence of ossicular development occurs at approximately 4 weeks. An interbranchial mesenchymal bridge appears between the first and second pharyngeal arches. Specifically, the bridge connects the upper end of a part of the first arch (referred to as the mandibular visceral bar) with the central region of the second pharyngeal arch (hyoid) visceral bar. Thus, this condensed mesenchymal bridge consists of both first and second pharyngeal arch elements, which ultimately undergoes cartilaginous differentiation that gives rise to the primordial malleus and incus. As for the stapes, all of its blastula derives from the hyoid visceral bar except for the medial surface of the footplate and the annular ligament, which are of otic capsular (lamina stapedialis) origin. Thus, the ossicles are derived from neural crest mesenchyme of the first and second branchial arches, with the only exception being the medial aspect of the stapes footplate and the annular ligament, which are derived from the mesenchyme of the otic capsule.

Over the following 11 weeks, the ossicles develop and grow as a cartilaginous model of the mandibular and hyoid arches. This process is bone formation from a cartilaginous framework and is referred to as endochondral ossification. The anterior process of the malleus is unique in that it develops by membranous ossification without a cartilaginous model. Although controversy exists as to the exact contribution of each arch to the ossicular chain, it is believed that the head of the malleus as well as the body and short process of the incus are formed from Meckel's cartilage. Meanwhile, the long process of the incus, handle of the malleus, stapes super-

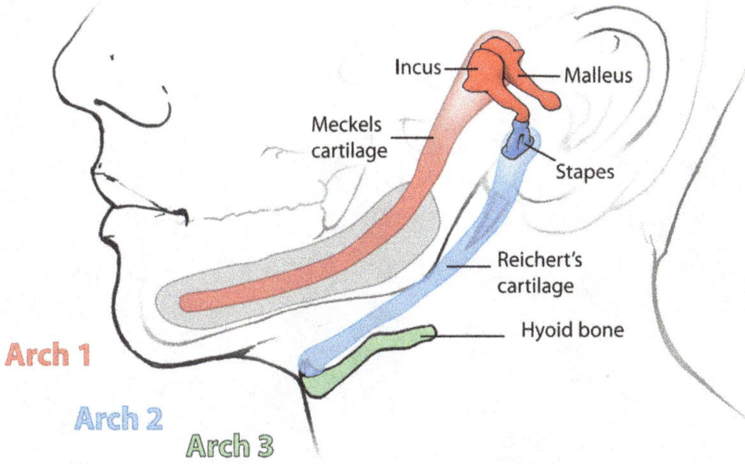

Fig. 2.7 Schematic diagram demonstrating the origin of ossicles and their relationship to the branchial arches

structure, and tympanic surface of the stapes footplate are derived from Reichert's cartilage. As previously mentioned, the medial surface of the footplate and the annular ligament are of otic capsular origin. Development of the stapes blastema involves progressive encirclement of the stapedial artery. The obturator foramen represents the completed ring left empty after the stapedial artery involutes.

By 15 weeks of gestation, the ossicles have already attained adult size, and the process of endochondral ossification soon begins. This process starts first in the incus, then in the malleus, and finally in the stapes. As the footplate attains adult size, the annular ligament is formed from the developing otic capsule. Paralleling this development, the tensor tympani and stapedius muscles develop. The tensor tympani muscle is innervated by the mandibular branch of the trigeminal nerve, the nerve of the first pharyngeal arch, while the stapedius muscle is innervated by the facial nerve, the nerve of the second pharyngeal arch. By 20 weeks gestation, the ossicles have assumed their adult configuration, and the endochondral bone of the ossicles, as with that of the otic capsule, undergoes little change over the lifetime of the individual. The exception to that is the stapes, which continues to lose bulk from its large structure well into the 32nd week of gestation. The stability of the ossicular bone explains the poor reparative capacity in response to trauma.

Although the ossicles appear during the first half of fetal life, they remain embedded in mesenchyme until the eighth month, when the surrounding tissue dissolves. As the mesenchyme surrounding the ossicles dissolves and the developing tympanic cavity expands, the endodermal epithelial lining of the primitive tympanic cavity then extends along the wall of the newly developing space to the epitympanic space and antrum and envelopes the developing ossicles. The tympanic cavity is now at least twice as large as before. When the ossicles are entirely free of surrounding mesenchyme, the endodermal epithelium connects them in a mesentery-like fashion to the wall of the cavity. The supporting ligaments of the ossicles develop later within these mesenteries.

During late fetal life, the tympanic cavity expands dorsally by vacuolization of surrounding tissue to form the tympanic antrum. After birth, epithelium of the tympanic cavity invades bone of the developing mastoid process, and epithelium-lined air sacs are formed (pneumatization). Later, most of the mastoid air sacs come in contact with the antrum and tympanic cavity.

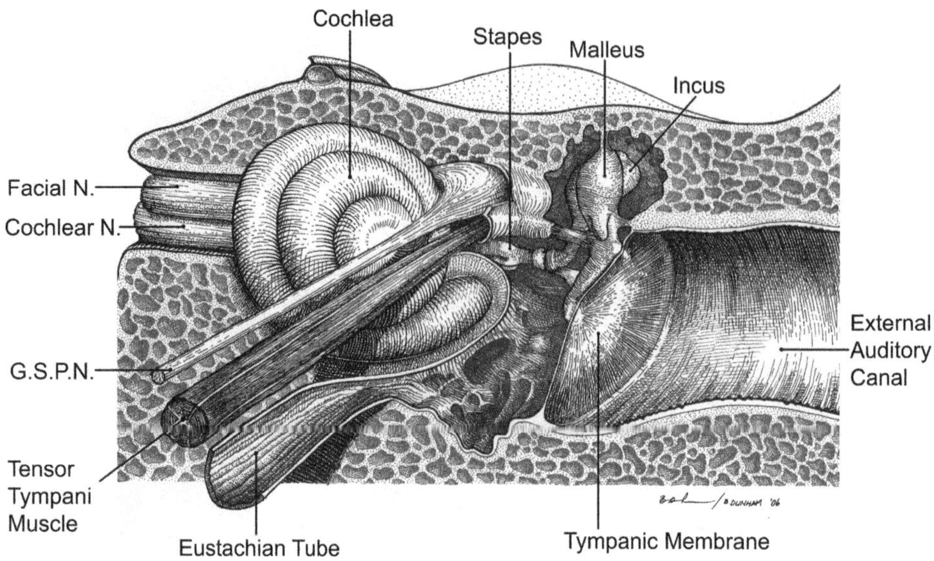

Fig. 2.8 Schematic of normal anatomy of middle ear

Ossicular Chain Malformations

Definition

Ossicular chain malformations describe a spectrum of anomalies that may include absence or maldevelopment of any of the ossicles (Fig. 2.8).

Incidence

Overall, isolated congenital ossicular anomalies are rare, with an incidence of less than 1 per 15,000 births [61]. In a study of 565 children with congenital hearing loss, 54 children (9.5 %) had CHL unrelated to otitis media and only 3 children (0.5 %) were found to have an isolated middle ear anomaly [62]. In a similar study of 687 children with congenital hearing loss, 8 children (0.1 %) had an isolated middle ear defect [42]. The most common congenital isolated ossicular anomalies in many series remain stapes fixation and incudostapedial discontinuity [63, 64], with isolated congenital stapes fixation representing 20–50 % of ossicular malformations [64–67].

Etiology

Etiologic factors related to ossicular chain abnormalities remain unclear. It would appear that most of these isolated anomalies arise from the lower part of the ossicular chain and are related to the second pharyngeal arch. It is yet unclear as to why anomalies are often restricted only to the stapes, or why other structures derived from the second arch are not affected with these ossicular anomalies. Congenital X-linked mixed deafness is a rare anomaly that occurs in males and is typified by progressive mixed hearing impairment from stapes fixation with perilymphatic gusher. It is inherited in an X-linked recessive pattern, and male patients tend to have severe mixed hearing loss at all frequencies, while female carriers have normal hearing or mild hearing loss. The condition is associated with anomalies of the vestibule and internal auditory canal (IAC). The gene defect has been localized to the Xq13–q21.1 region, which encodes the POU3F4 transcription factor [68]. The etiology of epitympanic fixation of the head of the malleus is rooted in the incomplete pneumatization of the epitympanum.

Associated Malformations

Because of the shared embryologic derivative, external ear abnormalities are often associated with middle ear abnormalities, and CAA can be associated not only with auricular but also with middle ear abnormalities. However, it is important to remember that the auricle, EAC, and ossicular chain originate from different segments of neural crest cells of the first and second pharyngeal arches and develop at different times in embryonic development. As such, a normally developed ossicular chain may be present despite a severe microtia with accompanying CAA.

Ossicular abnormalities may be associated with altered anatomy of middle ear structures. Jahrsdoerfer found the incidence of having an aberrant facial nerve course in ears with a congenital middle ear malformation was 24 % [69]. Ossicular chain abnormalities may also be seen in association with craniofacial anomalies. Many reports have found associations with congenital syndromes in approximately 20 % of middle ear malformations [70, 71]. The more common craniofacial syndromes involving conductive hearing losses are Treacher Collins, Crouzon, Apert, Goldenhar, BOR, Pfeiffer, Beckwith–Wiedemann and Klippel–Feil syndrome, as well as, CHARGE Association (coloboma, heart defects, atresia of the choanae, retarded growth or development of the central nervous system, genitourinary anomalies, and ear anomalies) syndromes.

Table 2.8 Cremers' classification of congenital middle ear anomalies

Class 1	Congenital stapes ankylosis without other deformities in the middle ear
Class 2	Congenital stapes ankylosis in combination with a congenital anomaly of the ossicular chain
Class 3	Congenital anomaly of the ossicular chain, but mobile footplate
3a	Discontinuity of the ossicular chain
3b	Epitympanic fixation
Class 4	Congenital aplasia or severe dysplasia of the oval or the round window

Table 2.9 Charachon's classification of congenital middle ear anomalies

Class 0	Normal ossicular chain, almost normal tympanic membrane but small atretic plate around malleus handle
Class 1	Fixation of the malleus head
Class 2	Normal ossicular chain but fixation of the footplate
2a	With abnormality of the facial nerve
2b	Without abnormality of the facial nerve
Class 3	Lack of a part of the ossicular chain with or without abnormality of the stapes
Class 4	Severe malformation of all the ossicular chain

Clinical Features

Congenital stapes fixation (SF) is often encountered in minor malformation cases and usually presents as a CHL with a patent EAC and normal TM. The differential diagnosis of stapes fixation includes other ossicular malformations, oval or round window atresia, congenital cholesteatoma, middle ear tumors including vascular lesions, and ossicular trauma. SF is bilateral in 70–90 % of patients [67, 71]. SF should be distinguished from juvenile stapes otosclerosis, which is defined by a progressive CHL. Furthermore, congenital SF presents at an earlier age than does juvenile otosclerosis (age 3 years vs. 10 years) [72]. Half of the children with juvenile otosclerosis have a positive family history; only 10 % of those children with congenital SF have other family members with CHL.

Classification

Classification of ossicular abnormalities can be divided into major and minor. Minor congenital ossicular anomalies are restricted to the middle ear, while major congenital ossicular anomalies can involve the auricle, EAC, and middle ear cleft. Different classifications are based on anatomic findings and/or embryologic malformations; however, none are universally accepted. Cremers' [73] and Charachon's [74] classifications are amongst the most commonly used (Tables 2.8 and 2.9).

Diagnosis

The diagnosis is suspected in a patient who presents with stable hearing loss present since birth without a history of recurrent ear infections or trauma. Otomicroscopy is often normal, but it may reveal an abnormality of the TM, malleus, or incus. An audiogram, in most cases, may demonstrate CHL in the 40–60 dB range. Impedance testing may be useful in the evaluation of some of these pathologies, as in congenital footplate fixation where typically there is absence of acoustic reflexes and a type A-shallow tympanogram. The hearing loss does not worsen with time, unless there is an associated Eustachian tube dysfunction, which is often seen in syndromic cases, and can lead to diagnostic difficulties. Generally, the diagnosis is easier and made earlier when the malformation is bilateral; in unilateral cases, a diagnosis is typically established at the age of 6 years. High-resolution CT scan may reveal the presence of various ossicular anomalies. Surgery in the form of exploratory tympanotomy offers a means for definitive diagnosis and the option of surgical correction at the same time.

Management

It is reasonable to offer hearing aids and defer surgical exploration until the child is older, when a series of hearing tests are available, and the child is more able to share in the consent-making process. A CT scan should be obtained at some point during the child's follow-up period. Imaging is useful in that it can provide essential diagnostic information to elucidate the cause of the CHL and identify associated middle or inner ear abnormalities. Concerning inner ear findings include an enlarged vestibular aqueduct, dilated IAC fundus, and an abnormal communication between the inner ear and intracranial space.

Given the nonprogressive nature of the hearing loss, amplification is a reasonable option in managing patients with isolated congenital ossicular anomalies. If surgery is contemplated, a comprehensive discussion with the family is essential and waiting until the child is capable of weighing the associated surgical risks, including sensorineural hearing loss, against the potential benefits of surgery. The rate of severe SNHL in patients with fixed stapes has been reported to be between 0 and 30 % in the literature [65, 75, 76]. With regard to patient age, many studies have found no correlation between the patient's age at the time of stapedectomy for congenital SF and postoperative audiometric results [77]. Many studies have reported good results following stapedectomies for congenital SF [67, 71, 74, 78]; however, hearing outcomes tend to be worse compared with the results for otosclerosis [79–81]. This may be attributable to the higher incidence of coexisting middle ear anomalies with congenital SF. The reported success rate of ossicular chain reconstruction is usually lower than that of stapedectomy and varies widely between series. Ossiculoplasty for combined ossicular anomalies yields an air–bone gap (ABG) of less than 30 dB in about 70 % of patients.

Congenital Cholesteatoma

Definition

Cholesteatoma refers to a collection of keratinizing squamous epithelium that can be trapped within the temporal bone and grows into a destructive lesion. Left untreated, a cholesteatoma can be a significant source of morbidity as it eventually erodes into critical structures, including the ossicles, facial nerve canal, inner ear, and tegmen. The latter may result in severe intracranial complications and even death. Cholesteatomas may be congenital or acquired. In the past, the diagnosis of congenital cholesteatoma (CC) depended only on the presence of a white mass behind an intact tympanic membrane in a child with no previous history of otitis media. The mass is often found within the anterior-superior portion of the middle ear. However, due to the high incidence of acute otitis media (60–80 % by 1 year of age, and 80–90 % by 2–3 years) [82, 83], the criteria have been modified to define a CC as a whitish mass behind an intact TM, with the absence of otorrhea or perforation and no previous otologic procedures, including myringotomy or insertion of ventilation tubes. Studies have since shown that the diagnosis should also not be excluded in cases of otorrhea or myringotomy [84].

Incidence

CC accounts for approximately 4 % of childhood cholesteatoma [84]. The number of reported cases of CC has increased dramatically over the last three decades, and this may be related to a better understanding and awareness of the disease entity, leading to timely diagnosis as well as improved otomicroscopic diagnostic tools. Improved medical management of otitis media may have led to a decrease in the number of acquired cholesteatomas and a relative increase in the percentage of the congenital type.

Etiology

The most popular theory of CC formation states that squamous inclusion cysts arise from epithelial rests (epidermoid formations) in the middle ear. These epidermoid formations have been demonstrated histologically in fetal temporal bones, and they may be single or multiple. They typically disappear in the third trimester of gestation. Failed involution leads to cholesteatoma formation behind an intact TM. Alternative but less supported theories include seeding of the middle ear by squamous cells in the amniotic fluid or from the surface epithelium of the TM after infection and microperforation.

Associated Malformations

CC has been associated with congenital ossicular malformations, including defects of the long process of the incus and the stapes superstructure. CC has also been associated with cholesterol granuloma and abnormal vestibular anatomy (dilated endolymphatic fossa, large vestibular aqueduct, and hypoplastic vestibule).

Clinical Features

The average age of presentation of children with CC is 3–5 years [84, 85]. The chief presenting symptom varies depending on the stage of the cholesteatoma. Asymptomatic cases are most prevalent. In symptomatic cases, hearing loss is the most prevalent symptom. Less common presenting symptoms include aural fullness, otalgia, tinnitus, dizziness, or headache. Facial nerve paralysis is rare and constitutes less than 1 % [84, 86]. CC may be found incidentally at myringotomy for serous otitis media.

Classification

Potsic et al. [84] proposed staging system for CC based on preoperative CT scans (Table 2.10). This system takes into consideration middle ear and mastoid extension as well as ossicular involvement. Nelson et al. [87] proposed a three-stage classification system based on the presumed natural history of these lesions, tracking them as they start in the anterior-superior quadrant, then extend to the anterior-inferior quadrant before progressing into the posterior-superior quadrant, the attic, and finally into the mastoid (Table 2.11).

Table 2.10 Potsic staging system for congenital cholesteatoma

Stage I	Single quadrant: No ossicular involvement or mastoid extension
Stage II	Multiple quadrants: No ossicular involvement or mastoid extension
Stage III	Ossicular involvement: Includes erosion of ossicles and surgical removal for eradication of disease; no mastoid extension
Stage IV	Mastoid extension (regardless of findings elsewhere)

Table 2.11 Nelson classification system for congenital cholesteatoma

Type I	Confined to the middle ear but does not involve the ossicles, except for the manubrium
Type II	Involvement of the ossicular mass in the posterior superior quadrant and the attic
Type III	Mastoid extension

In their series, this classification system correlated with the degree of CHL and the risk of recurrence as well as escalating complexity of surgical approach.

Diagnosis

CC may be diagnosed on otomicroscopy of an asymptomatic child or one being evaluated for hearing or other otologic symptoms. Early on, the cyst is hard to appreciate, appearing as a subtle whitish discoloration behind an otherwise normal TM (Fig. 2.9a). As the lesion grows, it becomes more evident as it contacts the medial aspect of the TM, which it may displace laterally. If the lesion obstructs the Eustachian tube (ET), it may result in a middle ear effusion, and this may complicate the diagnosis. With further progression, the cyst may impinge or erode the ossicles, worsening the conductive hearing loss. A thorough history should detail previous otologic procedures, ear infections, or temporal bone trauma. Complete audiometric assessment assesses for the presence and degree of CHL, and a preoperative CT scan is used to delineate disease extent, assess for temporal bone anatomy that may be used as a roadmap during surgery, and identify any alteration including scutum erosion and facial nerve dehiscence (Fig. 2.9b and c).

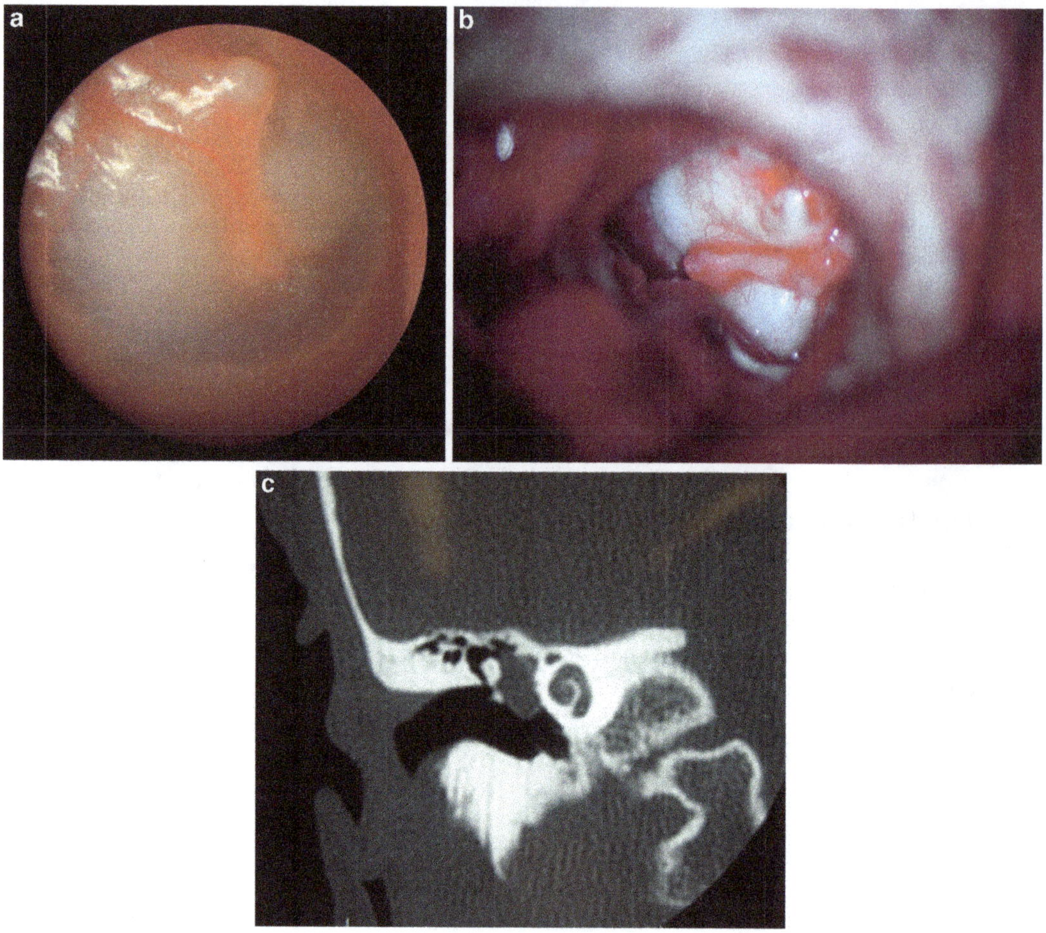

Fig. 2.9 (**a**) Photograph of child with congenital cholesteatoma behind an intact, bulging eardrum. (**b**) Intraoperative photograph of middle ear with elevated eardrum demonstrating ossicles and cholesteatoma. (**c**) CT scan demonstrating opacity in middle ear (congenital cholesteatoma) and intact ossicles (all images courtesy of John A. Germiller, MD, PhD)

Management

Management of cholesteatoma is surgical. In order of priority, the goals of surgery are prompt treatment of any complications evident on initial assessment, complete and safe removal of diseased tissue, attainment of a dry ear, preservation of as much normal ear anatomy as possible, and hearing restoration. The progression of surgical approaches generally follows the disease stage, dictated by disease size and extension. A small lesion confined to the middle ear space is readily managed via a transcanal approach. With further progression of the disease process, an endaural atticotomy or canal wall up tympanomastoidectomy may be required. There remains controversy as to the indications for taking down the posterior canal wall. While it is advisable to avoid a canal wall down mastoidectomy (CWD) procedure if possible, there are cases when it should be considered to optimize the chances of attaining a safe ear. These include cases where there is destruction of the posterior canal wall, labyrinthine involvement, petrous apex extension, disease in an only hearing ear, or concern about the reliability of follow-up. Depending on the chosen approach, a hearing restoration procedure may be performed at the same setting or part of a second-stage procedure, typically 6 months later. The

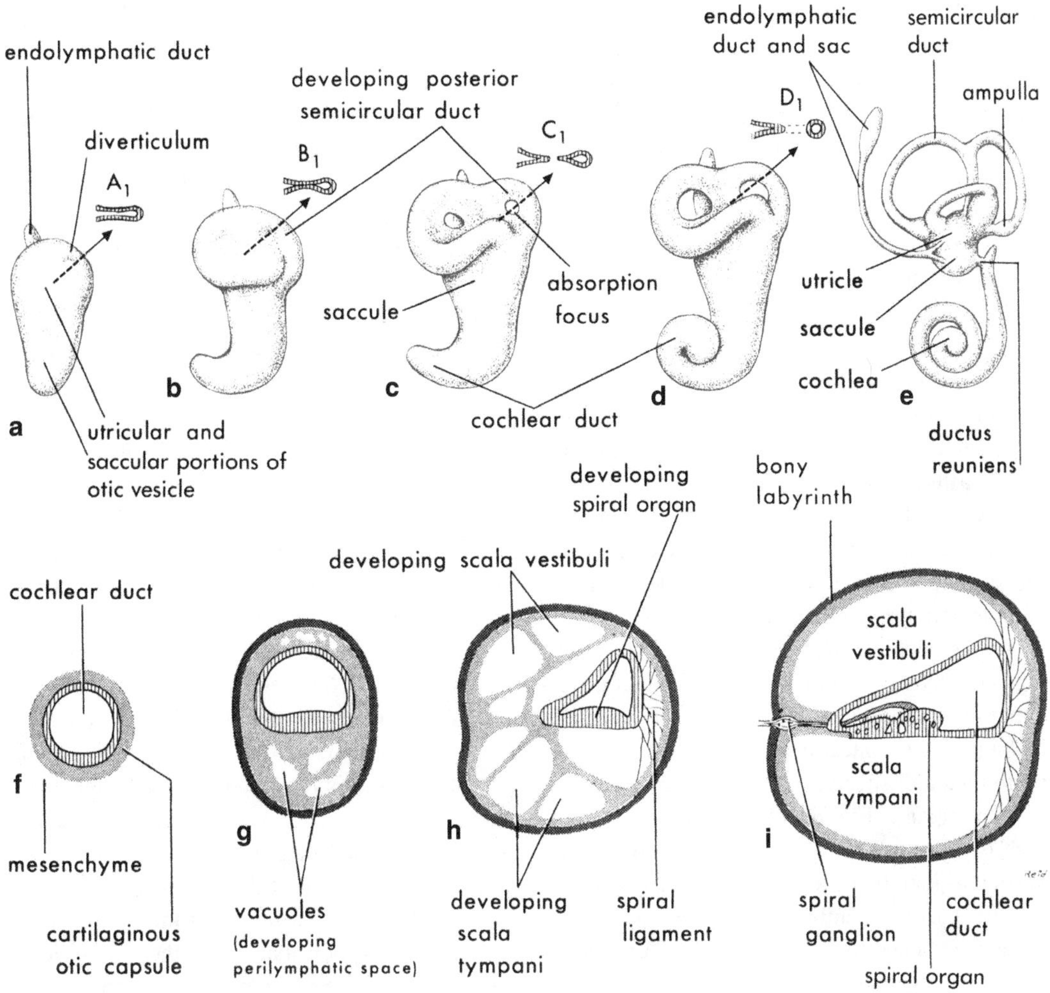

Fig. 2.10 Schematic diagram of embryology of the inner ear and of the scala tympani development (reprinted with permission from Moore KL, Persaud TVN. The Developing Human: Clinically Oriented Embryology. 5th ed. Philadelphia: W.B. Saunders; 1993)

need for ongoing follow-up is important given the risk of recurrence with cholesteatoma, which increases with the size of the lesion upon initial presentation.

Inner Ear

Embryology

Unlike the external and middle ear, the inner ear is not a pharyngeal arch derivative and is fairly unique in deriving all end organ structures and neural innervations from one common otic anlagen (the otocyst). At approximately 22 days of gestation, the first sign of the developing inner ear appears as thickening of the ectoderm on each side of the rhombencephalon, dorsal to the first branchial groove [88]. Within days, these bilateral ectodermal thickenings (the otic placodes) invaginate into the underlying mesenchyme to form the otic pit. Further invagination of the otic pit and fusion of overlying epithelium yield the otocyst or otic vesicle [89] (Fig. 2.10).

The otocyst begins to differentiate by week 5. One of the first elements to differentiate from the otocyst is a small diverticulum from the medial wall of the vesicle, extending above the dorsal pole; this eventually gives rise to the endolymphatic duct and sac. From the dorsal region of the otocyst, the pars utriculovestibularis grows dorsocranially, destined to become the utricle and semicircular canals. From the ventral region of the otocyst, the pars sacculocochlearis grows ventrocaudally, eventually giving rise to the cochlear duct and saccule.

By the sixth week of gestation, the ventral component has developed a more prominent outpouching (the cochlear duct) that elongates as it is penetrates the surrounding mesenchyme in a spiral fashion. The cochlear duct grows rapidly and by the eighth to tenth week has completed two-and-a-half turns [89, 90]. Its connection with the saccule at this point is reduced to a narrow confinement termed the ductus reunions.

As the cochlear duct elongates, the surrounding mesenchyme begins its cartilaginous differentiation. By the tenth week, this shell of cartilage had undergone vacuolization to form the two perilymphatic spaces, the scala vestibuli and scala tympani. The endolymph-filled cochlear duct is separated from the scala vestibuli by the vestibular membrane and from the scala tympani by the basilar membrane. The cochlear duct remains attached to the surrounding cartilage by the spiral ligament. The medial wall of the cochlear duct is partially supported by a long cartilaginous process, the modiolus. This represents the future central axis of the bony cochlea.

By the ninth gestational week, the first sign of a developing organ of Corti appears within the cochlear duct as a ridge of polygonal cells [91, 92]. While initially these cells appear alike, they soon form two ridges. The inner ridge represents the future spiral limbus. The outer ridge has cells that, on their surface, display a kinocilium and many hairlike microvilli. Over the next 3 weeks, hair cells are transformed by a progressive loss of microvilli and a developing array of stereocilia on their upper surface. At this point, it becomes evident that there is a single row of inner hair cells and three to four rows of outer hair cells. During this developmental period (9th to 12th week), a fibrillar gelatinous substance attached to the spiral limbus begins to form. This tectorial membrane, together with the sensory cells, constitutes the organ of Corti.

By the 15th gestational week, all the hair cells have developed an array of stereocilia, which is more advanced near the base of the cochlea than the apex. The development of stereocilia arrays occurs earlier on inner than on outer hair cells, and as such inner hair cells appear more mature displaying fewer microvilli. Their stereocilia are graduated upward in length toward the kinocilium and form a roughly U-shaped array. Outer hair cells follow the same trends, but their arrays are less geometric, showing a W pattern that is clearer toward the base of the cochlea than the apex. By the 22nd gestational week, the cochlear duct is larger in caliber. The stria vascularis demonstrates three cellular layers, and the tectorial membrane acquires a more adult appearance. The cochlear appearance continues to mature so that by the 24th to 26th gestational week, hair cells have fewer microvilli, and the V or W pattern of hair cell stereocilia is fully developed [90].

Paralleling this development, the semicircular canals start to appear during the sixth gestational week as flattened outpouchings from the dorsal (utricula) component of the otic vesicle. As these canals dilate, their central portions undergo an apoptotic resorption that yields the mature looplike semicircular canal. One end of each developing canal widens to form the crus ampullare. Two of the non-dilated ends from the superior and posterior semicircular canals fuse together to form the crus nonampullare (common crus). As such, only five crura enter the utricle, three with an ampulla and two without. Cells in the ampullae form a crest, the crista ampullaris, which contains sensory cells involved in rotary equilibrium. Similar sensory areas, the maculae, develop in the walls of the utricle and saccule. These cells convey information pertaining to horizontal and vertical bodily motion, respectively. Impulses generated in sensory cells of the cristae and maculae triggered by a change in body position are carried to the brain by vestibular fibers of cranial nerve VIII.

By the fourth week, a group of cells separate from the otic vesicle and become the statoacoustic ganglion [93]. Other cells of this ganglion are derived from the neural crest. The statoacoustic ganglion will proceed to develop the eighth cranial nerve. The ganglion cells destined to become the cochlear division of the nerve migrate to the developing cochlea where they wind around its central post, the modiolus, to form the spiral ganglion [90]. Once there, these neuronal cells begin to extend axonal processes in two directions: one toward the developing organ of Corti, and the other toward the brainstem. The processes directed to the brainstem reach there by the fifth to sixth gestational week. Those processes targeted toward the organ of Corti enter its base at the ninth gestational week. By the 10th to 12th week, these axonal branches form rounded synaptic terminals contacting the bases of the developing hair cells [94].

Congenital Inner Ear Anomalies

Definition

Congenital inner ear anomalies refer to the spectrum of malformations of the inner ear arising from an arrest of development of the labyrinth at a particular stage.

Embryology

As previously discussed, the bony labyrinth evolves early on between the 4th and 8th week of gestation, while the development of the sensory epithelium proceeds until the 25th week. As such, inner ear malformations evident on imaging studies are usually due to insults between the fourth and eighth week, whereas later injuries affect the sensory epithelium.

Etiology

In the current era of immunization, about 50 % of infants found to have congenital hearing loss are estimated to be genetic, with the remainder of cases attributed to environmental causes such as congenital infection, fetal ototoxic drug exposure, trauma, or other causes [95].

Classification

Inner ear anomalies can be classified as involving the membranous portion of the labyrinth only or the bony and the membranous components. Currently, the most common classification system of labyrinthine malformations is that introduced by Jackler et al. [96] in 1987 (Table 2.12). Based on radiographic and histologic studies, it was noted that most inner ear malformations resemble histologic sections of the inner ear taken at different points in development between the fourth and eighth week. Thus, Jackler's proposed classification of inner ear anomalies is based on an arrest in development at a specific point in embryogenesis (Fig. 2.11a, b).

The evolution of better imaging techniques, particularly with reference to magnetic resonance imaging (MRI) scanning, has resulted in the description of further divisions of cochlear anomalies. Jackler's classification system has since been expanded and modified by Sennaroglu [97], who differentiated five main categories: malformations of the cochlea, vestibule, semicircular canals, internal auditory canal, and vestibular or cochlear aqueduct (Table 2.13). Cochlear malformations were further divided into six categories of severity based on the timeline of developmental arrest. While more comprehensive, some observed inner ear malformations still cannot necessarily be categorized in any one subset. Furthermore, several inner ear structures, such as the cochlea and the semicircular canals, may share a common developmental timeline, yet have specific genes on which their development is dependent. As such, isolated arrest in the development of these structures can occur.

Table 2.12 Jackler's classification of inner ear malformations

Classification	Description
Category A: Cochlear aplasia or malformation	1. Michel aplasia (labyrinthine aplasia) 2. Cochlear aplasia, vestibule, and semicircular canals present 3. Cochlear hypoplasia 4. Incomplete cochlea 5. Common cavity *Note*: Enlarged vestibular aqueduct possible
Category B: Normal cochlea	1. Dysplasia of the vestibule and lateral semicircular canal 2. Large vestibular aqueduct

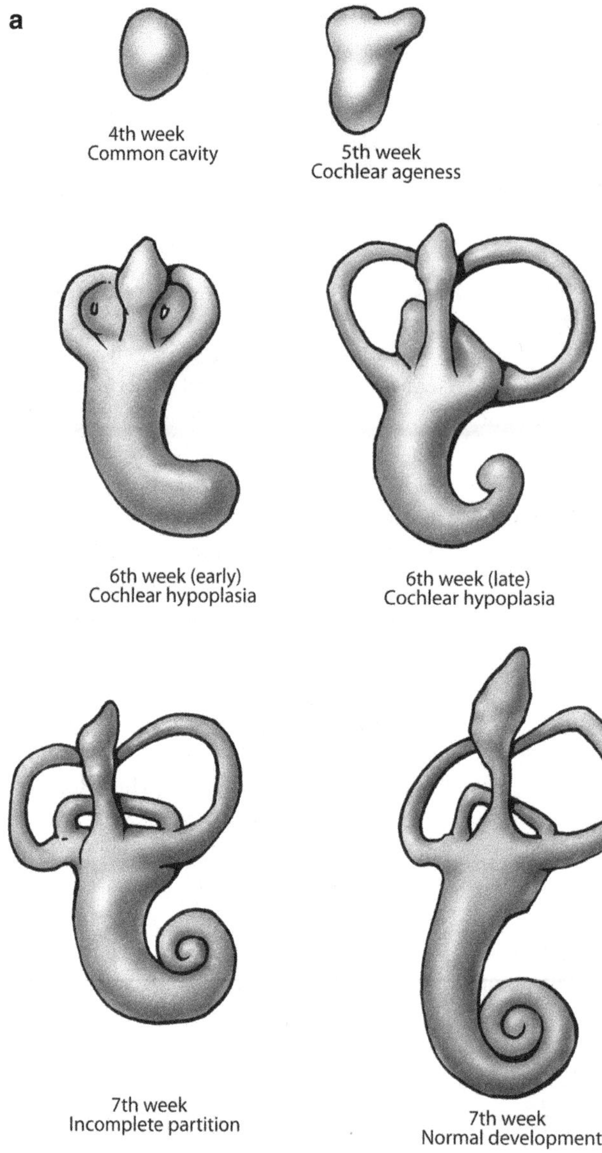

Fig. 2.11 (**a**, **b**) Schematic diagrams of the embryogenesis and more common anomalies of the inner ear (adapted from Jackler RK, Luxford WM, House WF. Congenital malformations of the inner ear: a classification based on organogenesis. Laryngoscope. 1987;97(Suppl 40):2)

Clinical Features

Inner ear anomalies are frequently found in patients who have SNHL. Combined malformations of the inner ear and the middle ear (with the external ear) are rare, reflecting their different embryologic origins. Only in 10–15 % of cases are combined malformations of the external, middle, and inner ear observed [98]. One plausible explanation for this finding is the participation of mesenchymal components in the development of all three parts of the ear. If these mesenchymal structures are altered by genetic or nongenetic triggers of developmental defects, all domains of the ear can be involved.

Diagnosis

In the United States, almost 90 % of newborns are screened for hearing impairment prior to

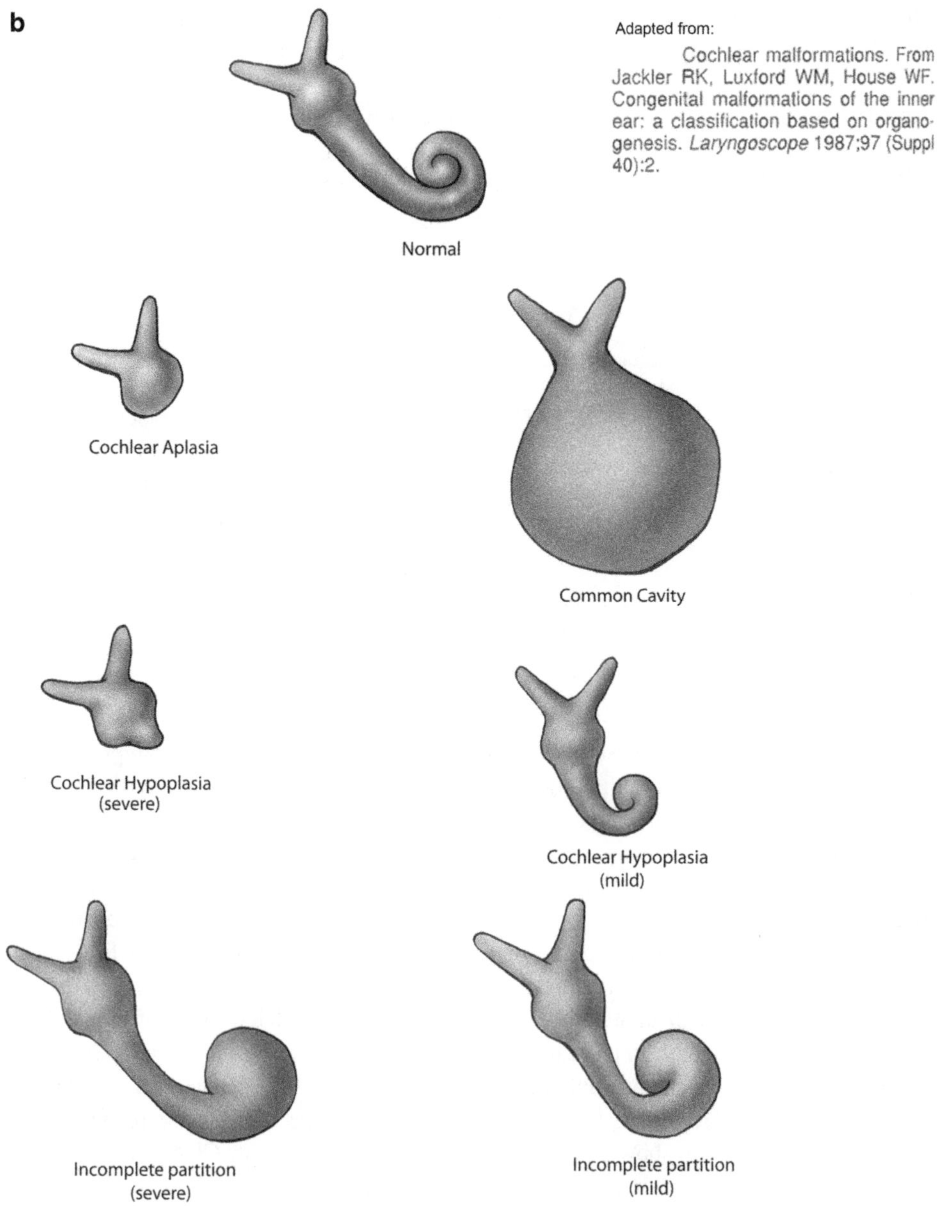

Fig. 2.11 (continued)

leaving the hospital [99]. Infants found to have abnormal screening results should be referred for formal audiologic testing. When indicated, consultation with a geneticist for chromosomal analysis and evaluation for specific syndromes related to hearing loss should also be obtained. A high-resolution CT scan or MRI scan of the inner ear should be obtained in all patients with suspected inner ear malformation, including all children with unexplained SNHL based on negative examination as well as laboratory and genetic testing. The timing of the scan should be early on in the work-up when the hearing loss is first realized. It is important to remember, however, that the majority of patients with congenital SNHL have defects limited to the membranous labyrinth, which are beyond the resolution of current imaging techniques and can only be seen

Table 2.13 Sennaroglu's classification of inner ear malformations

Category	Subgroups
A = Incomplete embryonic development	Complete aplasia of inner ear (Michel deformity) Common cavity Aplasia/hypoplasia of cochlea (normal posterior labyrinth) Aplasia/hypoplasia of posterior labyrinth (normal cochlea) Hypoplasia of entire labyrinth Mondini dysplasia
B = Aberrant embryonic development	Enlarged vestibular aqueduct Narrow internal auditory canal (intraosseous diameter less than 2 mm) Long crista transversa Internal auditory canal tripartitus Incomplete cochleomeatal separation
C = Isolated hereditary malformations	X-linked hearing loss
D	Malformations associated with syndromes

on histologic section. In large series, only approximately 20 % of patients with congenital hearing loss have anomalies visible on cross-sectional imaging [96, 100].

Management

While patients with unilateral SNHL and a normal ear may not need immediate intervention, the vast majority of children with bilateral hearing loss benefit from some form of amplification or assistive-listening device. Cochlear implantation is an option for children older than 1 year with bilateral profound SNHL who show only limited benefit from conventional amplification devices, although they may be used in patients younger than 1 year of age who have meningitis and may have resultant labyrinthitis ossificans, which can preclude implantation if allowed to progress prior to surgery.

Complete Labyrinthine Aplasia

Definition

Complete labyrinthine aplasia (CLA), or Michel aplasia, was first described by P. Michel in 1863. It refers to complete absence of development of inner ear structures.

Incidence

This deformity is rare and represents less than 1 % of all inner ear malformations.

Etiology

CLA is caused by early arrest of differentiation of the otic placode at the third gestational week.

Associated Malformations

Lack of development of the placode usually leads to disturbed development of the skeletal portion of the second arch. This leads to aplasia of the stapes and aberrance in the course of the facial nerve and the jugular vein. CLA has been associated with thalidomide exposure, anencephaly, Wildervanck syndrome, and Klippel–Feil syndrome [101].

Clinical Features

Patients with CLA present with profound SNHL.

Diagnosis

CT and MRI will show complete absence of the labyrinth. CLA must be differentiated from complete labyrinthine ossification secondary to meningitis, whereby the labyrinth is fully formed but obliterated by osteoneogenesis. In labyrinthine ossification, the lateral wall of the cochlea has a preserved convex form, while in CLA the promontory is flat [102]. In patients with labyrinthine ossification, the IAC can be recognized in contrast to patients with CLA. MRI may be more sensitive in the detection of neo-ossification of the cochlear duct compared with high-resolution CT [103]. This distinction between labyrinthine aplasia and labyrinthitis ossificans becomes important when considering a patient for cochlear implantation because aplasia is an absolute contraindication, whereas implantation has been successful in some patients who have labyrinthitis ossificans.

Management

There are currently no therapeutic options for patients with CLA, although these patients may

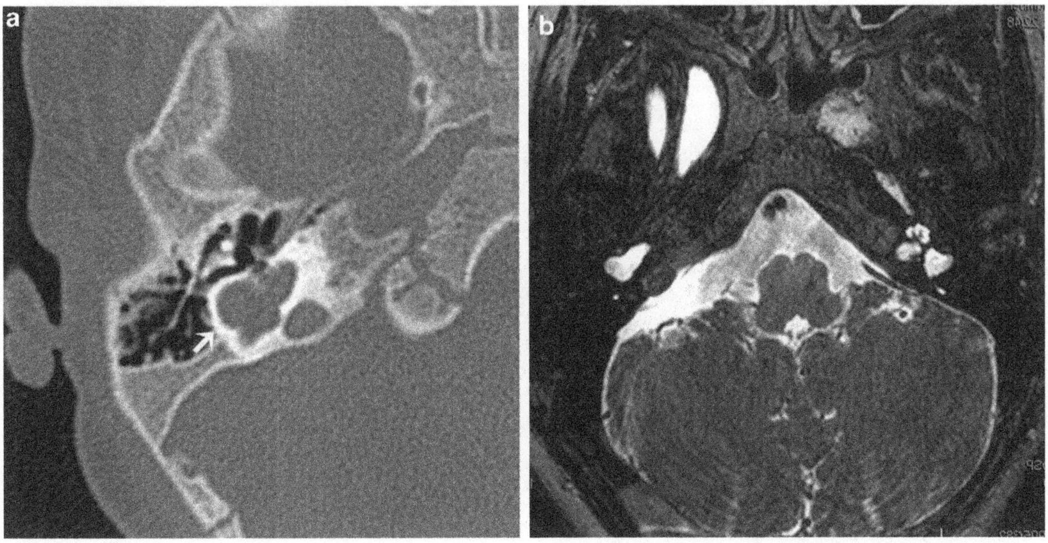

Fig. 2.12 (**a**) Axial computed tomography of right temporal bone demonstrating a common cavity malformation of the cochlea (*arrow*) (image courtesy of John A. Germiller MD, PhD). (**b**) Magnetic resonance image of right common cavity malformation

be candidates for brainstem implantation in the future [104].

Common Cavity Malformation

Definition

The common cavity malformation (CCM) refers to the abnormal differentiation of the otocyst into the inner ear structures, where a "common cavity" arises that represents the malformed cochlea and vestibule with a poorly differentiated membranous labyrinth within.

Incidence

The CCM represents approximately 25 % of all cochlear malformations.

Etiology

The CCM arises when development is arrested between the fourth and fifth weeks of gestation. During this developmental period, an otocyst is present; however, this otocyst has not differentiated yet into the primordia of the cochlea, vestibule, and semicircular canals.

Associated Malformations

CCM has been associated with an anteromedially displaced facial nerve course and possible cochlear nerve aplasia.

Clinical Features

Patients with CCM present with SNHL, generally in the severe to profound range.

Diagnosis

The "common cavity" appears as a single cavity in the region of the inner ear on CT and a fluid-filled cavity on MRI (Fig. 2.12a, b). The semicircular canals can be normal or may be malformed. In contrast to patients with CLA, the IAC can be identified in patients with the CCM. On axial CT, a CCM can be differentiated from lateral semicircular canal dysplasia by its anterior position with respect to the IAC [104].

Management

Cochlear implantation has been successfully performed in patients with CCM [105], although the results are less optimal compared to patients with an intact inner ear structure; results vary depending on the degree of membranous and neural development. An MRI and/or CT scan should be performed prior to proceeding with cochlear implantation given the risk of intraoperative cerebrospinal fluid and/or perilymphatic leaks as well as to assess for the position of the facial nerve and the presence of the cochlear nerve.

Cochlear Aplasia

Definition

Cochlear aplasia (CA) describes complete absence of development of the cochlea.

Incidence

CA contributes to only 3 % of cochlear malformations.

Etiology

CA results from arrest of development during the fifth fetal week.

Associated Malformations

Unknown.

Clinical Features

Patients with this anomaly present with profound SNHL.

Diagnosis

The abnormal cochlea is seen as a single cavity on radiologic imaging. The vestibule and semicircular canals can be normal; however, they are more commonly malformed and may have only remnants evident. These remnants can be distinguished from the cochlea by their position posterior to the IAC.

Management

Although cochlear implantation can be attempted, the procedure may be precluded by lack of an auditory nerve [106] (Fig. 2.13a–c).

Cochlear Hypoplasia

Definition

Cochlear hypoplasia refers to abnormal development of the cochlea, whereby it can be distinguished but has only one or fewer than one turn.

Incidence

CH represents 15 % of cochlear malformations.

Etiology

CH arises when the normal development of the cochlear duct is impaired during the sixth week of gestation.

Associated Malformations

CH is most often associated with BOR syndrome [107]. In severe cases, the labyrinthine segment of the facial nerve can be displaced anteromedially.

Clinical Features

Patients with CH present with variable degrees of hearing loss depending on the exact time of arrest within the sixth week, which reflects the degree of differentiation of the membranous labyrinth and neuroepithelial elements.

Diagnosis

On CT imaging, the cochlea may appear round and undeveloped, usually measuring 6 mm in height compared with a normal cochlea height of 10–12 mm. As with CA, the vestibule and semicircular canals can be normal, although most often they are malformed (Fig. 2.14).

Management

Cochlear implantation has been attempted, and the results of implantation depend on the degree of differentiation of the membranous labyrinth and neuroepithelial elements.

Incomplete Partitioning

Definition

Cochlear malformations classified as "incomplete partitioning" represent a spectrum of anomalies. At one end of the spectrum, a malformation may result such that a cystic cochlea lacks all interscalar septae and modiolus. This entity has been referred to as pseudo-Mondini malformation, cystic cochleovestibular malformation, or incomplete partition type I. On the other end of

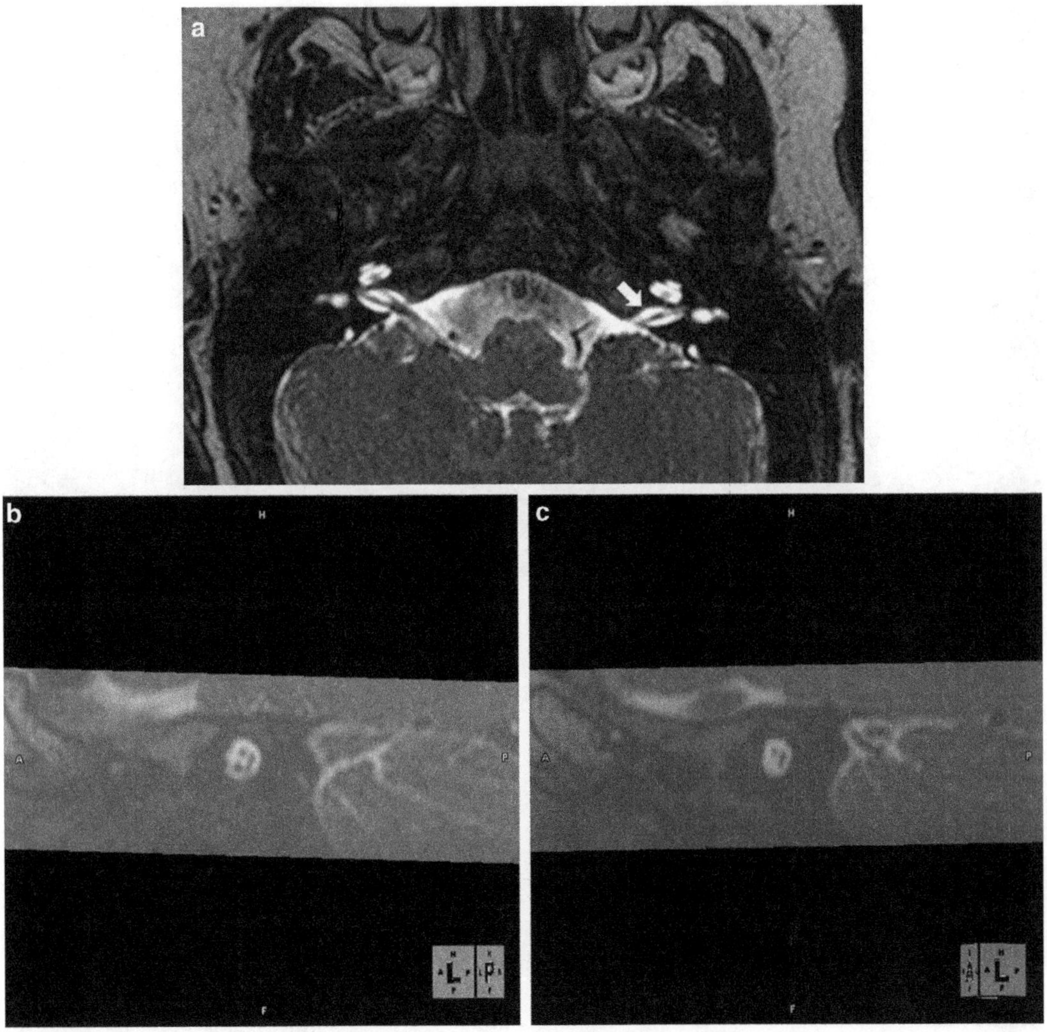

Fig. 2.13 (**a**) Axial magnetic resonance image of temporal bones demonstrating normal inner ears with a normal internal acoustic canal on the right compared with one that has no cochlear nerve on the left (*arrow*), respectively (image courtesy of John A. Germiller, MD, PhD). (**b**) Sagittal view of the right internal acoustic canal contents demonstrating normal nerve bundles (two vestibular nerves: one facial nerve and the cochlear nerve). (**c**) and demonstrating sagittal view of the left internal acoustic canal contents demonstrating that the cochlear nerve is absent (image courtesy of John A. Germiller, MD, PhD)

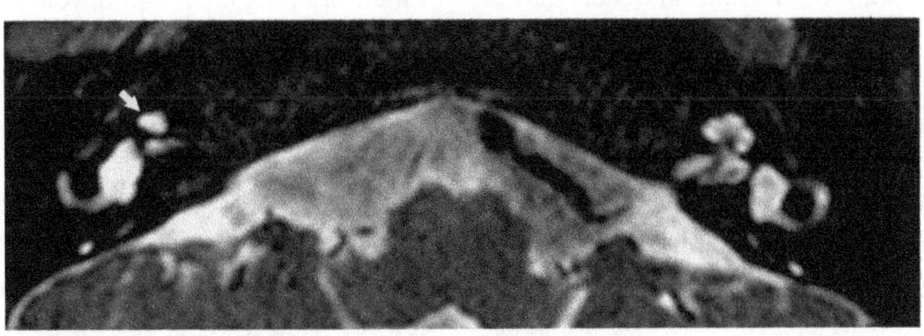

Fig. 2.14 Axial magnetic resonance image of temporal bone demonstrating cochlear hypoplasia (*arrow*) (image courtesy of John A. Germiller, MD, PhD)

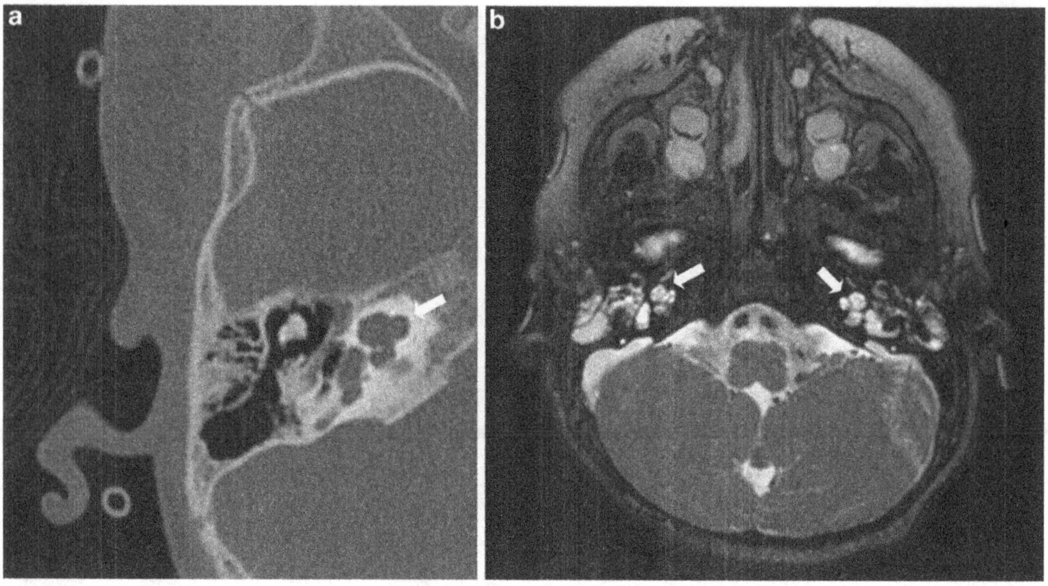

Fig. 2.15 (**a**, **b**) Right sided CT and bilateral magnetic resonance imaging of temporal bone demonstrating incomplete partitioning of the cochlea (Mondini malformation)

the spectrum, the cochlea may only demonstrate one-and-a-half turns; the basal turn of the cochlea is normal while the second and apical turn of the cochlea are fused. The interscalar septum between the middle and apical turn is typically normal. This refers to the classic Mondini malformation (MM) or incomplete partition type II.

Incidence

The MM is the most common cochlear malformation seen on imaging, and it accounts for 55 % of all cochlear malformations [108].

Etiology

The MM arises as a result of arrest of inner ear development during the seventh week of gestation. The pseudo-Mondini malformation occurs earlier in the seventh week than the more developed MM.

Associated Conditions

MM has also been associated with stapes footplate anomalies; in these cases, the second genu of the facial nerve can be displaced anteriorly and inferiorly [109]. Incomplete partition is often associated with a large vestibular aqueduct as well as a large endolymphatic duct [110, 111]. Overall, malformations involving the vestibule, semicircular canals, and endolymphatic duct and sac are found in 20 % of these patients [110]. MM has been associated with several syndromes including Waardenburg, DiGeorge, and Pendred.

Clinical Features

Patients with incomplete partition present with variable degrees of hearing loss, and the degree of hearing loss in true Mondini malformation is typically less severe than in the cystic cochleovestibular malformation [97, 112]. Since the basal turn is developed, high-frequency hearing is usually preserved to a variable degree. Overall, the severity of hearing loss depends on the degree of membranous labyrinth development.

Diagnosis

The interscalar septal defect and absence of the osseous spiral lamina of the middle and apical turns can be seen on CT, but is best be demonstrated on heavily T2-weighted gradient-echo images (Fig. 2.15a, b). Patients with MM have been reported to be at risk of recurrent meningitis, attributable to spontaneous fistulas between the middle ear and the subarachnoid space [113, 114]. As such, a patient with a history of unilateral or bilateral hearing loss and recurrent meningitis must be evaluated for the presence of an MM, even in adult patients as this condition may remain undiagnosed for many years.

Management

Cochlear implantation is usually the management of choice. Caution should be paid in the preoperative evaluation, as MM may be associated with a defect of the modiolus. In this case, the intracerebral pressure can be transmitted to the cochlea, resulting in a gusher at the time of electrode insertion. Several studies have demonstrated that evaluation of the modiolus and measurement of its size are possible on MRI [115, 116].

Membranous Labyrinthine Anomalies

Definition

Membranous labyrinthine anomalies refer to malformations of the membranous portion of the inner ear, and they can occur in isolation or in combination with bony labyrinthine anomalies.

Incidence

Membranous malformations are thought to account for up to 90 % of congenital SNHL cases, although this number may be dropping as improved imaging modalities are detecting a wider spectrum of osseous anomalies [110].

Etiology

Membranous labyrinthine anomalies result from arrest of development of the sensory neuroepithelium, which proceeds from the 4th to the 25th gestational week. Development of the bony labyrinth is complete at a much earlier embryologic timeline; it is essentially complete by the eighth week of gestation.

Classification

The classification of membranous anomalies is based on the embryologic division of the membranous labyrinth, arising from two components: the pars superior and the pars inferior. The pars superior forms the semicircular canals, endolymphatic duct, and utricle; the pars inferior becomes the saccule and cochlear duct. Anomalies can involve an isolated portion of the membranous labyrinth, one division, or the entire labyrinth [117].

Clinical Features

Patients with membranous labyrinthine anomalies present with variable degrees of SNHL. The longer period of gestational development required for development of the membranous compared to that of the bony labyrinth may explain why membranous malformations account for a larger percentage of patients who have SNHL.

Diagnosis

The diagnosis of membranous labyrinthine anomalies can only be inferred without histologic sectioning due to limitations in imaging. Nevertheless, the algorithm for the diagnostic work-up follows that described earlier for cochlear anomalies. Infants found to have abnormal screening results should be referred for prompt formal audiologic testing, with appropriate genetics consultation as appropriate. A high-resolution CT scan or MRI scan of the inner ear should be obtained early on in the work-up of all patients with suspected inner ear malformation.

Management

The severity of hearing loss, as well as whether one or both ears are involved, dictates further management. Children with bilateral profound SNHL should be referred for cochlear implantation candidacy evaluation. The assumption of implantation is that some of the cochlear neural population survives despite the absence of hair cells. In congenital malformations of the inner ear, the auditory nerve population has been shown to be typically less than with other forms of sensory deafness, including ototoxicity and sudden SNHL [118]. This type of data would suggest that while patients with congenital inner ear malformations may benefit from implantation, the hearing outcomes might not be as favorable as those observed in patients with non-congenital malformations of the inner ear [108].

Bing–Siebenmann Malformation

Definition

The Bing–Siebenmann malformation is a complete membranous labyrinthine dysplasia first described in 1907. It is a rare membranous malformation associated with a well-formed bony capsule.

Etiology

The Bing–Siebenmann malformation arises from the complete arrest of development of the embryologic division of the membranous labyrinth.

Associated Malformations

Bing–Siebenmann malformation has been seen in patients diagnosed with Usher syndrome, Jervell and Lange-Nielsen syndrome [117], and the oculo-auriculo-vertebral spectrum.

Clinical Features

Patients who have Bing–Siebenmann malformation have profound SNHL.

Diagnosis

On histopathologic sectioning, the cochlear duct has a poorly developed organ of Corti with an abnormal stria vascularis and collapse of Reissner's membrane. The saccule and macula are also poorly developed.

Scheibe Malformation

Definition

Scheibe malformation, first described in 1892, is the most common histopathologic membranous inner ear malformation. It is commonly known as cochleosaccular dysplasia and results in a malformed organ of Corti and saccule.

Etiology

Scheibe malformation arises from incomplete development of the pars inferior division of the membranous labyrinth. Inheritance is in an autosomal recessive fashion. A gene defect on chromosome 1q32 has been demonstrated [101].

Associated Malformations

It is most often associated with Usher syndrome but is also seen with Jervell–Lange-Nielsen, Refsum disease, Waardenburg syndrome, trisomy 18 [117], and congenital rubella infection.

Clinical Features

Patients with Scheibe malformation have severe to profound SNHL.

Diagnosis

Histologically, there is a partial or a complete aplasia of the organ of Corti and collapse of the cochlear duct [108]. The saccule is usually collapsed with degenerated sensory neuroepithelium. The stria vascularis is typically degenerated, with characteristic changes consisting of aplasia alternating with regions of hyperplasia and gross deformity.

Alexander Malformation

Definition

Alexander malformation involves an otherwise normal labyrinth with the exception of a dysplastic basal turn of the cochlea.

Etiology

Alexander malformation arises due to aplasia of the membranous cochlear duct, primarily affecting the neural receptor cells of the basal turn of the cochlea.

Associated Malformations

Alexander malformation may be related to familial high-frequency SNHL.

Clinical Features

Alexander malformation may present with high-frequency SNHL. Some patients may be asymptomatic.

Diagnosis

Histologically, dysplastic changes are limited to the basal turn of the cochlea.

Management

Preservation of the lower frequency hearing justifies a trial of hearing aids, with cochlear implantation for more severe hearing loss. Current trials involving the combination of a short-electrode cochlear implant with a traditional hearing aid, or a hybrid cochlear implant, may provide an the option for low-frequency hearing preservation in the future.

Enlarged Vestibular Aqueduct

Definition

The vestibular aqueduct traverses the otic capsule between the posterior cranial fossa and an opening in the medial wall of the vestibule. It has an average length of 10 mm. The osseous portion extends from the medial wall of the vestibule to the posterior surface of the petrous pyramid. Enlarged vestibular aqueduct (EVA) was first described by Valvassori and Clemis in 1978 [119] as a radiographic entity pertaining to enlargement of this structure beyond the normal limits. Enlarged vestibular aqueduct syndrome has been defined as the presence of the anomaly of the inner ear in the clinical setting of SNHL [120].

Incidence

Many authors have reported different incidence rates depending on the patient population studied. EVA is the most common cause of congenital/developmental SNHL for which an imaging correlate is found [121, 122]. EVA was found in 0.64–7 % of children with an SNHL of unknown etiology [121, 123], in 1 % of patients with various otologic problems [124], in 2.25 % of patients referred for temporal bone CT scans [125], and in 4 % of children in a cochlear implant program [126].

Associated Malformations

EVA is most frequently associated with Pendred syndrome [127] but can be associated with other syndromes such as BOR syndrome [128], Noonan syndrome [129], Waardenburg syndrome [130], and distal renal tubular acidosis [131, 132]. EVA and Pendred syndrome are closely linked on the basis of a common genetic disorder causing varying phenotypes. In 1999, Abe et al. [133] determined that the gene locus of EVA is located between the flanking markers D7S501 and D7S2425 on chromosome 7q31. This gene region overlaps the gene locus for SLC26A4, the pendrin gene. Usami et al. [134] detected seven mutations in EVA patients, two of them being common for Pendred syndrome and EVA.

Clinical Features

Most patients with EVA present between 3 and 5 years of age [122, 135–137]. The most common presenting symptom is that of hearing loss. In 73–100 % of cases, EVA is found to be bilateral [120, 122, 136, 138], although hearing loss may only be evident in one ear. The hearing loss on initial audiometric assessment is typically a down-sloping SNHL [120, 136, 139]. The mean pure tone average is reported to be about 60 dB [120, 136]. If there is bilateral involvement, the hearing loss is most commonly asymmetric. At least one-third of EVA patients suffer from dizziness and typically develop it later than the hearing loss [140, 141]. A conductive component to the SNHL is variably present in 17–90 % of the reported cases [120, 124, 136, 138].

There is variability in the literature on the progression of SNHL in patients with EVA. The incidence of progressive hearing loss ranges between 10 and 65 % [120, 135], whereas stable hearing is reported between 61 and 81 % of the cases/ears [122, 124, 132]. In a systematic review of the literature yielding a total of 310 ears with EVA with a mean follow-up of 4 years, Mori et al. [142] found stable hearing in 67 % of which 34 % demonstrated fluctuations in hearing. In the 33 % with progression of hearing loss, 50 % demonstrated fluctuations in hearing. Most of the studies have never been able to find a significant correlation between the degree, type, or progression of the hearing loss, the volume or diameter of the endolymphatic duct and sac, the area of the modiolus, or the signal intensity of the endolymphatic sac [122, 123, 143–145].

Minor head trauma is known to cause an acute hearing loss in EVA patients [120, 121, 123, 143, 146]. Activities that result in a change

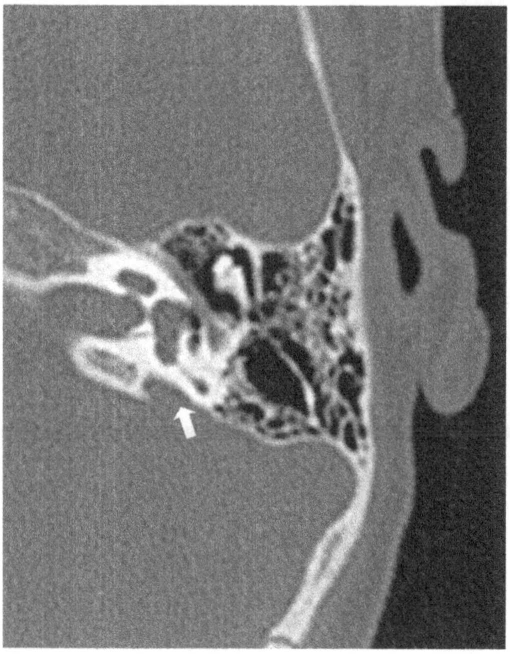

Fig. 2.16 Left temporal bone with enlarged vestibular aqueduct (*arrow*)

in barometric pressure, including scuba diving, lifting, playing a wind instrument, and airplane flights, have been reported to cause a sudden hearing loss [123, 147]. There remains debate as to the etiology of the sudden hearing loss with minor head trauma in EVA patients. The hearing loss following minor head trauma in EVA patients can spontaneously recover [136].

Diagnosis

The diagnosis of EVA is based on a CT scan or an MRI scan of the temporal bones in axial and/or coronal views (Fig. 2.16). There has been some variability noted in the literature regarding the criteria used for diagnosing EVA. In their original work, Valvassori and Clemis [119] diagnosed EVA to be present if the diameter of the vestibular aqueduct was greater than 1.5 mm, measured halfway between the external aperture and the common crus of the utricular and saccular duct. Others have diagnosed an EVA if the diameter is 2 mm or greater [120, 135] or if the midpoint diameter is more than double the diameter of the posterior semicircular canal [148]. Associated inner ear anomalies are noted, including a Mondini malformation. Complete audiometric assessment is undertaken to document any associated hearing loss. Some authors recommend routine genetic testing for the pendrin gene given the frequent association of EVA with Pendred syndrome.

Management

Children are fitted with hearing aid commensurate with their hearing loss and are followed on a regular basis with physical examinations and audiometric assessments to document the progression of hearing loss in one or both ears and to assess for the development of new symptoms, including vertigo. Many otologists recommend that patients with EVA avoid contact sports and the use of helmets in many activities, although there is no data demonstrating their efficacy.

In an effort to halt the progression of SNHL in EVA, surgical procedures, including endolymphatic sac decompression, shunt, or endolymphatic duct obliteration, have been attempted. None of these options are effective and may worsen the hearing loss [149–151]. Although Lin et al. [152] recommended corticosteroid therapy immediately after a sudden hearing loss in EVA patients, there is no evidence to support this recommendation. In patients who progress to severe or profound SNHL (with deterioration of word recognition scores), cochlear implantation evaluation is performed. Many authors have documented comparable results from implantation in patients with EVA compared to those with other etiologies of SNHL [126, 153–156]. There is a higher incidence of intraoperative perilymphatic gusher in patients with EVA undergoing implantation [126, 139, 153–155, 157].

Facial Nerve

Embryology

At about 4 weeks, the facial nerve and its geniculate ganglion begin development. The primordial tissue from which they arise is in the area of the rhombencephalon, abutting the deep aspect of the second pharyngeal arch epibranchial placode

[158]. The latter is a thickened area of surface ectoderm just caudal to the first pharyngeal groove. Neuroblasts in the region between the primordial facial nerve tissue and the epibranchial placode differentiate; this gives rise to the geniculate ganglion by 6 weeks of gestation. Paralleling this development, the facial motor nucleus appears in the future metencephalon [159, 160]. The first branch of the facial nerve, the chorda tympani nerve, also becomes evident at this point. As the abducens nucleus develops, it displaces the intramedullary fibers of the facial motor nucleus, creating the internal genu of the facial.

At approximately 6 weeks of gestation, the greater petrosal nerve, the second branch of the facial nerve to form, develops from the ventral aspect of the geniculate ganglion. By the seventh week, the chorda tympani and lingual nerves unite just proximal to the ganglion. Meanwhile, the nervus intermedius, the sensory fibers of the facial nerve, develops independently from the geniculate ganglion and extends to the brainstem between the motor root of the facial nerve and the eighth cranial nerve. The main trunk of the facial nerve establishes its intratemporal course within the developing otic capsule.

The next branches to develop are the posterior auricular nerve and the fibers to the posterior belly of the digastric muscle. Branches of the posterior auricular nerve communicate with nerves of the second and third cervical ganglia to form the transverse cervical and lesser occipital nerves. At approximately 7 weeks of gestation, a branch of the geniculate ganglion develops and travels to the glossopharyngeal ganglion; at 8 weeks, the tympanic plexus and the lesser petrosal nerve form along this branch. The nerve to the stapedius muscle develops at approximately the same time. The facial nerve develops peripheral branches that lie deep to the facial musculature. Most of these peripheral branches form anastomotic connections with other peripheral facial nerve fibers [159, 160].

Between the 12th and 13th weeks of gestation, Arnold's nerve (the auricular branch of the vagus) forms from the union of two branches that arise from the dorsomedial surface of the facial nerve (between the stapedius and the chorda tympani nerves). Arnold's nerve traverses the primitive tympanomastoid fissure to innervate the posterior aspect of the EAC. By 17 weeks, the various communications of the facial nerve, including those with the second and third cervical nerves and the trigeminal, vagus, and glossopharyngeal nerves, are well established.

The facial canal initially forms as a sulcus in the cartilaginous otic capsule, which later ossifies to form part of the fallopian canal, the remainder arising from Reichert's cartilage from the second branchial arch. The ossification of the tympanic segment of the fallopian canal involves two ossification centers [161]. The anterior segment develops at the apical cochlear ossification center at the end of 20 weeks, while the posterior segment develops at the pyramidal eminence at 25 weeks. Each ossification center projects two bony extensions that completely encircle the facial nerve. As the nerve continues to develop, the two centers extend from their origin, the anterior center posteriorly and the posterior center inferiorly, progressively lengthening to cover more of the nerve. Reichert's cartilage becomes attached to the otic capsule and provides the remaining cartilaginous circumference to the labyrinthine and tympanic segment of the facial canal [162]. By term, about 80 % of the tympanic segment of the fallopian canal is present. It is completely developed by about 3 months after birth. Failure of fusion of the two ossification centers or of their bony extensions is thought to be the cause of the surgically encountered facial canal dehiscences [161]. The mastoid process and tympanic ring grow postnatally, medially displacing and subsequently protecting the facial nerve [163].

Congenital Facial Palsy

Definition

Congenital facial palsy describes a developmental form of facial nerve paralysis, without a history of birth trauma. The paralysis can be unilateral or bilateral and may involve the entire nerve or only affect some of its branches

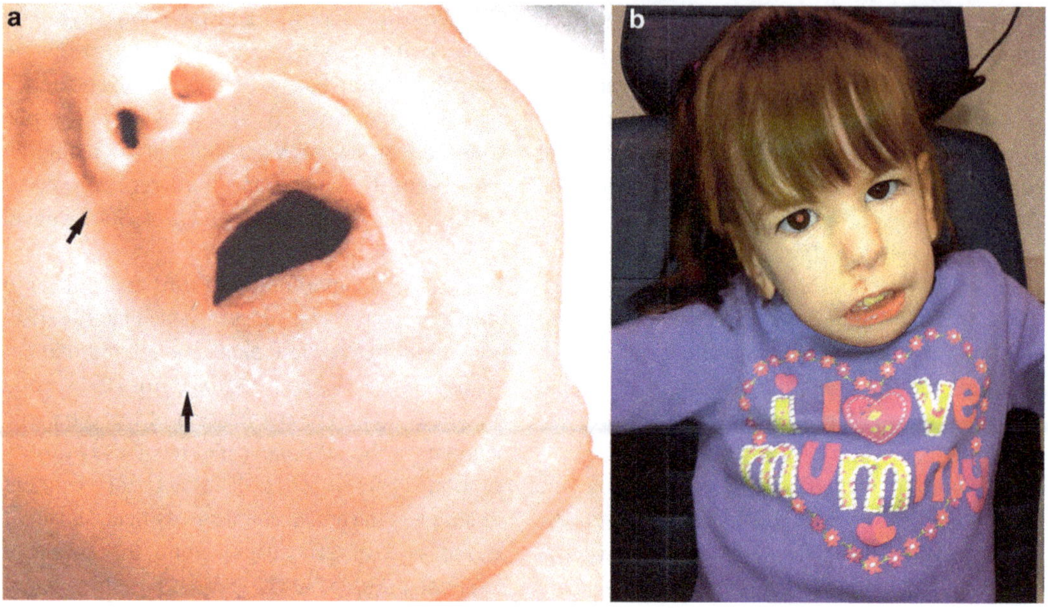

Fig. 2.17 (**a**) Photograph of infant with right facial nerve paralysis demonstrating lack of nasal flaring and asymmetric lower lip on crying. (**b**) Photography of child with bilateral facial nerve paralysis (Moebius syndrome)

(Fig. 2.17a). Moebius syndrome is perhaps the best known of the congenital facial palsy syndromes. It was first described by Paul Julius Moebius, a German neurologist, in 1892 as a clinical entity of bilateral combined palsies of the abducens and facial cranial nerves.

Incidence

Congenital facial palsy occurs with an incidence of approximately 1.4–2.1 per 1,000 live births [164, 165].

Etiology

Although sporadic cases of Moebius syndrome are thought to be most common, there have been pedigrees described, suggesting that some subgroups may be inherited via an autosomal dominant gene with variable expressivity and incomplete penetrance [166–168]. The etiology of Moebius syndrome is unknown. There are four general theories of pathogenesis [168–171]. The first describes aplasia or hypoplasia of affected cranial nerve nuclei, resulting in secondary muscle abnormalities [172]. The second theory hypothesizes foci of necrosis in the paramedian region of the pontine tegmentum with destruction of the VI and VII nuclei [167, 169, 171, 173, 174]. The third theory is based on the observation from cadaveric studies that have found absence or narrowing of the facial nerve in the fallopian canal, sometimes with normal nuclei [164, 175–177]. This may be related to vascular disruption and subsequent necrosis of the peripheral nerves [164, 177]. The fourth theory reflects primary myopathy based on autopsy studies on some patients showing normal neural components but atrophied and fibrotic facial muscles [178] (or absence of muscle in biopsies) [179, 180]. These muscle changes can occur secondary to prolonged muscle denervation or due to the lack of nerve development [181, 182]. If muscles fail to develop primarily, nerve fibers destined to innervate these muscles take on an aberrant course or fail to connect, retract, and atrophy [182].

Associated Malformations

Facial palsy can be associated with abnormalities of the EAC, middle ear, or mastoid. It may be a prominent feature in some infants with congenital muscle disorders, such as nemaline myopathy, congenital myotonic dystrophy, or congenital myasthenia. Congenital facial palsy is associated with several other syndromes, the most common of which is hemifacial microsomia. Other associated syndromes include Poland syndrome (absent pectoralis major muscle), Albers-Schoenberg disease, and the CHARGE Association.

Clinical Features

Moebius syndrome is characterized by sixth and seventh nerve palsies, which are its hallmark [183] (Fig. 2.17b). Congenital facial paralysis is usually noticed within the first few weeks of life and is often incomplete, with the upper face more severely affected [166, 184, 185]. Associated findings have included limb anomalies (e.g., webbed, absent, short, or deformed digits, club foot) [186–188], thoracic abnormalities (scoliosis, pectoral hypoplasia, or absence of the pectoral muscle) [186], and craniofacial deformities [189]. Lack of fine motor skills and poor coordination and balance performance are also highly associated with these patients. The syndrome can present profound psychological challenges as these children may have masklike facies; this may hinder parental attachment and can lead to social isolation, poor emotional development, and behavioral difficulties [190]. After infancy, children with Moebius syndrome experience difficulty with eating solid food and may develop a chronic drool. They are at risk of developing dental caries, enamel hypoplasia, and missing teeth. A child with an improper bite or difficulty swallowing probably will have micrognathia, and these children are at higher risk of developing sleep-disordered breathing. Speech development may be affected, secondary to incomplete lip closure coupled with the inability to use the tongue effectively. Ophthalmologic implications may include lack of lateral eye movement and reduced peripheral gaze. Irritation, corneal dryness, and even corneal ulceration can occur because of incomplete eyelid closure.

Classification

Abramson et al. [191] classified and graded Moebius syndrome on the basis of the clinical findings of cranial nerve palsies and musculoskeletal anomalies. They developed the acronym CLUFT (*c*ranial nerve, *l*ower limb, *u*pper limb, *f*ace, and *t*horax) to summarize the syndromal findings (Table 2.14). Recently, however, studies have defined and classified Moebius syndrome into two distinct neurophysiologic phenotypes. In one phenotype, patients have increased facial distal motor latencies (DML) and poor recruitment of small and polyphasic motor unit action potentials (MUAP). The second phenotype is characterized by normal facial DML and neuropathic MUAP [192].

Table 2.14 Abramson classification and grading system of Moebius syndrome

Features	Grade
C: Cranial nerves	
VII nerve partial	0
VI and VII nerve partial	1
VI and VII nerve complete	2
Additional nerve involvement	3
If bilateral and equal add	B
L: Lower extremity	
Normal	0
Talipes equinovarus, syndactyly, ankylosis	1
Absent phalanges	2
Longitudinal or transverse deficits	3
U: Upper extremity	
Normal	0
Digital hypoplasia or failure of differentiation	1
Ectrodactyly	2
Failure of formation, longitudinal or transverse	3
F: Facial structural anomaly	
Normal	0
Cleft palate	1
Micrognathia	2
Microtia, microphthalmia, abnormal joint, etc.	3
T: Thorax	
Normal	0
Scoliosis	1
Pectoral hypoplasia or breast anomaly	2
Chest wall deformity, breast or pectoral aplasia	3

Diagnosis

Initial assessment includes a detailed head and neck and microotoscopic examination to rule out an etiologic entity. Complete audiometric assessment is obtained, especially if associated ear anomalies are evident. Genetic testing is requested in accordance with clinical findings if an identifiable syndromal pattern is suspected. Imaging modalities are helpful in assessing the brainstem and the course of the lower cranial nerves. These studies are valuable if surgical intervention is contemplated.

Management

Management of children with Moebius syndrome requires a multidisciplinary approach. Psychological support and family counseling and support are important to alleviate the emotional burden on the child and caregivers. Afflicted children are unable to breastfeed or suck from a regular nipple and must be fed with a specialized device. Aspiration is a constant concern, and insufficient weight gain can occur. Regular dental appointments are important, and some may require orthodontic or orthognathic work. Speech and language pathologists are indispensable in assisting the child with proper enunciation, the use of appropriate body language to augment their spoken language, and adoption of vocal techniques. Ophthalmologic consultation with emphasis on proper eye care, including the use of artificial tears and eye ointment, is paramount. Children with Moebius syndrome may have other cranial nerves involved besides CN VI and VII that may necessitate further management. Other associated anomalies and problems, including autism, tongue and jaw deformities (e.g., cleft palate, Pierre Robin syndrome), and delayed gross motor development, will require involvement of subspecialty services.

Surgical intervention is a viable option in the management of children with Moebius syndrome. Some ophthalmologists place small gold weights into the upper eyelids to help effect eye closure. The lack of facial movement has been addressed using various forms of static and active supports and slings. With the advent of microsurgery, facial paralysis reconstruction with the use of nerve grafts and muscle transplants has been performed. These include a cross-facial nerve graft, free gracilis muscle transfer, as well as ipsilateral hypoglossal, motor trigeminal, and accessory nerve grafts.

Conclusion

Congenital ear anomalies present a diverse spectrum of clinical entities, either in isolation or in association with a multitude of anomalies. The treating otolaryngologist may be challenged with potential esthetic and functional limitations, some of which may have a significant impact on a child's development from a speech and language, cognitive, and psychosocial perspective. In managing these patients, a thorough understanding of the underlying embryologic basis as well as a team approach that involves the family and members of the various involved disciplines will enhance management and optimize favorable outcomes.

References

1. De la cruz A, Hansen MR. Reconstruction surgery of the ear: auditory canal and tympanum. In: Cummings CW, Flint PW, Harker LA, et al., editors. Otolaryngology head and neck surgery. Philadelphia: Mosby; 2004. p. 4439–44.
2. Cunningham MJ, Aguilar E. Congenital auricular malformation. In: Johnson JT, Bailey BJ, Newlands SD, editors. Otolaryngology head and neck surgery. Philadelphia: Lippincott Williams and Wilkins; 2006. p. 2691–700.
3. Lee KJ. Essentials of otolaryngology. 5th ed. New York: McGraw-Hill; 2003.
4. Davis J. Otoplasty: aesthetic and reconstructive techniques. Berlin: Springer; 1987.
5. Beahm EK, Walton RL. Auricular reconstruction for microtia: part I. Anatomy, embryology, and clinical evaluation. Plast Reconstr Surg. 2002;109(7): 2473–82.
6. Murakami CS, Quatela VC. Reconstruction surgery of the ear: microtia reconstruction. In: Cummings CW, Flint PW, Harker LA, et al., editors. Otolaryngology head and neck surgery. Philadelphia: Mosby; 2004. p. 4422–8.
7. Zim SA. Microtia reconstruction: an update. Curr Opin Otolaryngol Head Neck Surg. 2003;11(4): 275–81.
8. Chami RG, Apesos J. Treatment of asymptomatic preauricular sinuses: challenging conventional wisdom. Ann Plast Surg. 1989;23(5):406–11.
9. Scheinfeld NS, Silverberg NB, Weinberg JM, et al. The preauricular sinus: a review of its clinical pre-

sentation, treatment, and associations. Pediatr Dermatol. 2004;21(3):191–6.
10. Huang XY, Tay GS, Wansaicheong GK, et al. Preauricular sinus: clinical course and associations. Arch Otolaryngol Head Neck Surg. 2007;133(1):65–8.
11. Meggyessy V, Mehes K. Preauricular pits in Hungary: epidemiologic and clinical observations. J Craniofac Genet Dev Biol. 1982;2(3):215–8.
12. Ewing MR. Congenital sinuses of the external ear. J Laryngol Otol. 1946;61:18–23.
13. Tsai FJ, Tsai CH. Birthmarks and congenital skin lesions in Chinese newborns. J Formos Med Assoc. 1993;92(9):838–41.
14. Leung AK, Robson WL. Association of preauricular sinuses and renal anomalies. Urology. 1992;40(3):259–61.
15. Smith PG, Dyches TJ, Loomis RA. Clinical aspects of the branchio-oto-renal syndrome. Otolaryngol Head Neck Surg. 1984;92(4):468–75.
16. Clementi M, Mammi I, Tenconi R. Family with branchial arch anomalies, hearing loss, ear and commissural lip pits, and rib anomalies. A new autosomal recessive condition: branchio-oto-costal syndrome? Am J Med Genet. 1997;68(1):91–3.
17. Magenis RE, Sheehy RR, Brown MG, et al. Parental origin of the extra chromosome in the cat eye syndrome: evidence from heteromorphism and in situ hybridization analysis. Am J Med Genet. 1988; 29(1):9–19.
18. Zelig S, Deutsch E, Eilon A. Waardenburg syndrome with associated multiple anomalies. ORL J Otorhinolaryngol Relat Spec. 1984;46(1):34–7.
19. Petersen MB, Hansen M, Djernes BW. Full trisomy 22 in a newborn infant. Ann Genet. 1987;30(2):101–4.
20. Lessick ML, Szego K, Wong PW. Trisomy 22 mosaicism with normal blood chromosomes. Case report with literature review. Clin Pediatr (Phila). 1988;27(9):451–4.
21. Wang RY, Earl DL, Ruder RO, et al. Syndromic ear anomalies and renal ultrasounds. Pediatrics. 2001;108(2):E32.
22. Firat Y, Sireci S, Yakinci C, et al. Isolated preauricular pits and tags: is it necessary to investigate renal abnormalities and hearing impairment? Eur Arch Otorhinolaryngol. 2008;265(9):1057–60.
23. Islam MA, Habib MA. Branchial cleft anomalies – a study of 20 cases. Bangladesh Med Res Counc Bull. 1995;21(3):104–7.
24. Rodriguez SJ. Branchio-oto-renal syndrome. J Nephrol. 2003;16(4):603–5.
25. Izzedine H, Tankere F, Launay-Vacher V, et al. Ear and kidney syndromes: molecular versus clinical approach. Kidney Int. 2004;65(2):369–85.
26. Kugelman A, Tubi A, Bader D, et al. Pre-auricular tags and pits in the newborn: the role of renal ultrasonography. J Pediatr. 2002;141(3):388–91.
27. O'Mara W, Guarisco L. Management of the preauricular sinus. J La State Med Soc. 1999;151(9):447–50.
28. Tan T, Constantinides H, Mitchell TE. The preauricular sinus: a review of its aetiology, clinical presentation and management. Int J Pediatr Otorhinolaryngol. 2005;69(11):1469–74.
29. Emery PJ, Salama NY. Congenital pre-auricular sinus. A study of 31 cases seen over a ten year period. Int J Pediatr Otorhinolaryngol. 1981;3(3):205–12.
30. Kugelman A, Hadad B, Ben-David J, et al. Preauricular tags and pits in the newborn: the role of hearing tests. Acta Paediatr. 1997;86(2):170–2.
31. Zou F, Peng Y, Wang X, et al. A locus for congenital preauricular fistula maps to chromosome 8q11.1-q13.3. J Hum Genet. 2003;48(3):155–8.
32. Coatesworth AP, Patmore H, Jose J. Management of an infected preauricular sinus, using a lacrimal probe. J Laryngol Otol. 2003;117(12):983–4.
33. Currie AR, King WW, Vlantis AC, et al. Pitfalls in the management of preauricular sinuses. Br J Surg. 1996;83(12):1722–4.
34. Prasad S, Grundfast K, Milmoe G. Management of congenital preauricular pit and sinus tract in children. Laryngoscope. 1990;100(3):320–1.
35. Lam HC, Soo G, Woemald PJ, et al. Excision of the preauricular sinus: a comparison of two surgical techniques. Laryngoscope. 2001;111(2):317–9.
36. Baatenburg de Jong RJ. A new surgical technique for treatment of preauricular sinus. Surgery. 2005;137(5):567–70.
37. Ahuja AT, Marshall JN, Roebuck DJ, et al. Sonographic appearances of preauricular sinus. Clin Radiol. 2000;55(7):528–32.
38. Lau JT. Towards better delineation and complete excision of preauricular sinus. Aust N Z J Surg. 1983;53(3):267–9.
39. Declau F, Van De Heyning P, Cremers C. Diagnosis and management strategies in congenital middle and external ear anomalies. In: Scadding GK, Graham JM, Bull PD, editors. Pediatric ENT. Heidelberg: Springer; 2007. p. 361–75.
40. Kelley PE, Scholes MA. Microtia and congenital aural atresia. Otolaryngol Clin North Am. 2007;40(1):61–80. vi.
41. Shaw GM, Carmichael SL, Kaidarova Z, et al. Epidemiologic characteristics of anotia and microtia in California, 1989–1997. Birth Defects Res A Clin Mol Teratol. 2004;70(7):472–5.
42. Klaiber S, Weerda H. [BAHA (bone-anchored hearing aid) in bilateral external ear dysplasia and congenital ear atresia]. HNO. 2002;50(10):949–59.
43. Murphy TP, Burstein F, Cohen S. Management of congenital atresia of the external auditory canal. Otolaryngol Head Neck Surg. 1997;116(6 Pt 1):580–4.
44. Veltman JA, Jonkers Y, Nuijten I, et al. Definition of a critical region on chromosome 18 for congenital aural atresia by arrayCGH. Am J Hum Genet. 2003;72(6):1578–84.
45. Swartz JD, Faerber EN. Congenital malformations of the external and middle ear: high-resolution CT

findings of surgical import. AJR Am J Roentgenol. 1985;144(3):501–6.
46. Kosling S, Omenzetter M, Bartel-Friedrich S. Congenital malformations of the external and middle ear. Eur J Radiol. 2009;69(2):269–79.
47. Weerda H. Chirurgie der ohrmuschel: verletzungen, defekte und anomalien. Stuttgart: Thieme; 2004. p. 105–226.
48. Altmann F. Congenital atresia of the ear in man and animals. Ann Otol Rhinol Laryngol. 1955;64(3): 824–58.
49. Declau F, Offeciers F, Van de Heyning P. Classification of the non-syndromal type of meatal atresia. In: Devranoglu I, editor. Proceedings of the XVth world congress of otorhinolaryngology head and neck surgery: panel discussions. Istanbul, Turkey. 1999. p. 135–7.
50. Walton RL, Beahm EK. Auricular reconstruction for microtia: part II. Surgical techniques. Plast Reconstr Surg. 2002;110(1):234–49. quiz 250–1, 387.
51. Jahrsdoerfer RA, Yeakley JW, Aguilar EA, et al. Grading system for the selection of patients with congenital aural atresia. Am J Otol. 1992;13(1): 6–12.
52. Jahrsdoerfer RA. Congenital atresia of the ear. Laryngoscope. 1978;88(9 Pt 3 Suppl 13):1–48.
53. Vendramini-Pittoli S, Kokitsu-Nakata NM. Oculoauriculovertebral spectrum: report of nine familial cases with evidence of autosomal dominant inheritance and review of the literature. Clin Dysmorphol. 2009;18(2):67–77.
54. Harris J, Kallen B, Robert E. The epidemiology of anotia and microtia. J Med Genet. 1996;33(10): 809–13.
55. Nelson SM, Berry RI. Ear disease and hearing loss among Navajo children – a mass survey. Laryngoscope. 1984;94(3):316–23.
56. Novacek MJ. Patterns of diversity in the reptilian skull. In: Hall BK, Hanken J, editors. The skull, vol. 2. Chicago: University of Chicago Press; 1993. p. 438–545.
57. Rieppel O. Patterns of diversity in the reptilian skull. In: Hall BK, Hanken J, editors. The skull, vol. 2. Chicago: University of Chicago Press; 1993. p. 344–90.
58. Rowe T. Coevolution of the mammalian middle ear and neocortex. Science. 1996;273(5275):651–4.
59. Allin EF. Evolution of the mammalian middle ear. J Morphol. 1975;147(4):403–37.
60. Hopson JA. The origin of the mammalian middle ear. Am Zool. 1966;6(3):437–50.
61. Farrior JB. Surgical management of congenital conductive deafness. South Med J. 1987;80(4):450–3.
62. Stewart JM, Downs MP. Congenital conductive hearing loss: the need for early identification and intervention. Pediatrics. 1993;91(2):355–9.
63. Yuen HY, Ahuja AT, Wong KT, et al. Computed tomography of common congenital lesions of the temporal bone. Clin Radiol. 2003;58(9):687–93.
64. Park HY, Han DH, Lee JB, et al. Congenital stapes anomalies with normal eardrum. Clin Exp Otorhinolaryngol. 2009;2(1):33–8.
65. Raveh E, Hu W, Papsin BC, et al. Congenital conductive hearing loss. J Laryngol Otol. 2002;116(2):92–6.
66. Hung KL, Tu TY, Tsai TL, et al. Congenital ossicular anomalies. J Chin Med Assoc. 2003;66(8):474–9.
67. Teunissen B, Cremers WR, Huygen PL, et al. Isolated congenital stapes ankylosis: surgical results in 32 ears and a review of the literature. Laryngoscope. 1990;100(12):1331–6.
68. Vore AP, Chang EH, Hoppe JE, et al. Deletion of and novel missense mutation in POU3F4 in 2 families segregating X-linked nonsyndromic deafness. Arch Otolaryngol Head Neck Surg. 2005;131(12): 1057–63.
69. Jahrsdoerfer RA. The facial nerve in congenital middle ear malformations. Laryngoscope. 1981;91(8): 1217–25.
70. Cremers CW, Teunissen E. The impact of a syndromal diagnosis on surgery for congenital minor ear anomalies. Int J Pediatr Otorhinolaryngol. 1991;22(1):59–74.
71. Albert S, Roger G, Rouillon I, et al. Congenital stapes ankylosis: study of 28 cases and surgical results. Laryngoscope. 2006;116(7):1153–7.
72. De la Cruz A, Angeli S, Slattery WH. Stapedectomy in children. Otolaryngol Head Neck Surg. 1999;120(4):487–92.
73. Teunissen EB, Cremers WR. Classification of congenital middle ear anomalies. Report on 144 ears. Ann Otorhinolaryngol. 1993;102(8 Pt 1):606–12.
74. Charachon R, Barthez M, Lavieille JP. Minor malformations of the ear ossicles. New classification and therapeutic results. Ann Otolaryngol Chir Cervicofac. 1994;111(2):69–74.
75. von Haacke NP. Juvenile stapedectomy. Clin Otolaryngol Allied Sci. 1985;10(1):9–13.
76. Tange RA. Ossicular reconstruction in cases of absent or inadequate incus, congenital malformation of the middle ear and epitympanic fixation of the incus and malleus. ORL J Otorhinolaryngol Relat Spec. 1996;58(3):143–6.
77. House JW, Sheehy JL, Antunez JC. Stapedectomy in children. Laryngoscope. 1980;90(11 Pt 1):1804–9.
78. Dornhoffer JL, Helms J, Hoehmann DH. Stapedectomy for congenital fixation of the stapes. Am J Otol. 1995;16(3):382–6.
79. Massey BL, Hillman TA, Shelton C. Stapedectomy in congenital stapes fixation: are hearing outcomes poorer? Otolaryngol Head Neck Surg. 2006;134(5):816–8.
80. Bachor E, Just T, Wright CG, et al. Fixation of the stapes footplate in children: a clinical and temporal bone histopathologic study. Otol Neurotol. 2005;26(5):866–73.
81. Kisilevsky VE, Bailie NA, Dutt SN, et al. Hearing results of stapedotomy and malleo-vestibulopexy in

congenital hearing loss. Int J Pediatr Otorhinolaryngol. 2009;73(12):1712–7.
82. Teele DW, Klein JO, Rosner B. Epidemiology of otitis media during the first seven years of life in children in greater Boston: a prospective, cohort study. J Infect Dis. 1989;160(1):83–94.
83. Paradise JL, Rockette HE, Colborn DK, et al. Otitis media in 2253 Pittsburgh-area infants: prevalence and risk factors during the first two years of life. Pediatrics. 1997;99(3):318–33.
84. Nelson M, Roger G, Koltai PJ, et al. Congenital cholesteatoma: classification, management, and outcome. Arch Otolaryngol Head Neck Surg. 2002;128(7):810–4.
85. Potsic WP, Korman SB, Samadi DS, et al. Congenital cholesteatoma: 20 years' experience at The Children's Hospital of Philadelphia. Otolaryngol Head Neck Surg. 2002;126(4):409–14.
86. Parisier SC, Weiss MH. Recidivism in congenital cholesteatoma surgery. Ear Nose Throat J. 1991;70(6):362–4.
87. Lazard DS, Roger G, Denoyelle F, et al. Congenital cholesteatoma: risk factors for residual disease and retraction pockets – a report on 117 cases. Laryngoscope. 2007;117(4):634–7.
88. Baker CV, Bronner-Fraser M. Vertebrate cranial placodes I. Embryonic induction. Dev Biol. 2001;232(1):1–61.
89. O'Rahilly R. The early development of the otic vesicle in staged human embryos. J Embryol Exp Morphol. 1963;11:741–55.
90. Moore JK, Linthicum Jr FH. The human auditory system: a timeline of development. Int J Audiol. 2007;46(9):460–78.
91. Bredberg G. Cellular pattern and nerve supply of the human organ of Corti. Acta Otolaryngol. 1968;Suppl 236:1+.
92. Lavigne-Rebillard M, Pujol R. Surface aspects of the developing human organ of Corti. Acta Otolaryngol Suppl. 1987;436:43–50.
93. Cooper HR. The development of the human auditory pathway from the cochlear ganglion to the medial geniculate body. Acta Anat (Basel). 1948;5(1–2): 99–122.
94. Pujol R, Lavigne-Rebillard M. Early stages of innervation and sensory cell differentiation in the human fetal organ of Corti. Acta Otolaryngol Suppl. 1985;423:43–50.
95. Robson CD. Congenital hearing impairment. Pediatr Radiol. 2006;36(4):309–24.
96. Jackler RK, Luxford WM, House WF. Congenital malformations of the inner ear: a classification based on embryogenesis. Laryngoscope. 1987;97(3 Pt 2 Suppl 40):2–14.
97. Sennaroglu L, Saatci I. A new classification for cochleovestibular malformations. Laryngoscope. 2002;112(12):2230–41.
98. Krombach GA, Honnef D, Westhofen M, et al. Imaging of congenital anomalies and acquired lesions of the inner ear. Eur Radiol. 2008;18(2):319–30.
99. White KR. Early hearing detection and intervention programs: opportunities for genetic services. Am J Med Genet A. 2004;130A(1):29–36.
100. Bamiou DE, Phelps P, Sirimanna T. Temporal bone computed tomography findings in bilateral sensorineural hearing loss. Arch Dis Child. 2000;82(3):257–60.
101. Reilly GP, Lalwani AK, Jackler RK. Congenital anomalies of the inner ear. In: Grundfast KM, Lalwani AK, editors. Pediatric otology and neurotology. Philadelphia: Lippincott-Raven; 1998. p. 201–10.
102. Eelkema EA, Curtin HD. Congenital anomalies of the temporal bone. Semin Ultrasound CT MR. 1989;10(3):195–212.
103. Parry DA, Booth T, Roland PS. Advantages of magnetic resonance imaging over computed tomography in preoperative evaluation of pediatric cochlear implant candidates. Otol Neurotol. 2005;26(5): 976–82.
104. Colletti V, Carner M, Fiorino F, et al. Hearing restoration with auditory brainstem implant in three children with cochlear nerve aplasia. Otol Neurotol. 2002;23(5):682–93.
105. Graham JM, Phelps PD, Michaels L. Congenital malformations of the ear and cochlear implantation in children: review and temporal bone report of common cavity. J Laryngol Otol Suppl. 2000;25:1–14.
106. Mylanus EA, Rotteveel LJ, Leeuw RL. Congenital malformation of the inner ear and pediatric cochlear implantation. Otol Neurotol. 2004;25(3):308–17.
107. Smith RJ, Schwartz C. Branchio-oto-renal syndrome. J Commun Disord. 1998;31(5):411–20. quiz 421.
108. Jackler RK. Congenital malformations of the inner ear. In: Cummings CS, editor. Otolaryngology—head and neck surgery. Chicago: Mosby-Yearbook; 1993.
109. Papsin BC. Cochlear implantation in children with anomalous cochleovestibular anatomy. Laryngoscope. 2005;115(1 Pt 2 Suppl 106):1–26.
110. Casselman JW, Offeciers EF, De Foer B, et al. CT and MR imaging of congential abnormalities of the inner ear and internal auditory canal. Eur J Radiol. 2001;40(2):94–104.
111. Atkin JS, Grimmer JF, Hedlund G, et al. Cochlear abnormalities associated with enlarged vestibular aqueduct anomaly. Int J Pediatr Otorhinolaryngol. 2009;73(12):1682–5.
112. Phelps PD. Mondini and 'pseudo Mondini'. Clin Otolaryngol Allied Sci. 1990;15(2):99–101.
113. Wilson JT, Leivy SW, Sofferman RA, et al. Mondini dysplasia: spontaneous cerebrospinal fluid otorrhea. New perspectives in management. Pediatr Neurosurg. 1990;16(4–5):260–4.
114. Ohlms LA, Edwards MS, Mason EO, et al. Recurrent meningitis and Mondini dysplasia. Arch Otolaryngol Head Neck Surg. 1990;116(5):608–12.
115. Naganawa S, Ito T, Iwayama E, et al. MR imaging of the cochlear modiolus: area measurement in

healthy subjects and in patients with a large endolymphatic duct and sac. Radiology. 1999;213(3):819–23.
116. Kendi TK, Arikan OK, Koc C. Magnetic resonance imaging of cochlear modiolus: determination of mid-modiolar area and modiolar volume. J Laryngol Otol. 2004;118(7):496–9.
117. Rodriguez K, Shah RK, Kenna M. Anomalies of the middle and inner ear. Otolaryngol Clin North Am. 2007;40(1):81–96. vi.
118. Nadol Jr JB, Young YS, Glynn RJ. Survival of spiral ganglion cells in profound sensorineural hearing loss: implications for cochlear implantation. Ann Otol Rhinol Laryngol. 1989;98(6):411–6.
119. Valvassori GE, Clemis JD. The large vestibular aqueduct syndrome. Laryngoscope. 1978;88(5): 723–8.
120. Jackler RK, De La Cruz A. The large vestibular aqueduct syndrome. Laryngoscope. 1989;99(12):1238–42. discussion 1242–3.
121. Okumura T, Takahashi H, Honjo I, et al. Sensorineural hearing loss in patients with large vestibular aqueduct. Laryngoscope. 1995;105(3 Pt 1):289–93. discussion 293–4.
122. Zalzal GH, Tomaski SM, Vezina LG, et al. Enlarged vestibular aqueduct and sensorineural hearing loss in childhood. Arch Otolaryngol Head Neck Surg. 1995;121(1):23–8.
123. Levenson MJ, Parisier SC, Jacobs M, et al. The large vestibular aqueduct syndrome in children. A review of 12 cases and the description of a new clinical entity. Arch Otolaryngol Head Neck Surg. 1989;115(1):54–8.
124. Emmett JR. The large vestibular aqueduct syndrome. Am J Otol. 1985;6(5):387–415.
125. Valvassori GE. The large vestibular aqueduct and associated anomalies of the inner ear. Otolaryngol Clin North Am. 1983;16(1):95–101.
126. Fahy CP, Carney AS, Nikolopoulos TP, et al. Cochlear implantation in children with large vestibular aqueduct syndrome and a review of the syndrome. Int J Pediatr Otorhinolaryngol. 2001;59(3):207–15.
127. Phelps PD, Coffey RA, Trembath RC, et al. Radiological malformations of the ear in Pendred syndrome. Clin Radiol. 1998;53(4):268–73.
128. Stinckens C, Standaert L, Casselman JW, et al. The presence of a widened vestibular aqueduct and progressive sensorineural hearing loss in the branchio-oto-renal syndrome. A family study. Int J Pediatr Otorhinolaryngol. 2001;59(3):163–72.
129. Miura M, Sando I, Orita Y, et al. Temporal bone histopathological study of Noonan syndrome. Int J Pediatr Otorhinolaryngol. 2001;60(1):73–82.
130. Madden C, Halsted MJ, Hopkin RJ, et al. Temporal bone abnormalities associated with hearing loss in Waardenburg syndrome. Laryngoscope. 2003;113(11):2035–41.
131. Berrettini S, Forli F, Franceschini SS, et al. Distal renal tubular acidosis associated with isolated large vestibular aqueduct and sensorineural hearing loss. Ann Otol Rhinol Laryngol. 2002;111(5 Pt 1):385–91.
132. Shinjo Y, Kaga K, Igarashi T. Distal renal tubular acidosis associated with large vestibular aqueduct and sensorineural hearing loss. Acta Otolaryngol. 2005;125(6):667–70.
133. Abe S, Usami S, Hoover DM, et al. Fluctuating sensorineural hearing loss associated with enlarged vestibular aqueduct maps to 7q31, the region containing the Pendred gene. Am J Med Genet. 1999;82(4):322–8.
134. Usami S, Abe S, Weston MD, et al. Non-syndromic hearing loss associated with enlarged vestibular aqueduct is caused by PDS mutations. Hum Genet. 1999;104(2):188–92.
135. Arcand P, Desrosiers M, Dube J, et al. The large vestibular aqueduct syndrome and sensorineural hearing loss in the pediatric population. J Otolaryngol. 1991;20(4):247–50.
136. Govaerts PJ, Casselman J, Daemers K, et al. Audiological findings in large vestibular aqueduct syndrome. Int J Pediatr Otorhinolaryngol. 1999;51(3):157–64.
137. Belenky WM, Madgy DN, Leider JS, et al. The enlarged vestibular aqueduct syndrome (EVA syndrome). Ear Nose Throat J. 1993;72(11):746–51.
138. Lai CC, Shiao AS. Chronological changes of hearing in pediatric patients with large vestibular aqueduct syndrome. Laryngoscope. 2004;114(5):832–8.
139. Steinbach S, Brockmeier SJ, Kiefer J. The large vestibular aqueduct – case report and review of the literature. Acta Otolaryngol. 2006;126(8):788–95.
140. Walsh RM, Ayshford CA, Chavda SV, et al. Large vestibular aqueduct syndrome. ORL J Otorhinolaryngol Relat Spec. 1999;61(1):41–4.
141. Oh AK, Ishiyama A, Baloh RW. Vertigo and the enlarged vestibular aqueduct syndrome. J Neurol. 2001;248(11):971–4.
142. Mori T, Westerberg BD, Atashband S, et al. Natural history of hearing loss in children with enlarged vestibular aqueduct syndrome. J Otolaryngol Head Neck Surg. 2008;37(1):112–8.
143. Dahlen RT, Harnsberger HR, Gray SD, et al. Overlapping thin-section fast spin-echo MR of the large vestibular aqueduct syndrome. AJNR Am J Neuroradiol. 1997;18(1):67–75.
144. Naganawa S, Koshikawa T, Iwayama E, et al. MR imaging of the enlarged endolymphatic duct and sac syndrome by use of a 3D fast asymmetric spin-echo sequence: volume and signal-intensity measurement of the endolymphatic duct and sac and area measurement of the cochlear modiolus. AJNR Am J Neuroradiol. 2000;21(9):1664–9.
145. Berrettini S, Forli F, Bogazzi F, et al. Large vestibular aqueduct syndrome: audiological, radiological, clinical, and genetic features. Am J Otolaryngol. 2005;26(6):363–71.
146. Harker LA, Vanderheiden S, Veazry D, et al. Multichannel cochlear implantation in children with large vestibular aqueduct syndrome. Ann Otol Rhinol Laryngol Suppl. 1999;177:39–43.

147. Nowak KC, Messner AH. Isolated large vestibular aqueduct syndrome in a family. Ann Otol Rhinol Laryngol. 2000;109(1):40–4.
148. Wilson DF, Hodgson RS, Talbot JM. Endolymphatic sac obliteration for large vestibular aqueduct syndrome. Am J Otol. 1997;18(1):101–6. discussion 106–7.
149. Reussner LA, Dutcher PO, House WF. Large vestibular aqueduct syndrome with massive endolymphatic sacs. Otolaryngol Head Neck Surg. 1995;113(5):606–10.
150. Welling DB, et al. Endolymphatic sac occlusion for the enlarged vestibular aqueduct syndrome. Am J Otol. 1998;19(2):145–51.
151. Welling DB, Slater PW, Martyn MD, et al. Sensorineural hearing loss after occlusion of the enlarged vestibular aqueduct. Am J Otol. 1999;20(3):338–43.
152. Lin CY, Lin SL, Kao CC, et al. The remediation of hearing deterioration in children with large vestibular aqueduct syndrome. Auris Nasus Larynx. 2005;32(2):99–105.
153. Aschendorff A, Marangos N, Laszig R. Large vestibular aqueduct syndrome and its implication for cochlear implant surgery. Am J Otol. 1997;18(6 Suppl):S57.
154. Miyamoto RT, Bichey BG, Wynne MK, et al. Cochlear implantation with large vestibular aqueduct syndrome. Laryngoscope. 2002;112(7 Pt 1):1178–82.
155. Au G, Gibson W. Cochlear implantation in children with large vestibular aqueduct syndrome. Am J Otol. 1999;20(2):183–6.
156. Slattery 3rd WH, Luxford WM. Cochlear implantation in the congenital malformed cochlea. Laryngoscope. 1995;105(11):1184–7.
157. Bent 3rd JP, Chute P, Parisier SC. Cochlear implantation in children with enlarged vestibular aqueducts. Laryngoscope. 1999;109(7 Pt 1):1019–22.
158. Gasser RF, Shigihara S, Shimada K. Three-dimensional development of the facial nerve path through the ear region in human embryos. Ann Otol Rhinol Laryngol. 1994;103(5 Pt 1):395–403.
159. Gasser RF. The development of the facial nerve in man. Ann Otol Rhinol Laryngol. 1967;76(1): 37–56.
160. Gasser RF, Maya M. Embryonic development of the facial nerve. In: May M, editor. The facial nerve. New York: Thieme; 1986. p. 3–19.
161. Spector JG, Ge X. Ossification patterns of the tympanic facial canal in the human fetus and neonate. Laryngoscope. 1993;103(9):1052–65.
162. Caparosa RJ, Klassen D. Congenital anomalies of the stapes and facial nerve. Arch Otolaryngol. 1966;83(5):420–1.
163. Gulya AJ. Developmental anatomy of the temporal bone and skull base. In: Gulya AJ, Glasscock ME, editors. Ear surgery. Hamilton: BC Decker; 2003. p. 24–5.
164. Saito H, Takeda T, Kishimoto S. Neonatal facial nerve defect. Acta Otolaryngol Suppl. 1994;510: 77–81.
165. Falco NA, Eriksson E. Facial nerve palsy in the newborn: incidence and outcome. Plast Reconstr Surg. 1990;85(1):1–4.
166. Evans PR. Nuclear agenesis: Mobius' syndrome: the congenital facial diplegia syndrome. Arch Dis Child. 1955;30(151):237–43.
167. Legum C, Godel V, Nemet P. Heterogeneity and pleiotropism in the Moebius syndrome. Clin Genet. 1981;20(4):254–9.
168. MacDermot KD, et al. Oculofacialbulbar palsy in mother and son: review of 26 reports of familial transmission within the 'Mobius spectrum of defects'. J Med Genet. 1991;28(1):18–26.
169. Kuhn MJ, Clark HB, Morales A, et al. Group III Mobius syndrome: CT and MR findings. AJNR Am J Neuroradiol. 1990;11(5):903–4.
170. Sudarshan A, Goldie WD. The spectrum of congenital facial diplegia (Moebius syndrome). Pediatr Neurol. 1985;1(3):180–4.
171. Towfighi J, Marks K, Palmer E, et al. Mobius syndrome. Neuropathologic observations. Acta Neuropathol. 1979;48(1):11–7.
172. Heubner O. Uber angeborenen Kernmangel (infantiler Kernschwund, Moebius). Charite Annaien. 1900;25:211–43.
173. D'Cruz OF, Swisher CN, Jaradeh S, et al. Mobius syndrome: evidence for a vascular etiology. J Child Neurol. 1993;8(3):260–5.
174. Thakkar N, O'Neil W, Duvally J, et al. Mobius syndrome due to brain stem tegmental necrosis. Arch Neurol. 1977;34(2):124–6.
175. Harris JP, Davidson TM, May M, et al. Evaluation and treatment of congenital facial paralysis. Arch Otolaryngol. 1983;109(3):145–51.
176. Hanissian AS, Fuste F, Hayes WT, et al. Mobius syndrome in twins. Am J Dis Child. 1970;120(5): 472–5.
177. Saito H, Kishimoto S, Furuta M. Temporal bone findings in a patient with Mobius syndrome. Ann Otol Rhinol Laryngol. 1981;90(1 Pt 1):80–4.
178. Reed H, Grant W. Mobius's syndrome. Br J Ophthalmol. 1957;41(12):731–40.
179. Richards RN. The Mobius syndrome. J Bone Joint Surg Am. 1953;35-A(2):437–44.
180. McHugh HE, Sowden KA, Levitt MN. Facial paralysis and muscle agenesis in the newborn. Arch Otolaryngol. 1969;89(1):131–43.
181. Sunderland S. Nerve injuries and their repair: a critical appraisal. Edinburgh: Churchill Livingstone; 1991.
182. Carlson BM. The development of facial muscles and nerves in relation to the Mobius syndrome. Otolaryngol Head Neck Surg. 1981;89(6):903–6.
183. Carr MM, Ross DA, Zuker RM. Cranial nerve defects in congenital facial palsy. J Otolaryngol. 1997;26(2):80–7.

184. Van Allen MW, Blodi FC. Neurologic aspects of the Mobius syndrome. A case study with electromyography of the extraocular and facial muscles. Neurology. 1960;10:249–59.
185. Hanson PA, Rowland LP. Mobius syndrome and facioscapulohumeral muscular dystrophy. Arch Neurol. 1971;24(1):31–9.
186. Ouanounou S, Saigal G, Birchansky S. Mobius syndrome. AJNR Am J Neuroradiol. 2005;26(2): 430–2.
187. Verzijl HT, van den Helm B, Veldman B, et al. A second gene for autosomal dominant Mobius syndrome is localized to chromosome 10q, in a Dutch family. Am J Hum Genet. 1999;65(3):752–6.
188. Rizos M, Negron RJ, Serman N. Mobius syndrome with dental involvement: a case report and literature review. Cleft Palate Craniofac J. 1998;35(3):262–8.
189. Sugarman GI, Stark HH. Mobius syndrome with Poland's anomaly. J Med Genet. 1973;10(2):192–6.
190. Pedraza S, Gamez J, Rovira A, et al. MRI findings in Mobius syndrome: correlation with clinical features. Neurology. 2000;55(7):1058–60.
191. Abramson DL, Cohen Jr MM, Mulliken JB. Mobius syndrome: classification and grading system. Plast Reconstr Surg. 1998;102(4):961–7.
192. Cattaneo L, Chierici E, Bianchi B, et al. The localization of facial motor impairment in sporadic Mobius syndrome. Neurology. 2006;66(12):1907–12.

Congenital Malformations of the Nose and Nasopharynx

3

Mark D. Rizzi and Brian P. Dunham

Abstract

This chapter provides embryologic and clinical descriptions, photographs, and illustrations of the more common congenital anomalies of the nose and nasopharynx. The authors present the topics in sections based on the underlying pathology. These sections include malformations that occur because the nose failed to form properly (such as arhinia, polyrhinia, and nasal colomboma), those that resulted in midline nasal and nasopharyngeal malformations (such as choanal atresia and craniopharyngioma), and those that resulted in congenital nasopharyngeal or nasal midline masses (such as epignathi, Thornwaldt cysts, dermoids, gliomas, and encephaloceles).

Keywords

Arhinia • Bifid nose • Proboscis • Choanal atresia • Epignathis • Nasal pyriform stenosis • Dermoid • Glioma • Encephalocele

Nasal Embryology

The development of a functional nasal architecture requires the careful and precise orchestration of mesenchymal components. Any interruption or disruption of these delicate processes will lead to nasal malformation.

By the end of the fourth week of gestation, bilateral oval thickenings of the surface ectoderm called nasal placodes appear. These are the primordia of the nose and nasal cavities. Initially, the placodes are convex but as they stretch later, they produce a flat depression in each placode. The placodes then invaginate to form nasal pits, which are the primordia of the nares and nasal cavities (Fig. 3.1). The proliferating mesenchyme in the margins of the placodes produces

M.D. Rizzi, M.D. (✉) • B.P. Dunham, M.D.
Division of Pediatric Otolaryngology, The Children's Hospital of Philadelphia, 3400 Civic Center Boulevard, Wood Building, 1st Floor, Philadelphia, PA 19104, USA

Department of Otolaryngology: Head and Neck Surgery, Perelman School of Medicine at the University of Pennsylvania, Philadelphia, PA, USA
e-mail: rizzim@email.chop.edu; dunhamb@email.chop.edu

L.M. Elden and K.B. Zur (eds.), *Congenital Malformations of the Head and Neck*,
DOI 10.1007/978-1-4419-1714-0_3, © Springer Science+Business Media New York 2014

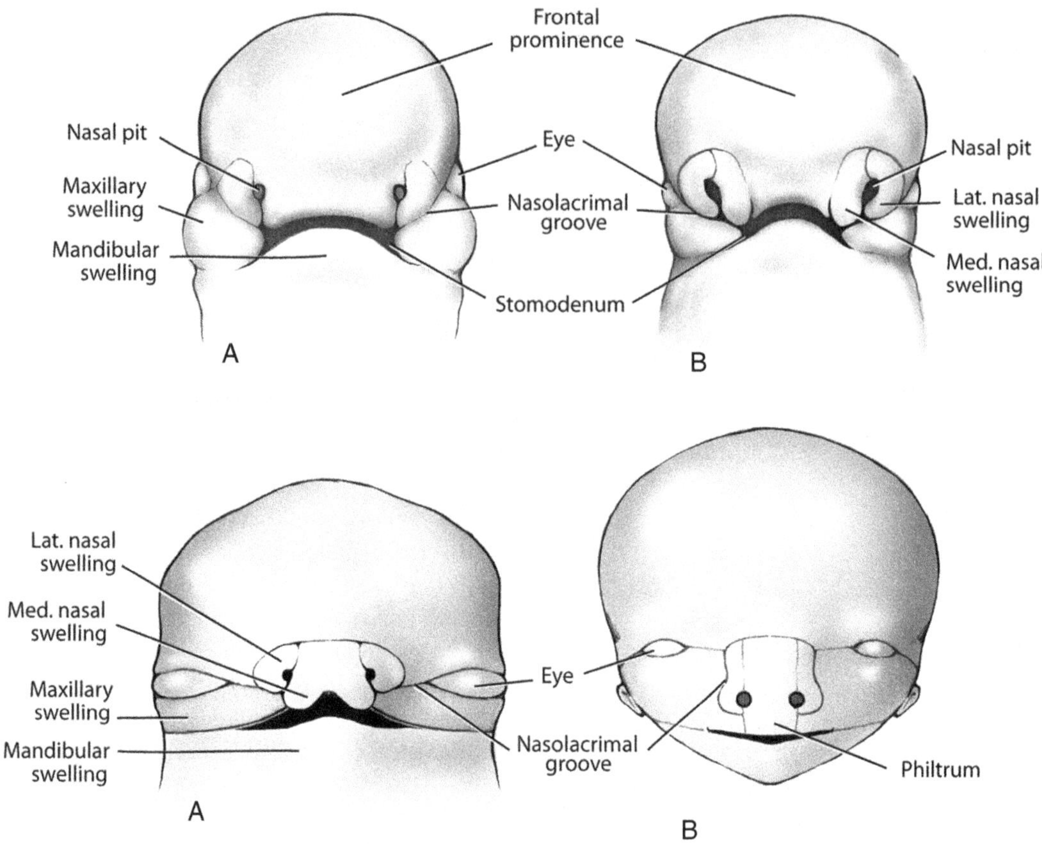

Fig. 3.1 Embryology of the development of the nose

horseshoe-shaped elevations—the medial and lateral nasal prominences; their cooperative interaction with the developing maxillary processes eventually creates multiple paramedian structures: the nasal aperture, the nasolacrimal ducts, and the upper lip. The nasolacrimal groove forms at the junction of the nasal and maxillary prominences. As the groove subsequently invaginates, the epithelium within resorbs leading the formation of the nasolacrimal duct. The medial nasal prominences grow faster than the lateral processes, and extend anteriorly to form the ridge, tip, and columella of the nose and toward the oral plate to form the philtrum and medial portion of the upper lip. The lateral nasal prominences eventually form the nasal bones, the upper lateral cartilages, and the lateral crus of the lower lateral cartilage [1–3].

The deepening of the nasal pits leads to the formation of the primordial nasal sacs, which grow dorsally. The oronasal membrane, which first separates the nasal sacs from the oral cavity, ruptures by the end of the sixth week forming an open communication between the nasal and oral cavities. A temporary epithelial plug is formed in the nasal cavity from the expansion of cells lining it; this plug resorbs between the 13th and 15th weeks. The primordial choanae lie posterior to the primary palate. After the secondary palate develops, the choanae position themselves at the junction of the nasal cavity and the pharynx. As the maxillary palatal shelves lengthen and grow medially, they fuse with each other and the septum, effectively separating the nasal cavities from the oral cavity [4]. Eruption of the nasal pits into the choanae, fusion of the palatal shelves and growth of the nasal septum and soft palate coincide with the development of the lateral nasal wall and primitive sinus anatomy.

Congenitally Malformed Nose

Arhinia

Definition

Arhinia is defined as the congenital absence of a nose (Fig. 3.2).

Incidence

Arhinia is an extremely rare condition. All cases are thought to be sporadic.

Etiology

The pathogenesis of arhinia is poorly understood. It has been postulated that lack of development of the nose results from failure of the medial and lateral nasal processes to grow, but it is also possible that overgrowth and premature fusion of the nasal medial processes result in formation of an atretic plate. Arhinia may also result from lack of resorption of the nasal epithelial plugs during the 13th–15th weeks of gestation. Another explanation may be related to abnormal migration of neural crest cells to this region, resulting in aberrant flow of the multiple mesodermal structures required to establish the nose and its cavities normally [5].

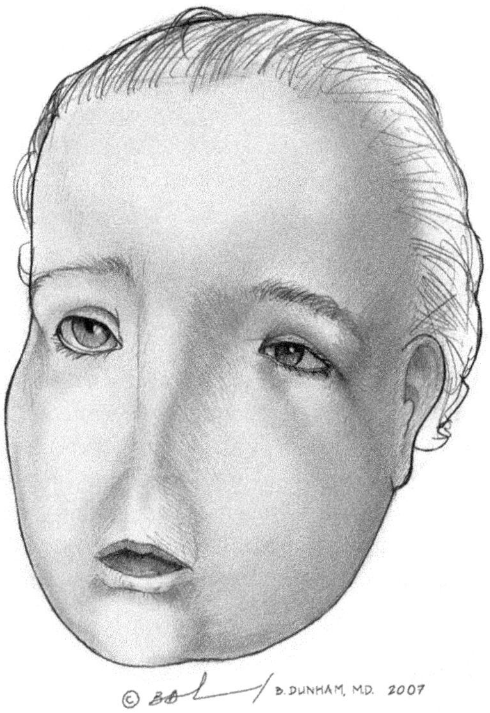

Fig. 3.2 Diagram of a child with arhinia

Associated Malformations

Microphthalmia, iris coloboma, hypertelorism, submucous cleft palate, and meningocele occasionally associate with this condition. Intelligence is usually normal.

Clinical Features

Neonates are obligate nasal breathers and become symptomatic with respiratory distress and cyanosis when the nasal passages are blocked, especially during feeding. Affected infants, however, can survive and adapt to oral breathing. The site of the external nose is flat, covered with normal appearing skin. Occasionally, a blind dimple is present in lieu of the nostrils. While the upper lip is normal, the palate is high-arched and the maxilla hypoplastic. The nasal cavity fails to form and there is bilateral bony choanal atresia [2].

Diagnosis

Diagnosis is based on visual inspection. Computed tomography imaging of the nose and midface is recommended to evaluate the underlying structure. Evaluation of the thickness of the atretic bony plate is an important preoperative consideration.

Management

An oral airway is often used in the neonatal setting. A surgically created nasal airway or a tracheostomy tube is an important part of early management, as either allows the infant to feed orally and precludes the complications associated with orogastric tubes. Most authors agree that surgical reconstruction of the external nose and inner cavities should be delayed at least until preschool years, when facial development is nearly complete [6, 7].

Unilateral Arhinia, Heminasal Aplasia

Definition

Unilateral arhinia is the unilateral absence of one nostril. Occasionally, a blind dimple is present in lieu of a nostril. It differs from cebocephaly, which presents as a single midline nostril. Cebocephaly is a congenital condition with monkey-like facial features with closely set eyes, a defective or absent nose, and a tendency towards cyclopedia (Fig. 3.3).

Incidence

Unilateral arhinia is extremely rare and is sporadic.

Associated Malformations

The condition may be associated with a blind dimple, skin tag, or a proboscis [8]. There are a significant number of bony abnormalities associated including an absent cribriform plate, nasal septal deviation towards the affected side, malformation of the ipsilateral lateral nasal wall, absence of the nasal bones, and disruption of the lacrimal bone. The ipsilateral olfactory tract and bulb are typically absent. The ipsilateral eye may be microphthalmic, absent, or anomalous. Orofacial clefting has been seen in some cases. In the absence of associated central nervous malformations, intelligence is usually normal.

Diagnosis

The diagnosis is based on visual inspection and computed tomography of the midface.

Management

Treatment consists of reconstructive operations as well as prostheses [2].

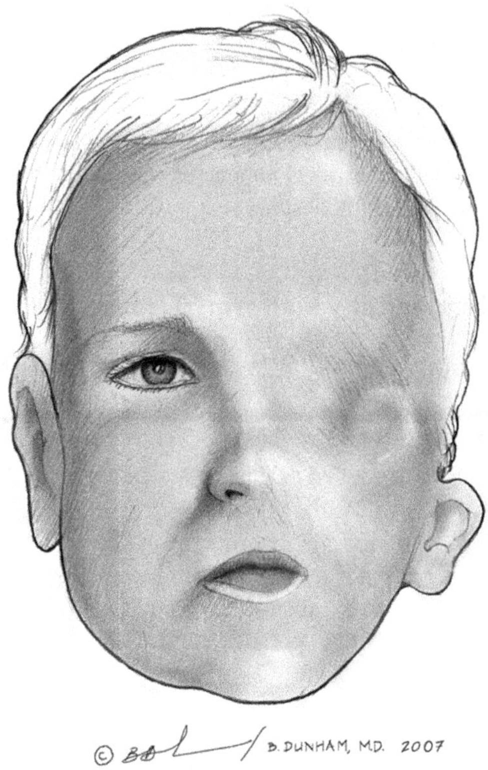

Fig. 3.3 Diagram of a child with unilateral arhinia

Nostril Coloboma

Definition

A nostril coloboma is a triangular cleft of the nasal ala (Fig. 3.4).

Incidence

Unilateral nostril coloboma is rare and sporadic. Bilateral nasal colobomas occur even less frequently.

Associated Malformations

Unilateral anophthalmia, lower lid coloboma, frontal glioma, and ocular hypertelorism can occur simultaneously.

Diagnosis

Its diagnosis is made by visual inspection. The defect is typically unilateral.

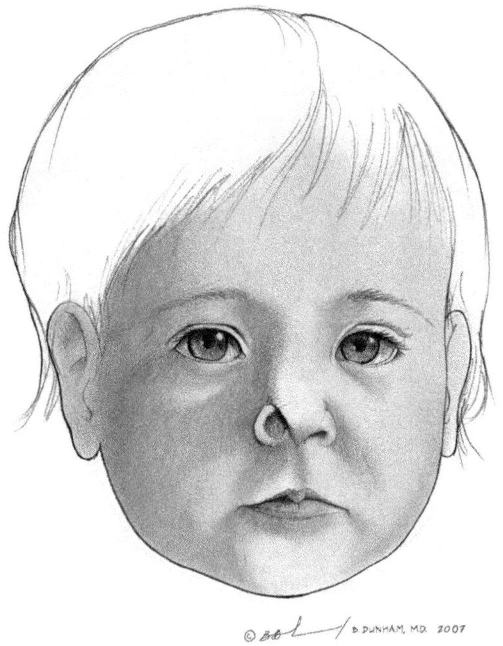

Fig. 3.4 Diagram of a child with a nostril colomba

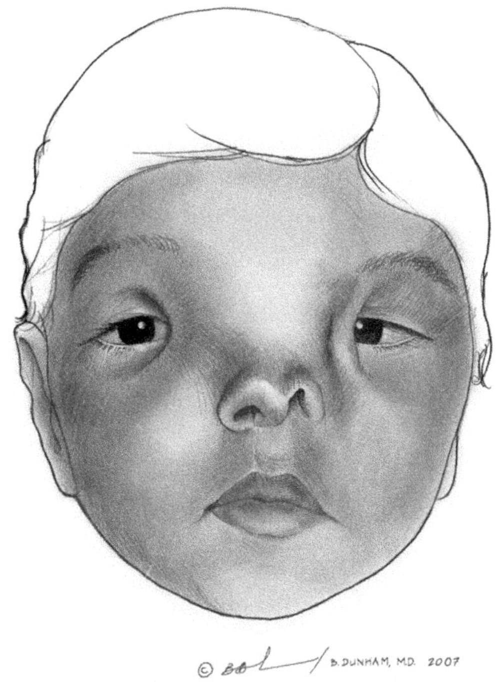

Fig. 3.5 Diagram of a child with a bifid nose

Management

Surgical repair is the treatment of choice [2].

Bifid Nose

Definition

In this rare and sporadic condition, a central groove bifurcates the nose. The condition may result from an anomalous infolding of the median nasal processes (Fig. 3.5).

Incidence

The incidence of these rare clefts has been estimated at 1.43–4.85 per 100,000 births [9].

Associated Malformations

Ocular hypertelorism often occurs concurrently. The upper lip may also have a median cleft. Pseudohypertelorism can also occur as a result of an optical illusion. This illusion is produced by the wide spacing of the components of the face adjacent to the eyes.

Diagnosis

Visual inspection is the basis for diagnosis. The presentation of a bifid nose ranges from a minimally noticeable midline nasal tip central groove to a complete clefting of the osteocartilaginous framework, resulting in two complete half noses [10].

Management

Surgical repair is the treatment of choice. The rarity of these types of cleft makes any surgeon relatively inexperienced. Not surprisingly, as with many of these malformations, no true consensus exists as to the best approach for repair [9].

Polyrhinia

Definition

Polyrhinia is characterized by either a partial or a complete duplication of the nose (Fig. 3.6).

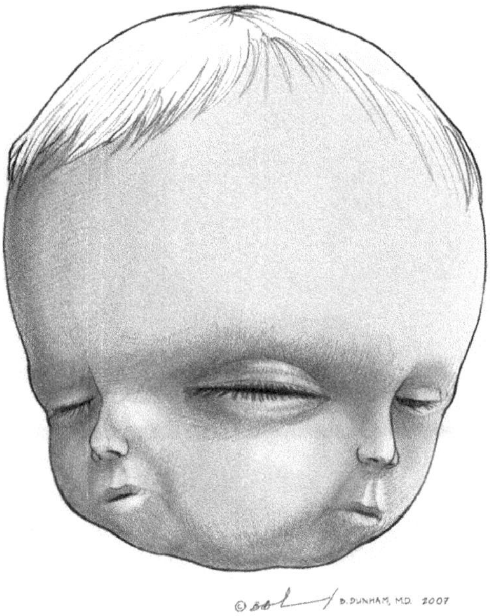

Fig. 3.6 Diagram of a child with polyrhinia and partial facial duplication

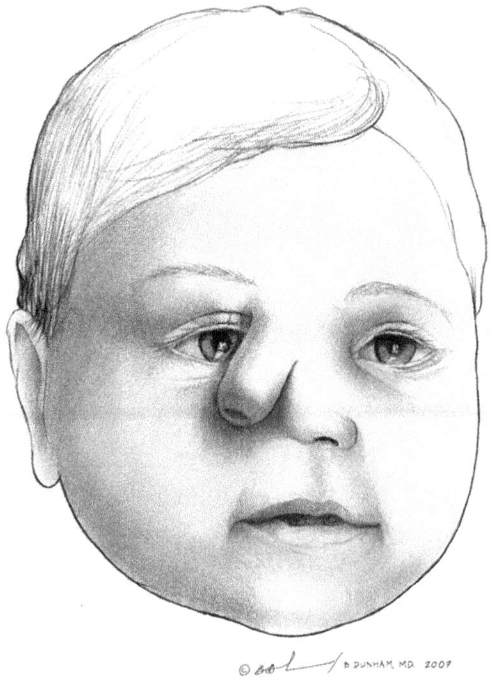

Fig. 3.7 Diagram of a child with proboscis

Incidence

This is an extremely rare and sporadic condition.

Associated Malformations

Choanal atresia is commonly found in association with polyrhinia. Two separate noses each with a pair of nostrils can occur with diprosopia, a condition of partial facial duplication. Some cases of facial duplication are incompatible with life.

Diagnosis

Clinical inspection provides the diagnosis.

Management

If the child does survive, however, treatment is surgical [2]. In the absence of facial duplication, treatment involves correcting the associated choanal atresia and then removing the medial portions of both noses and anastomosing their lateral counterparts in the midline.

Proboscis

Definition and Associated Malformations

A proboscis is a snout-like tubular structure arising from the midface (Fig. 3.7). There are four different types: lateral nasal proboscis, supernumerary proboscis, disruptive proboscis, and holoprosencephaly proboscis.

Lateral nasal proboscis results from the incomplete formation of one side of the nose, including an ipsilateral absence of the nostril, nasal cavity, paranasal sinuses, and olfactory tract and bulb. Typically the proboscis emanates from the medial canthus on the affected side. A supernumerary proboscis occurs in the setting of two nostrils as an accessory structure and is thought to arise from a supernumerary nasal placode. Disruptive proboscis occurs in the setting of an early embryonic hamartoneoplastic lesion in the primitive prosencephalon.

Holoprosencephaly is a failure of the forebrain to divide into lobes; cyclopia occurs in its most severe form. Proboscises occur in many but not all cases of cyclopia. Ethmocephaly, also caused by holoprosencephaly, consists of a proboscis in lieu of a nose in between narrowly set microphthalmic eyes. Prognosis depends on the associated anomalies. Holoprosencephaly forecasts a poor prognosis [2].

Incidence

Proboscis is a rare anomaly. The incidence of proboscis lateralis is less than 1 in 100,000 [11].

Etiology

Proboscis represents a failure of the lateral nasal process to fuse with both the medial nasal process and the maxillary process. The etiology and pathogenesis of proboscises is heterogeneous.

Diagnosis

Clinical inspection provides the diagnosis.

Management

Isolated proboscis formation is amenable to surgical correction. Preoperative imaging with both computed tomography (CT) and magnetic resonance (MR) scans is imperative. Given the high degree of variability of associated anomalies, an individualized approach is suggested when addressing the surgical correction of a proboscis. In general surgical repair can be undertaken as early as the surgeon is comfortable without affecting the cosmetic outcome [12, 13].

Congenital Midline Nasal and Nasopharyngeal Malformations

Choanal Atresia

Definition

Choanal atresia is an uncommon congenital obstruction of one or both of the posterior choanae. The choanae are the spaces that separate the most posterior aspect of the nose from the nasopharynx. About 30 % are purely bony while the remaining 70 % are thought to have mixed bony and membranous atresias [14]. Choanal stenosis may be considered a milder variation of atresia.

History

Roederer was first to describe the condition of congenital choanal atresia in 1755 and Emmert reported the first successful surgical dilation using curved trocars transnasally in 1854 [15].

Incidence

In a review of over five million births, the prevalence at birth varied between 0.54 and 1.13 per 10,000 with an equal sex distribution and without evidence of side predilection [16]. The frequency of unilateral versus bilateral, while it had traditionally been thought to be 2:1, has more recently shown to be closer to 1:1 [17].

Etiology

During development, the nasal cavities extend posteriorly as the palatal processes fuse to form a single closed palate. Failure of the posterior rupture of the buccopharyngeal membrane that separates the nose from the nasopharynx or abnormal growth of the palatine bone may be responsible for choanal atresia. The bony narrowing can result from narrowing of the pterygoid plates laterally, the vomer medially or the sphenoid superiorly.

Associated Malformations

Forty-seven percent of cases have been reported to be associated with other major congenital malformations and should alert physicians to look for other anomalies. Some syndromes associated with choanal atresia include Apert syndrome, Crouzon syndrome, DiGeorge sequence, Pfeiffer syndrome, Treacher-Collins syndrome, and CHARGE association [16]. Choanal atresia is a common finding in CHARGE Association, which is a nonrandom association of malformations whose acronym stands for coloboma, heart defects, and atresia of the choanae, retarded growth or development of the central nervous system (CNS), genitourinary anomalies, and ear anomalies. A child has to have three or more of the cardinal malformations (excluding growth/mental retardation) to meet diagnostic criteria.

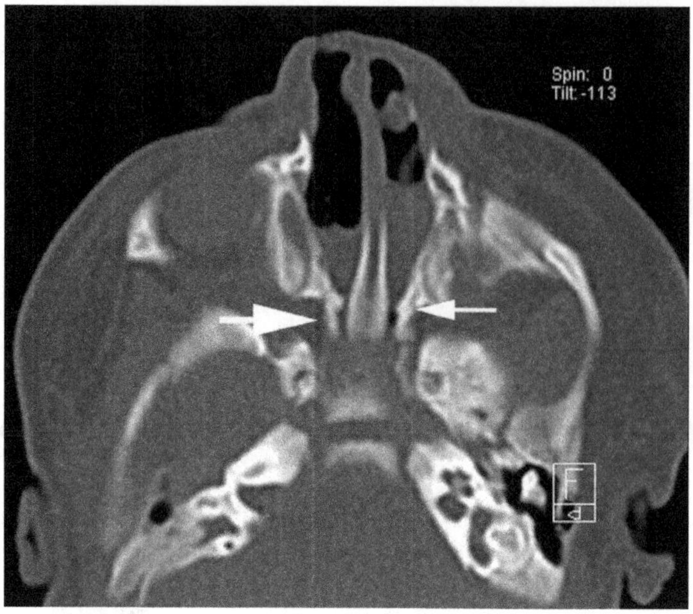

Fig. 3.8 Computed tomography demonstrating choanal atresia (see *arrows*)

By those criteria, approximately 7 % of children with choanal atresia belong to the CHARGE constellation [16].

Clinical Features

Bilateral choanal atresia presents very differently than its unilateral counterpart. Because an infant is typically an obligate nasal breather, bilateral obstruction often presents with immediate respiratory distress during the newborn period. The resulting distress is typically cyclical. During the inspiratory effort, the infant's tongue apposes the palate, occluding the oral airway. Increased inspiratory effort leads to marked retractions. The occlusion is broken if and when the child cries or opens his/her mouth. Asphyxia can and does occur with bilateral atresia.

Diagnosis

The suspected diagnosis is clinically supported by the inability to pass a 6 French suction catheter through the nasal cavity and can be confirmed with a diagnostic flexible nasopharyngoscopy. Computed tomography of the nose can also confirm the diagnosis; furthermore it shows what type of atresia it is, purely bony or membranous and bony (Fig. 3.8). Unilateral atresia rarely causes respiratory distress and often escapes detection until later in childhood when a thick unilateral mucoid discharge is noted; it is not uncommon for it to be diagnosed as sinusitis.

Management

Treatment of choanal atresia is surgical. In the case of bilateral atresia, the immediate distress can often be temporarily addressed with either an oral airway or a McGovern nipple, which has either a single enlarged hole or two additional lateral holes at its tip. There are three basics approaches for the repair: transpalatal, transeptal, and transnasal. The transpalatal approach, while it provides great visualization of the surgical field, is typically reserved for older patients as it can result in malocclusion in up to 50 % of patients, a consequence of disrupting the palate before it has completely grown [18]. The transeptal approach is typically reserved for unilateral cases. Endoscopic transnasal repair is the most common approach today; it can address either membranous or bony defects. Endoscopes can be used transnasally and through the oropharynx (Fig. 3.9) demonstrates the endoscopic appearance of the bilateral atresia taken from the nasopharynx. Revision surgery is commonly needed to dilate the passages as the child grows.

Craniopharyngioma

Definition

Craniopharyngiomas are benign-appearing dysodontogenic epithelial tumors; the great majority of these affect intradural suprasellar anatomy but they can and do extend into infrasellar regions.

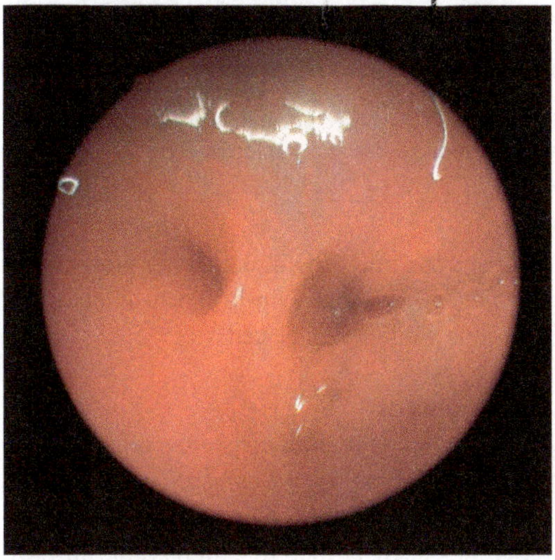

Fig. 3.9 Endoscopic photograph of bilateral choanal atresia taken from the nasopharynx

Incidence

The overall incidence of craniopharyngiomas is approximately 0.13 per 100,000 person years and is not gender or race dependent. Craniopharyngiomas comprise approximately 1.5–11.6 % of all intracranial tumors. A bimodal distribution places peak incidence rates in children (aged 5–14 years) and adults (aged 50–74). Approximately 338 cases of this disease occur annually in the United States, with 96 occurring in children from 0 to 14 years of age [19].

Etiology/Embryology

Craniopharyngiomas are thought to arise from the remnants of Rathke's pouch, which arises during the fourth week of gestation from the oral stomodeum and projects dorsally towards the brain, eventually forming the anterior lobe and pars intermedia of the pituitary gland (Fig. 3.10). By the eighth week, Rathke's pouch has typically lost its contact with the stomodeum [4]. By the 12th week, the craniopharyngeal duct, the cellular tract formed by the dorsal ascension of Rathke's pouch disappears, leaving an obliterated tract between the sphenoid cavity to the junction of the palate and posterior nasal septum. Most craniopharyngiomas occur in and/or above the sella turcica. Only occasionally do they

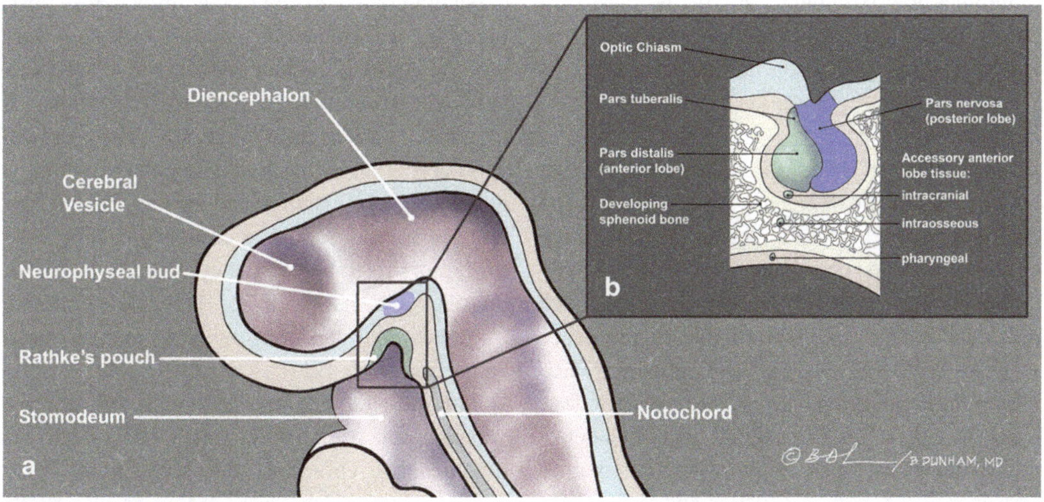

Fig. 3.10 Schematic diagram demonstrating the possible mechanism of formation of a craniopharyngioma

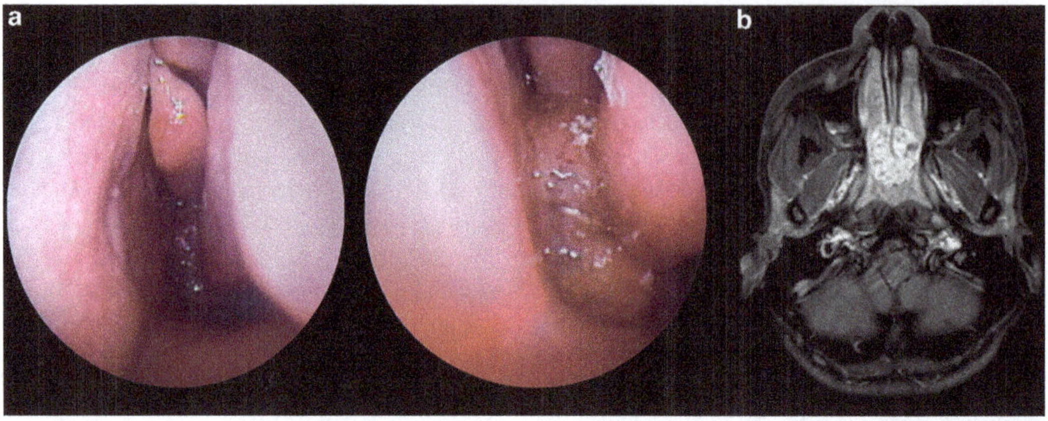

Fig. 3.11 (**a**) Two Endoscopic photographs of a right nostril with a mass diagnosed as craniopharyngioma. (**b**) Axial cuts of an MRI demonstrating a mass in the sphenoid sinus, which was diagnosed as a craniopharyngioma

develop in the basisphenoid or pharynx, presumably from rest of cells in an incompletely obliterated tract.

Associated Malformations

If there is a suprasellar/intracranial component, then visual field defects, varying degrees of pituitary insufficiency and signs of increasing intracranial pressure may appear.

Clinical Features

Craniopharyngiomas' symptomatology results from local expansion and impingement on surrounding structures; metastases from craniopharyngiomas are extremely rare. In the case of a purely infrasellar mass, nasal obstruction, epistaxis, sinusitis, and headaches predominate.

Diagnosis

Initial suspicion of an intranasal mass is made either by nasal endoscopy or imaging (Fig. 3.11a, b). The final diagnosis relies on histopathology. The work up should include general and neurologic examination (including visual field evaluation), a thorough nasal endoscopy, and both magnetic resonance imaging with and without angiography (MRI/MRA) and CT imaging with and without contrast of the brain and sinuses. CT imaging will often detect the calcifications found in the adamantinomatous variant as well as bony destruction and remodeling. MRI imaging best delineates soft tissue involvement and is particularly important for preoperative planning. If intracranial involvement is noted, an endocrine workup is indicated.

Management

To date, there is no true consensus regarding the optimal treatment of craniopharyngiomas. In the case of uniquely infrasellar tumors, only case reports exist. It is therefore impossible to have true evidence-based recommendations regarding treatment and prognosis. From the gathered case reports of infrasellar tumors, the primary treatment has historically been complete surgical excision with or without postoperative radiation depending on the extent of the tumor. Close postoperative surveillance is warranted for these rare tumors; it should include postoperative MRI surveillance at regulated intervals (3 months, 6 months, 1 year, and 2 years). The surgical approach to an infrasellar craniopharyngioma is dictated by its location and extent. Lateral rhinotomy or endoscopic approaches can be used for tumors restricted to the confined to the nasopharynx and nasal cavity. For larger tumors, transphenoidal and transcranial trajectories may be necessary.

For intracranial tumors, though still controversial, radical excision is still considered the treatment of choice if the tumor's size and involvement with the surrounding tissue permits it [20]. If not, then subtotal resection is usually

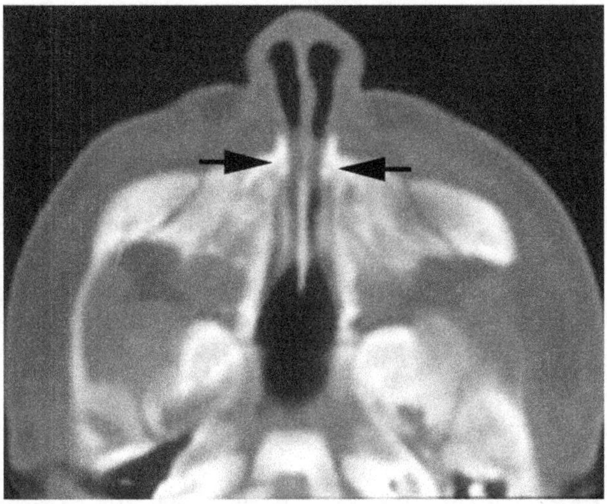

Fig. 3.12 Axial cuts of a CT demonstrating bony narrowing at the level of the anterior pyriform process (see *arrows*)

accompanied by radiation therapy; without radiation, recurrence rates may be as high as 73 % and is likely to occur regardless of tumor variant [21, 22]. Some authors have reported success in treatment of cystic craniopharyngiomas with intracystic chemotherapeutic therapy using bleomycin as well as intracavitary radiotherapy [23–25].

Nasal Pyriform Aperture Stenosis

Definition

Congenital nasal piriform aperture stenosis (CNPAS) consists of narrowing of the anterior nasal cavity due to the medial displacement of the maxillary prominences bilaterally. A width of 10 mm or less of the piriform aperture on CT scan in a term infant has been suggested as diagnostic by Belden and others [26] (Fig. 3.12). Furthermore, each naris should allow the passage of a 5 French catheter [27]. The resulting nasal obstruction associated with CNPAS leads to respiratory distress that can be life threatening in a neonate and is similar in presentation to choanal atresia.

History

First described in a series of six patients treated for nasal obstruction by Brown et al. in 1989 [28].

Incidence

The true incidence is unknown although it is thought to be less common than choanal atresia.

Etiology

The etiology is unknown although it has been postulated that CNPAS is due to an overgrowth of the nasal process of the maxilla that occurs at 4 months in utero [29].

Associated Malformations

Associated craniofacial anomalies occur in up to 40 % of cases and include: agenesis of the pituitary gland, the presence of a prominent central "mega incisor," holoprosencephaly, and midface hypoplasia [29].

Clinical Features

Infants are obligate nasal breathers for the first 6–8 weeks of life and, therefore, CNPAS results in newborn respiratory distress. As mentioned, CNPAS is similar in presentation to choanal atresia and results in respiratory distress which worsens with feeding and improves with crying. Additionally, infants with CNPAS may manifest increased distress with upper respiratory infection that causes increased nasal obstruction due to mucosal edema.

Diagnosis

Early diagnosis of neonatal nasal obstruction is essential. Axial thin cut CT scanning is diagnostic and requires a piriform aperture width of less than 11 mm in a term infant. The average width of symptomatic patients, however, is often much less and may be as low as 1–2 mm.

Management

Most patients with CNPAS can be managed expectantly once the diagnosis is established. Placement of an oral airway, the use of small frequent feedings (with the possible need for gavage feeding), humidification, frequent nasal suctioning, and the use of topical decongestants are often adequate. In children who fail conservative management and are unable to thrive, surgery is indicated. Repair is best performed via a sublabial approach with drilling or curetting to widen the lateral dimensions of the piriform aperture. Care must be taken to avoid injury to the nasolacrimal ducts posterolaterally or the tooth buds inferiorly. The allowance of a 3.5 mm endotracheal tube as a stent to be placed at surgery denotes adequate widening.

Epignathi

Definition

Epignathi are rare teratomas that arise in the oral cavity and consequently are composed of ectodermal, mesodermal, and endodermal tissues. They commonly emanate from the skull base, palate or pharyngeal walls but may also arise from alveolar bone. When they are large, they may be associated with life-threatening airway obstruction. Prenatal diagnosis of these tumors, especially when large, is critical in determining optimal and timely management of the airway.

Incidence

1:35,000 to 1:200,000 live births and represents 3–9 % of all teratomas [30].

Etiology

The etiology of epignathi is unknown although it has been postulated to arise from the pluripotential cells of Rathke's pouch region [31].

Clinical Features

The oropharyngeal obstruction associated with epignathi commonly leads to polyhydramnios in utero. Ultrasound examination of the fetus reveals the mass which can then be further characterized by magnetic resonance imaging. The tumors may be very large and can be highly differentiated, with evidence of intact vertebral columns, evidence of organ or limb development.

Management

Optimal management of epignathi requires early prenatal diagnosis and a multidisciplinary approach. When prenatally diagnosed, and life-threatening airway obstruction is anticipated, an EXIT (ex utero intrapartum treatment) procedure is often electively performed. This approach allows the airway to be secured via tracheotomy, while placental blood flow is maintained. Thereafter, surgical excision of the tumor can be undertaken. Massive lesions are often removed in a staged manner by first debulking the mass on day of life one and considering further resection or repair of associated cleft palate remotely [32].

Thornwaldt Cyst

Definition

Thornwaldt (or Tornwaldt) cysts are congenital, cystic masses located in the posterior midline wall of the nasopharynx. They form just cranial to the superior border of the superior constrictor muscle and are usually noted only incidentally, although they may become symptomatic when infected.

History

The first description of Thornwaldt cysts was offered by Mayer when he described the lesion in autopsy specimens [33]. They were later characterized further by Tornwaldt [34] in the mid-nineteenth century.

Incidence

Studies analyzing the incidental finding of a Thornwaldt cyst based on radiological examinations and autopsy specimens estimate the incidence to be 1.5–5 % [35, 36].

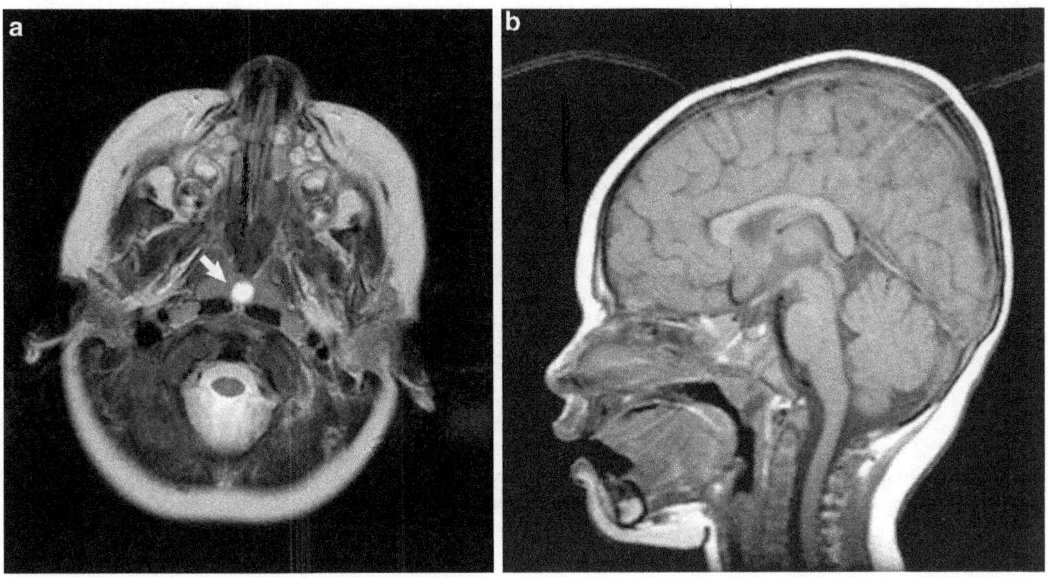

Fig. 3.13 (**a**, **b**) Thornwald cysts (*arrow*)

Etiology

Thornwaldt cysts result from an abnormally persistent connection between the cranial aspect of the notochord and the endoderm of the developing pharynx. This connection leads to the formation of a potential space between the two layers that is often called a pharyngeal bursa. A majority of patients with Thornwaldt cysts have had a previous adenoidectomy, leading to speculation that trauma or inflammation may prevent drainage of the nasopharyngeal bursa.

Clinical Features

Thornwaldt cysts are most commonly asymptomatic. However, they may become acutely or chronically infected leading to symptoms of pain, which is often worse with head turning, headache, chronic posterior nasal drainage, otalgia, otitis media, and halitosis [37]. Diagnosis is aided by endoscopic visualization of the nasopharynx. The acquisition of subsequent imaging studies is advised to better characterize the lesion and differentiate it from invasive neoplastic masses. Thornwaldt cysts are hyperintense on both T_1- and T_2-weighted MR images (Fig. 3.13a, b).

Management

Small, asymptomatic lesions can often be observed without the need for surgery. However, if they become significantly large or infected, surgical removal is indicated. This procedure after any apparent infection has been treated with antibiotics where appropriate. Wide marsupialization of the cyst can usually be accomplished by a transnasal endoscopic approach.

Hairy Polyp

Definition

Hairy polyps are congenital masses that arise in the nasopharynx or oropharynx. Because they are usually composed of ectodermal and mesodermal elements, some authors classify them as dermoids [37]. However, some authors have objected to this nosology and prefer to designate hairy polyps as choristomas because they represent aberrant rests of normal tissue and not neoplastic masses [38–40].

Clinical Features

Hairy polyps commonly present as fleshy, sausage-shaped masses that are often covered with thin hairs. Symptoms often depend on their location. They may be large enough to cause neonatal respiratory distress. When based laterally in the nasopharynx, they may cause eustachian tube dysfunction and actual growth into the middle ear

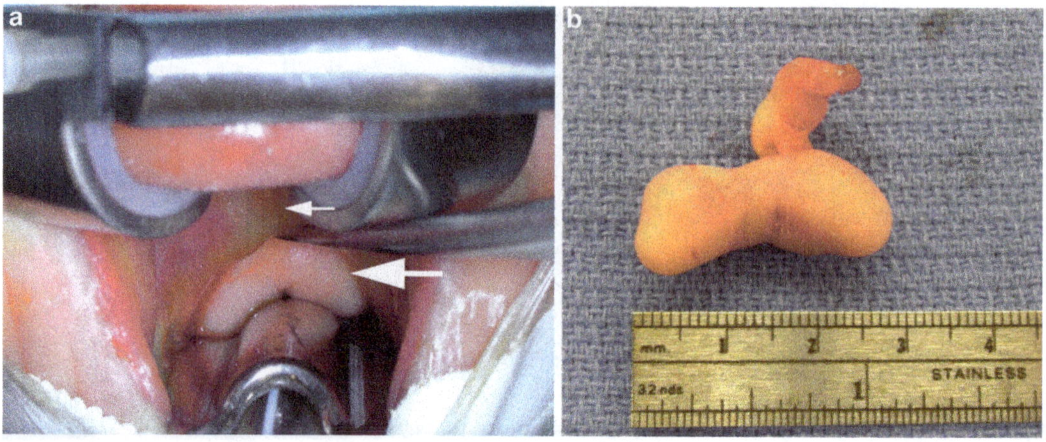

Fig. 3.14 (**a**) Intraoperative photograph of an hairy polyp located in the nasopharynx (*large arrow*: horseshoe-shaped mass; *small arrow*: palate). (**b**) Specimen of excised hairy polyp (note the finger-like characteristic of the mass)

through the eustachian tube has been described [41, 42].

Incidence

Hairy polyps are the most common congenital masses arising in the nasopharynx. They are six times more common in females [43]. They are not associated with any particular syndrome and there is no known genetic basis for their development [37].

Management

Treatment of hairy polyps is similar to the treatment of epignathi described above. Like epignathi, these lesions may cause complete neonatal airway obstruction and management may involve prenatal diagnosis. Usually, transoral resection is possible and may be aided by the use of angled telescopes [42] (Fig. 3.14a, b).

Nasal Dermoids, Gliomas, and Encephaloceles

Definition

Nasal dermoids, gliomas, and encephaloceles present as midline nasal masses. Of these, nasal dermoid cysts are the most common. These three entities are often grouped together in light of their similarities in presentation, etiology, and management.

Nasal Dermoids

Nasal dermoids account for 3 % of all dermoid cysts and approximately 10 % of dermoids of the head and neck [44]. They are comprised of ectodermal and mesodermal embryonic elements and as such may contain epidermal tissue, hair follicles, sweat glands, or sebaceous glands. As is detailed below in the etiology section, the existence of a nasal dermoid represents a failure of the developing dura to separate from the skin in utero. Accordingly, the contents of nasal dermoids may maintain some degree of connection to the CNS. They most commonly present as a noncompressible mass with an associated overlying pit or sinus tract anywhere from the glabella to the columella (Fig. 3.15). They do not transilluminate or expand with crying or with compression of the internal jugular vein (negative Furstenberg test). The presence of hair emanating from the cutaneous sinus punctum can be considered pathognomonic for dermoids [45] (Fig. 3.16a). Approximately two-thirds are situated along the lower nasal dorsum. The mass associated with these lesions may be primarily external or intranasal. Thirty percent of dermoids present first as intranasal masses (Fig. 3.16b).

Widening of the nasal dorsum may be seen from extension through the nasal bones.

Glioma

When used to describe a congenital nasal mass, the term glioma is a misnomer because these lesions do not represent neoplastic tissue. Gliomas are composed of heterotopic glial tissue that forms as a result of the same failure of separation from intracranial and extracranial tissue elements that is responsible for dermoid formation. As is the case with nasal dermoids, comprehension of the etiology of nasal gliomas requires a thorough understanding of the developmental anatomy of the anterior skull base. Like dermoids, gliomas present as smooth, firm, noncompressible masses along the midline aspect of the nasal dorsum or glabella. The overlying skin often takes on a blue or red hue, and there is not typically an associated cutaneous pit. In approximately 15 % of cases, they maintain a fibrous connection to the dura [46]. Approximately 30 % of gliomas are entirely intranasal. In these cases, they are usually situated on the lateral nasal wall and are more likely to have and intracranial connection.

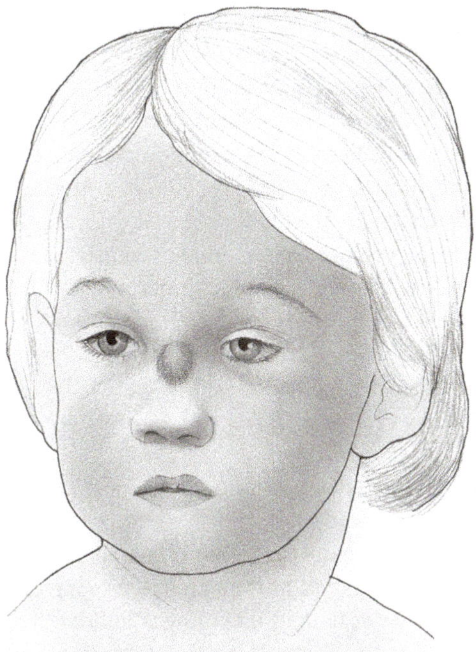

Fig. 3.15 Diagram of a child demonstrating a nasal dermoid on the dorsum of the nose

Encephalocele

Encephaloceles result from herniation of intracranial contents through a defect in the skull base. The presentation and etiology of congenital nasal encephaloceles is similar to that of dermoids and gliomas with several exceptions. Encephaloceles are usually compressible and enlarge with crying or compression of the internal jugular veins (positive Furstenburg test). The location of the mass will depend on the

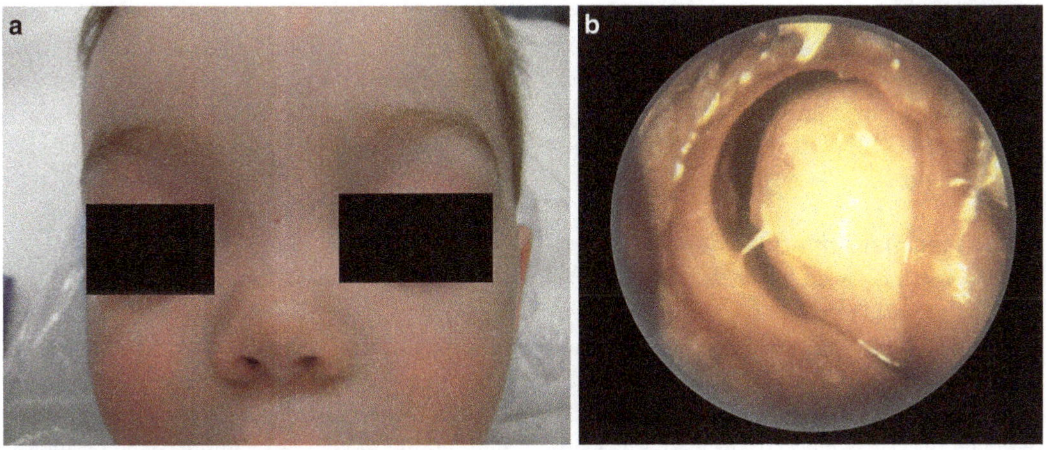

Fig. 3.16 (**a**) Photography of a child with a nasal dermoid presenting as a pit on the bony dorsum of the nose. (**b**) Endoscopic photograph of a nasal dermoid presenting within the nasal cavity

location of the defect and may be on the lower forehead, medial orbit, or nasal dorsum. If the lesion is predominantly intranasal, it may be misdiagnosed as a nasal polyp. A cerebrospinal fluid leak may be present concomitantly or may be caused by biopsy of the lesion.

Etiology

Multiple theories for the development of midline nasal masses have been proposed with the most widely excepted mechanism being the one described by Pratt [47]. Normally, at approximately 8 weeks gestation, a dural diverticulum exists between the nasal bones and the cartilaginous nasal capsule in a region known as the prenasal space. During this time of separation of the frontal bone and skull base, the nasal and frontal bones are also not yet fused at a region known as the fonticulus frontalis. During this time, the dura is in contact with the dermis via the prenasal space and perhaps through the more anterior and superior fonticulus. The nasal processes of the frontal bone then develop further until only a small surrounding an area just anterior to the crista galli that will be known as the foramen cecum. Simultaneously, the nasal and frontal bones fuse to obliterate the fonticulus. During this time of development, the dural–dermal connection normally separates and any remaining connective tract is obliterated. The formation of nasal dermoid cysts is thought to involve the trapping of ectodermal elements that occur as the dura involutes. Gliomas and encephaloceles represent entrapment of cranial contents during this process. Depending on whether this persistent communication involves the prenasal space or the fonticulus, these lesions may present as a nasal mass or in the glabellar region, respectively.

Associated Malformations

Midline nasal masses are not necessarily associated with any specific craniofacial syndrome. However, various reports have reported the existence of associated congenital anomalies in up to 40 % of patients with nasal dermoid cysts [48]. Wardinsky et al. [49] have described a significantly increased incidence of intracranial involvement when there are other congenital malformations present.

Diagnosis

Intracranial extension occurs in approximately 20 % of cases [50] of nasal dermoids and is suggested on CT scanning by the presence of an enlarged foramen cecum, bifid crista galli, or bifid nasal septum. A confirmatory MRI should be obtained when the CT scan suggests intracranial extension to minimize the chance of an unnecessary craniotomy. It should be noted that, in most children, marrow within the crista galli has been replaced by fat by the age of 5 years. The resulting signal intensity on T1-weighted MRI can lead to the false impression that a dermoid cyst is present [51]. Gliomas maintain a connection to the dura in 15 % of cases and encephaloceles by definition are connected intracranially. As is the case with dermoids, CT and MRI are helpful in the characterization of gliomas and encephaloceles to optimally delineate these lesions' bony and soft tissue involvement, respectively.

Management

Nasal Dermoids

The treatment of nasal dermoids is complete surgical excision. Multiple surgical approaches have been described including a midline longitudinal incision along the nasal dorsum, external rhinoplasty approach, and endoscopic approaches (Fig. 3.17). Excision of any cutaneous sinus ostium on the nasal dorsum is necessary for complete removal of all dermal elements. Given the potential for intracranial involvement, a craniotomy is required in some cases. When necessary, a standard frontal craniotomy is typically used to access the lesion, although, more recently, the transglabellar, subcranial approach has been described and may carry less morbidity [52].

Encephaloceles and Gliomas

Excision of gliomas and encephaloceles adhere to the principles outlined above for dermoids except that, unlike dermoids, these lesions usually do not require resection of a cutaneous punctum. Furthermore, unlike gliomas and dermoids, intracranial communication can be assumed to be present in cases of nasal encephalocele.

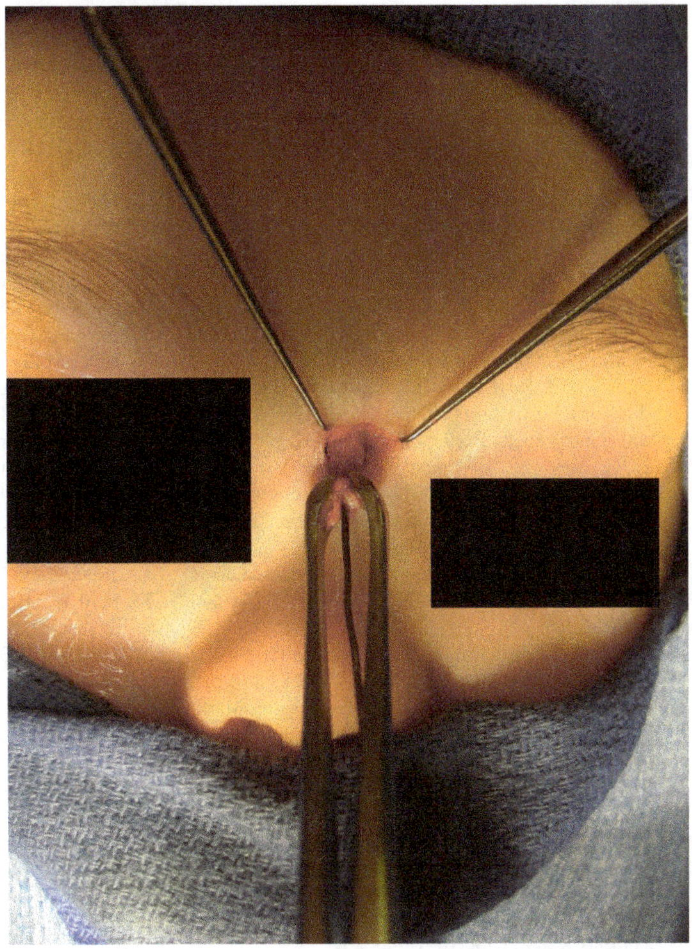

Fig. 3.17 Intraoperative photograph demonstrating the most common method of excising midline dermoid nasal malformations via vertical incision on dorsum of nose

References

1. Hengerer AS, Wein RO. Congenital malformations of the nose and paranasal sinuses. In: Bluestone CD, Casselbrant ML, Stool SE, et al., editors. Pediatric otolaryngology. Philadelphia, PA: Saunders; 2003. p. 979–94.
2. Cohen MM. Nose. In: Stevenson RE, Hall JG, editors. Human malformations and related anomalies. New York, NY: Oxford University Press; 2006. p. 373–87.
3. Moore KL. The branchial apparatus and the head and neck. In: The developing human: clinically oriented embryology. Philadelphia, PA: W. B. Saunders Company; 1988. p. 170–206.
4. Moore KL. The developing human—clinically oriented embryology. Philadelphia, PA: W.B. Saunders Company; 1988.
5. Albernaz VS, Castillo M, Mukherji SK, Ihmeidan IH. Congenital arhinia. AJNR Am J Neuroradiol. 1996;17:1312–4.
6. Weinberg A, Neuman A, Benmeir P, Lusthaus S, Wexler MR. A rare case of arhinia with severe airway obstruction: case report and review of the literature. Plast Reconstr Surg. 1993;91:146–9.
7. Cole RR, Myer 3rd CM, Bratcher GO. Congenital absence of the nose: a case report. Int J Pediatr Otorhinolaryngol. 1989;17:171–7.
8. Guion-Almeida ML, Machado-Paula LA, Richieri-Costa A. Newly recognized syndrome with heminasal aplasia and ocular anomalies or wider spectrum of heminasal aplasia/atypical clefting syndrome? Am J Med Genet A. 2004;129A:156–61.
9. Turkaslan T, Ozcan H, Genc B, Ozsoy Z. Combined intraoral and nasal approach to Tessier No: 0 cleft with bifid nose. Ann Plast Surg. 2005;54:207–10.

10. Miller PJ, Grinberg D, Wang TD. Midline cleft. Treatment of the bifid nose. Arch Fac Plast Surg. 1999;1:200–3.
11. English GM. Congenital anomalies of the nose, nasopharynx, and paranasal sinuses. Philadelphia, PA: Lippincott, Williams, and Wilkins; 1998.
12. Thorne MC, Ruiz RE, Carvalho J, Lesperance MM. Proboscis lateralis: case report and review. Arch Otolaryngol Head Neck Surg. 2007;133:1051–3.
13. Eroglu L, Uysal OA. Proboscis lateralis: report of two cases. Br J Plast Surg. 2003;56:704–8.
14. Brown OE, Pownell P, Manning SC. Choanal atresia: a new anatomic classification and clinical management applications. Laryngoscope. 1996;106:97–101.
15. Harney MS, Russell J. Choanal atresia. In: Puri P, Hollward ME, editors. Pediatric surgery: diagnosis and management. Berlin: Springer-Verlag; 2009. p. 223–8.
16. Harris J, Robert E, Kallen B. Epidemiology of choanal atresia with special reference to the CHARGE association. Pediatrics. 1997;99:363–7.
17. Leclerc JE, Fearon B. Choanal atresia and associated anomalies. Int J Pediatr Otorhinolaryngol. 1987;13:265–72.
18. Freng A. Surgical treatment of congenital choanal atresia. Ann Otol Rhinol Laryngol. 1978;87:346–50.
19. Bunin GR, Surawicz TS, Witman PA, Preston-Martin S, Davis F, Bruner JM. The descriptive epidemiology of craniopharyngioma. J Neurosurg. 1998;89: 547–51.
20. Savas A, Erdem A, Tun K, Kanpolat Y. Fatal toxic effect of bleomycin on brain tissue after intracystic chemotherapy for a craniopharyngioma: case report. Neurosurgery. 2000;46:213–6. discussion 6-7.
21. Sanford RA, Muhlbauer MS. Craniopharyngioma in children. Neurol Clin. 1991;9:453–65.
22. Weiner HL, Wisoff JH, Rosenberg ME, et al. Craniopharyngiomas: a clinicopathological analysis of factors predictive of recurrence and functional outcome. Neurosurgery. 1994;35:1001–10. discussion 10–1.
23. Hasegawa T, Kondziolka D, Hadjipanayis CG, Lunsford LD. Management of cystic craniopharyngiomas with phosphorus-32 intracavitary irradiation. Neurosurgery. 2004;54:813–20. discussion 20–2.
24. Broggi G, Franzini A. Bleomycin for cystic craniopharyngioma. J Neurosurg. 1996;84:1080–1.
25. Cavalheiro S, Sparapani FV, Franco JO, da Silva MC, Braga FM. Use of bleomycin in intratumoral chemotherapy for cystic craniopharyngioma. Case report. J Neurosurg. 1996;84:124–6.
26. Belden CJ, Mancuso AA, Schmalfuss IL. CT features of congenital nasal piriform aperture stenosis: initial experience. Radiology. 1999;213:495–501.
27. Hui Y, Friedberg J, Crysdale WS. Congenital nasal pyriform aperture stenosis as a presenting feature of holoprosencephaly. Int J Pediatr Otorhinolaryngol. 1995;31:263.
28. Brown OE, Myer CM, Manning SC. Congenital nasal pyriform aperture stenosis. Laryngoscope. 1989; 99:86.
29. Shikowitz MJ. Congenital nasal piriform aperture stenosis: diagnosis and treatment. Int J Pediatr Otorhinolaryngol. 2003;67:635–9.
30. Haghighi K, Milles M, Cleveland D, Ziccardi V. Epignathus teratoma with bifid tongue and median glossal salivary mass: report of a Case. J Oral Maxillofac Surg. 2004;62:379–84.
31. Hatzihaberis F, Stamatis D, Staurinos D. Giant epignathus. J Pediatr Surg. 1978;13:517–8.
32. Mayer AFCJ. Bursa seu Cystis tubae eustachianae bei eingen saugethieren. Neue Notizen aus dem Gebiete der Nature Heilkunde von Froeiep. 1840;14:1.
33. Dohman G, Sjovall A. A large epignathus teratoma, successfully operated on immediately after birth. Glassgow Med J. 1953;34(3):123–5.
34. Tornwaldt GL. Uber die Bedeutung der bursa pharygea fur die erkennung und behandlung gewisser nasenrauchenraum. Krankheiten. Weisbaden: J.F. Bergmann; 1885.
35. Battino RA, Khangure MS. Is that another Thornwaldt's cyst on M.R.I.? Australas Radiol. 1990;34:19–23.
36. Ford WJ, Brooks BS, el Gammal T. Thornwaldt cyst: an incidental MR diagnosis. Am J Neuroradiol. 1987;8:922–3.
37. Moody MW, Chi DH, Mason JC, et al. Tornwaldt's cyst: incidence and a case report. Ear Nose Throat J. 2007;86(3):129.
38. Kelly A, Bough Jr ID, Luft JD, Conard K, Reilly JS, Tuttle D. Hairy polyp of the oropharynx: case report and literature review. J Pediatr Surg. 1996;31:704–6.
39. Sexton M. Hairy polyp of the oropharynx: a case report with speculation on nosology. Am J Dermatopathol. 1990;12:294–8.
40. Yossuck P, Williams HJ, Polak MJ, Vaughan R. Oropharyngeal tumor in the newborn: a case report. Neonatology. 2007;91:69–72.
41. Chang SS, Halushka M, Meer JV, Goins M, Francis HW. Nasopharyngeal hairy polyp with recurrence in the middle ear. Int J Pediatr Otorhinolaryngol. 2008;72(2):261–4.
42. Roh JL. Transoral endoscopic resection of nasopharyngeal hairy polyp. Int J Pediatr Otorhinolaryngol. 2004;68:1087–90.
43. Burns BV, Axon PR, Pahade A. Hairy polyp of the pharynx in association with an ipsilateral branchial sinus: evidence that the "hairy polyp" is a second branchial arch malformation. J Laryngol Otol. 2001;115:145–8.
44. Crawford JK, Webster JP. Congenital dermoid cyst of the nose. Plast Reconstr Surg. 1952;9:235–40.
45. Kearns DB, Zapata S. Nasal dermoids. Curr Opin Otolaryngol Head Neck Surg. 2006;14:406–11.
46. Ma KJ, Cheung KL. Nasal glioma. Hong Kong Med J. 2006;12:477–9.
47. Pratt LW. Midline cyst of the nasal dorsum: Embryologic origin and treatment. Laryngoscope. 1985;75:968–75.
48. Denoyelle F, Ducroz V, Roger G, et al. Nasal dermoid sinus cysts in children. Laryngoscope. 1997;107: 795–800.

49. Wardinsky T, Pagon R, Kropp R, Hayden P, Clarren S. Nasal dermoid sinus cyst: association with intracranial extension and multiple malformations. Cleft Pal Craniofac J. 1991;28:87–95.
50. Hanikeri M, Waterhouse N, Kirkpatrick N, Peterson D, Macleod I. The management of midline transcranial nasal dermoid sinus cysts. Br J Plast Surg. 2005;58:1043–50.
51. Posnick JC, Bortoluzzi P, Armstrong DC, Drake JM. Intracranial nasal dermoid sinus cysts: computed tomographic scan findings and surgical results. Plast Reconstr Surg. 1994;93:745–54.
52. Goyal P, Kellman RM, Tatum SA. Transglabellar subcranial approach for the management of nasal masses with intracranial extension in pediatric patients. Arch Facial Plast Surg. 2007;9:314–7.

Congenital Malformations of the Oral Cavity and Oropharynx

4

Lisa M. Elden and Richard E. Kirschner

Abstract

The common congenital malformations of the oral cavity are presented in this chapter, along with photographs and schematic figures of each anomaly. Specific topics that are highlighted include benign tumors, hamartomas, dermoids, teratomas, vascular malformations, and hemangiomas of the oral cavity. In addition, other malformations are described including macroglossia, lingual thyroid, ankyloglossia, ranulas, and mucoceles.

Keywords

Macroglossia • Hamartoma • Lingual thyroid • Hemangioma • Ankyloglossia • Teratoma • Beckwith–Wiedemann syndrome

Malformations of the Oral Cavity and Oropharynx (Congenital Lesions/Benign Tumors)

Definition: The lesions or benign tumors that can form when the tongue develops can be grouped into categories listed below. Most of these lesions present within the mucosa or submucosa of the tongue or within the lining of the oral cavity. They usually are identified when they are small and can be treated by surgical excision. A pathologist should review the surgical specimens to ensure that they are benign and that they have been completely excised.

1. Hamartoma is a lesion consisting of benign tissue with components that are indigenous to the area in which it is located, i.e., normal tissue that forms in excess in normal locations. Examples of hamartomas in the oral cavity

L.M. Elden, M.S., M.D. (✉)
Division of Pediatric Otolaryngology, Department Surgery The Children's Hospital of Philadelphia, 34th Street and Civic Center Boulevard, 1 Wood Center, Philadelphia, PA 19104, USA

Otorhinolaryngology: Head and Neck Surgery, Perelman School of Medicine at the University of Pennsylvania, Philadelphia, PA, USA
e-mail: elden@email.chop.edu

R.E. Kirschner, M.D., F.A.C.S., F.A.A.P.
Section of Plastic and Reconstructive Surgery, Nationwide Children's Hospital,
700 Children's Drive, Columbus, OH 43205, USA
e-mail: Richard.Kirschner@nationwidechildrens.org

L.M. Elden and K.B. Zur (eds.), *Congenital Malformations of the Head and Neck*,
DOI 10.1007/978-1-4419-1714-0_4,

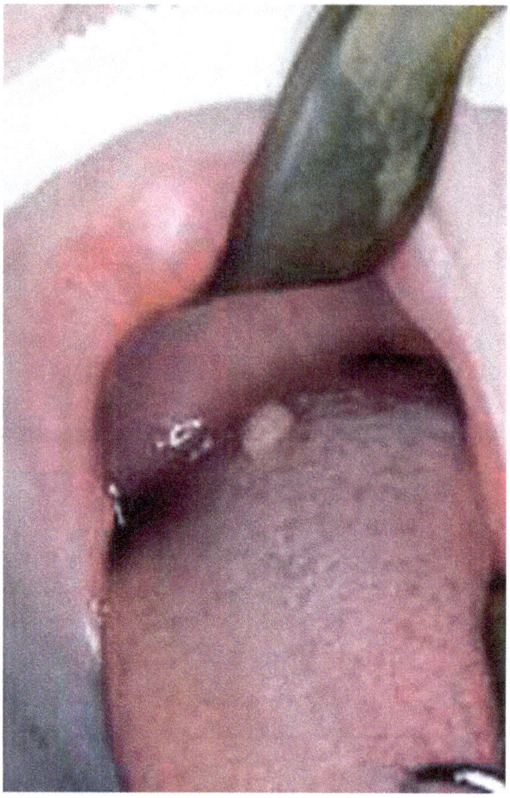

Fig. 4.1 Photograph of lipofibroma located in the midline posteriorly on the surface of the tongue

include fibromas and lipomas of the tongue (Fig. 4.1). Some authors describe hemangiomas as forms of hamartomas, but most consider them benign tumors because their rates of proliferation may differ from normal tissue.

2. Choristoma is a benign, well-organized heterotopic growth of tissue that forms in excess in areas in which it normally is not located, i.e., normal tissue that forms in excess in abnormal locations. In the oral cavity, choristomas may consist of a proliferation of an ectopic rest of bone, cartilage, fat, neural or glial tissue, thyroid tissue, respiratory tissue, gastric mucosa, or intestinal mucosa. They may or may not form a mass lesion and are not neoplastic. More common choristomas in the oral cavity include those that occur on the tongue, specifically gliomas, salivary tissue rests, and skin tissue (dermoids, see below) (Fig. 4.2).

Teratoma is a benign, haphazardly organized growth of tissue (or tumor) containing all three germ layers (endoderm, mesoderm, and ectoderm), which may be located anywhere in the body, especially in the head and neck. Teratomas may have malignant potential. Unlike hamartomas and choristomas, teratomas may also present as large obstructing masses of the head and neck. Smaller teratomas may be found anywhere within the oral cavity including the tonsil and are treated by surgical excision.

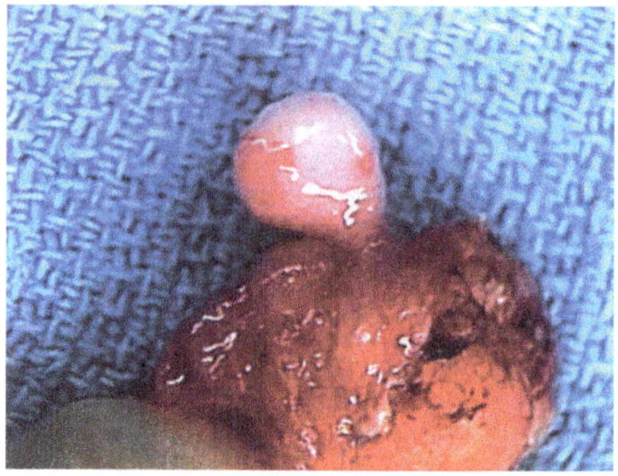

Fig. 4.2 Photograph of ectopic salivary tissue specimen

1. A hairy polyp is similar to a teratoma but consists of cells of only two germ cell lines (mesodermal and ectodermal tissue). These masses tend to originate in the oropharynx or nasopharynx and may stem from a malformed second branchial arch. Hairy polyps are more common in girls and usually are present at birth or within the first few years of life. They may be associated with other malformations of the head and neck, including cleft palate. The treatment for these tumors is complete surgical excision (refer Chap. 3, Fig. 14).
2. Dermoid is a lesion, which consists of mostly ectodermal tissue that forms a cyst filled with keratin or sebaceous material, and sometimes hair. It is most commonly found in planes of embryonic fusion. Common cutaneous locations include the regions lateral to the eyebrow, and in the midline of the neck, but they may be located anywhere within the oral cavity, including on the tongue or uvula. Treatment is excision.
3. Congenital epuli arise most often arise from the maxilla or mandible of the newborn. They are composed of cells derived from mesenchyme (granular cells with eosinophilic cytoplasm and

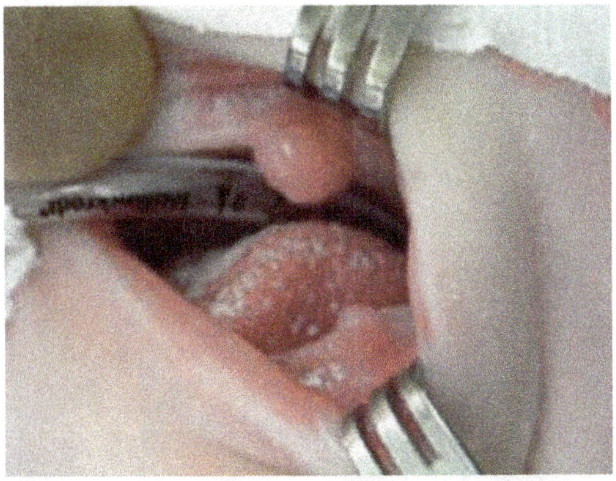

Fig. 4.3 Photograph of infant with two epuli: one on surface of mandible and one on surface of maxilla

small, eccentric nuclei). The lesions are more commonly found in girls and can present as small or very large lesions. Some have been found to regress with time, but they should be excised if they interfere with feeding or if they bleed (Fig. 4.3) [1].

Hemangiomas/Vascular Malformations

Definition

Vascular birthmarks are most commonly located in the skin and subcutaneous tissues, but they are also the most common congenital malformations found within the oral cavity and oropharynx. These lesions are usually located within the mucous membranes of the oral cavity and oropharynx, but they may also appear within the hypopharynx and the larynx. They may range in appearance from flat vascular mucosal patches to bulky lesions that can interfere with breathing or swallowing.

Vascular birthmarks are classified as either hemangiomas or vascular malformations. Infantile hemangiomas are the most common benign tumors of infancy. Thirty percent are seen at birth and the remaining form within the first few weeks of life. Eighty percent are focal and solitary in nature. The remaining may be multifocal or segmental. Segmental hemangiomas may involve large areas of skin and often associated with complications and associated malformations. Superficial hemangiomas involve the superficial dermis and consequently appear red in color, whereas deep hemangiomas reside in the deep dermis and subcutis, resulting in a blue color on the surface. Mixed hemangiomas involve both the superficial dermis and the deep dermis/subcutis. Infantile hemangiomas, which are not apparent at birth, must be distinguished from the less-common congenital hemangiomas. These lesions proliferate in utero and are fully formed at birth. They may be further categorized based on their pattern of involution after birth (RICH, rapidly involuting congenital hemangioma and NICH, non- involuting congenital hemangioma).

Vascular malformations are nonproliferative hamartomatous lesions that are usually present at birth and are classified as low-flow lesions (lymphatic, venous, capillary) or high-flow lesions (arteriovenous) [2].

Incidence

Infantile hemangiomas have been reported to occur in 2.5–10 % of infants (12 % of Caucasian infants, 1.4 % of African American infants, and 0.8 % of Asian infants, respectively). Fifty percent are located in the head and neck. Females are affected three times more often than male babies. The incidence is higher in preterm babies (up to 25–30 %), especially in those of extreme low birth weight and in multiple births (independent of birth weight) Vascular malformations are less common, have no gender predilection, and tend to grow proportionally with the affected child.

Heredity

Most hemangiomas and vascular malformations occur sporadically, although hemangiomas have been found to be familial in 12 % of cases. A linkage to chromosome 5q31–33 has been identified, but no specific gene has been implicated in their etiopathogenesis. DNA studies of some families who have multiple vascular malformations suggest that a genetic defect may exist in cells that form the smooth muscle lining of normal blood vessels.

Etiology

Infantile hemangiomas are neoplasms composed of proliferating endothelial cells that eventually form vascular spaces and channels, some filled with blood cells. There is limited basement membrane and as they grow they fill local potential spaces in the oral cavity and oropharynx. They eventually may appear as lobular, red structures extending beyond mucosal membranes. Congenital hemangiomas are composed of normal endothelial cells. Vascular malformations present as true structural anomalies, with normal rates of endothelial cell turnover. They lack muscular support and contain large vascular channels because they do not have smooth muscle lining cells that are normally present in blood vessels.

Multiple hypotheses exist to explain the underlying etiology of infantile hemangiomas, including the theory that they represent immature tissue, possibly similar to placental tissue, endothelial progenitor cells, or mesenchymal stem cells. These cells may maintain their proliferative capacity for a period of time postnatally. Various growth factors, including beta-fibroblast growth factor, vascular endothelial growth factor (VEGF) and proliferating cell nuclear antigen may induce proliferation. However as the endothelial cells differentiate, mast cells appear which produce transforming growth factors and other tissue inhibitors including interferon, which terminate the proliferation. Involution of the hemangioma tends to occur when these cells and factors are present [2, 3].

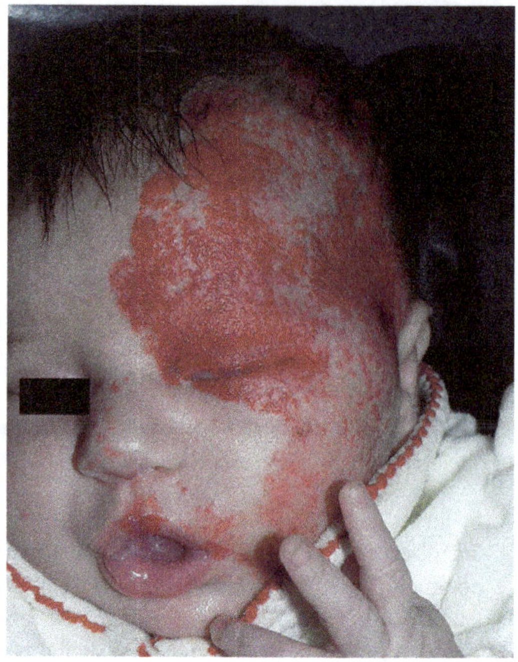

Fig. 4.4 Photograph of infant with PHACE syndrome of left face (Image courtesy of David W. Low, MD, Attending Surgeon, The Children's Hospital of Philadelphia; Associate Professor, Department of Plastic Surgery, University of Pennsylvania School of Medicine)

Associated Malformations

Most hemangiomas occur as isolated lesions, but the following associations have been recognized:

- PHACE association represents a neurocutaneous disorder most commonly presenting with large segmental facial hemangiomas and additional structural anomalies of cerebral vessels, eye vessels, and the aorta. The acronym stands for *p*osterior cranial fossa malformation(s) (including Dandy-Walker and Arnold Chiari malformations), large cervicofacial or laryngeal *h*emangiomas, *a*rterial anomalies of the head and neck (that can involve the carotid and cerebral vessels), *c*oarctation of the aorta and cardiac defects, and *e*ye anomalies. Sternal clefts or other ventral defects may also be present (PHACE(S)). The PHACE association affects female infants in 90 % of cases (Fig. 4.4) [3–5].
- Kasabach–Merritt Phenomenon is a rare, life-threatening condition which may occur if one of two specific benign vascular tumors is present (tufted angioma or kaposiform hemangioendothelioma). These lesions tend to be larger and cause thrombocytopenia by trapping and destroying platelets. This phenomenon does not occur in children with common infantile hemangiomas.

Several syndromes associated with vascular malformations include the following:

- Sturge–Weber (encephalotrigeminal angiomatosis): A rare congenital, usually unilateral phakomatoses (neural and skin disorder). It is associated with a facial port wine stain (or capillary malformation) located in the region of the first and second divisions of the trigeminal nerve (V1 and V_2 correlating to the regions of the forehead and cheek, respectively), along with ipsilateral leptomeningeal and brain angiomas (frequently leading to mental retardation and seizures). Glaucoma may be present caused by excess capillaries near the ophthalmic branch of the trigeminal nerve. This is a noninherited, nonfamilial syndrome (Fig. 4.5).

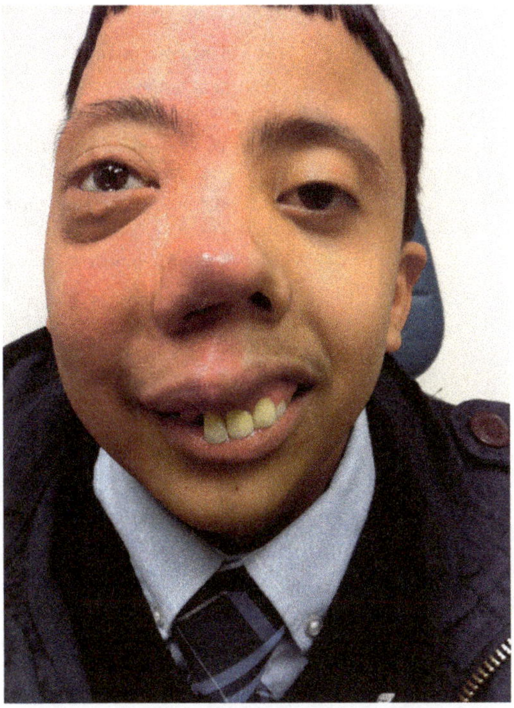

Fig. 4.5 Patient with Sturge Weber demonstrating port wine stain (capillary hemangioma of right face) and facial deformity due to changes in growth of these bones

- Klippel–Trenaunay: Capillary malformation of an extremity associated with deeper venous and lymphatic malformations and skeletal overgrowth.
- Parkes–Weber: Capillary malformation of an extremity associated with a deeper arteriovenous malformation.
- Osler–Weber–Rendu (hereditary hemorrhagic telangiectasia): An inherited disorder of blood vessels resulting in arterial venous malformations (AVMs) within the skin and mucous membranes. Affected individuals have diffuse cutaneous and visceral telangectasias and small AVMs. It may be associated with epistaxis, oral or gastrointestinal bleeding, hematuria, and CNS hemorrhage. This syndrome may be inherited in an auto-dominant pattern.

Clinical Features

Infantile hemangiomas are rarely visible at birth, but are recognized within days to weeks of delivery. In the oropharynx, these benign vascular proliferative lesions initially appear as flat red or bluish areas of mucosal discoloration. Most undergo rapid proliferation in the first 6–12 months of life, with the majority of proliferation occurring within the first 5 months. After reaching a plateau, hemangiomas slowly regress, or involute, a process that may continue for many years (50 % by 5 years, 70 % by 7 years and 90 % by 9 years of age) (Table 4.1). Complications of proliferative hemangiomas include ulceration and bleeding, airway obstruction, visual compromise, feeding impairment, and, in very large lesions, high-output congestive heart failure. Hemangiomas of the lip, neck, and diaper area are most prone to ulceration. Facial hemangiomas may cause cosmetic disfigurement and may necessitate surgical reconstruction after involution (Fig. 4.6).

Children who are at higher risk of developing complications from their hemangiomas include those with large hemangiomas, multiple cutaneous hemangiomas, or segmental hemangiomas. Infants with more than five cutaneous hemangiomas are more likely to have visceral hemangiomas, including those of the liver, gastrointestinal tract, liver, lungs, and brain. Larger hemangiomas and segmental hemangiomas are more likely to cause cosmetic disfigurement and are more likely to ulcerate and bleed as they grow. Airway lesions involving the subglottis, larynx, or oral cavity may be present in up to 29 % of those with segmental hemangiomas of the face (including patients who do not have PHACE(S) syndrome), especially in those with hemangiomas that are located within the beard or mandible distribution [5]. In most instances, the complications described above are apparent within the first 6 months of life during the phase of rapid proliferation (Fig. 4.7a) [3].

Unlike hemangiomas, vascular malformations are usually present at birth and do not undergo rapid proliferation or involution. Low flow vascular malformations typically demonstrate growth that is proportional to that of the patient. Venous malformations are soft, easily compressible, and are usually blue or purple in color (Table 4.1). Although usually small and asymptomatic, venous malformations of the oropharynx, oral cavity, or tongue may expand to compromise the

Table 4.1 Comparisons of characteristics of infantile hemangiomas vs. vascular malformations

	Infantile hemangioma	Vascular malformation
Onset	Only one-third present at birth Most appear within first few weeks of life	Present at birth Not always obvious
Growth pattern	Rapid in first year Regress over early childhood	Grow proportionately to child Never regress
Gender	Affects girls more than boys (3:1)	Girls and boys equally affected
Color/consistency	Red, less often bluish Raised with distinct border Doughy texture	Purple to blue Flatter, often submucosal Usually soft

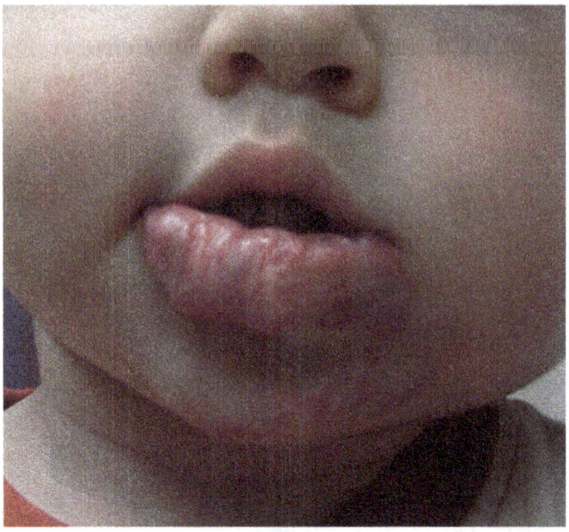

Fig. 4.6 Photograph of oral and lip hemangioma in infant (Image courtesy of David W. Low, MD, Attending Surgeon, The Children's Hospital of Philadelphia; Associate Professor, Department of Plastic Surgery, University of Pennsylvania School of Medicine)

airway, interfere with speech or cause failure to thrive secondary to poor feeding (Fig. 4.7b).

Capillary malformations (also known as port wine stains) usually present at birth as pink, macular discoloration of the skin. With time, untreated capillary malformations may darken and hypertrophy. Patients with capillary malformations of the head and neck may also have involvement of the oropharyngeal or oral mucosa (Fig. 4.7b).

Arteriovenous malformations (AVMs) are high-flow congenital vascular anomalies that may be found within the tongue or oral/oropharyngeal submucosa. The blood vessels appear as a tangled mass of arteries and veins without an interposed capillary bed. Although most are present at birth, they often remain undetected for many years. On physical examination, arteriovenous malformations frequently appear similar to venous malformations, but they may be associated with an audible bruit, a palpable thrill, or visible pulsations. Complications of AVMs include potentially life-threatening hemorrhage. Larger AVMs may extend to include surrounding soft tissue and bone causing distortion of the face and oral cavity (Fig. 4.7c).

Diagnosis

In most cases, the diagnosis of hemangioma or vascular malformation is made by correlating the pattern and timing of emergence of the lesion along with the physical findings. In the oral cavity and oropharynx, both direct exam and flexible nasopharyngoscopy and laryngoscopy are helpful to determine the extent of the lesion. Magnetic resonance imaging (MRI) with gadolidium contrast-enhanced computed tomography (CT) may be warranted to further determine the extent and depth of the lesion (Fig. 4.8). Biopsy is indicated in patients when the growth appears atypical or when malignancy is suspected. Angiography may be helpful in the assessment of AVM.

Patients with multiple cutaneous hemangiomas (more than 5 before age 6 months) may benefit from abdominal ultrasound or MRI to rule out the presence of visceral hemangiomas. Those with suspected PHACE(S) syndrome should undergo MRI/MRA (magnetic resonance angiography) of the brain and intracranial vasculature, assessment of the upper airway, cardiac evaluation, and ophthalmologic examination.

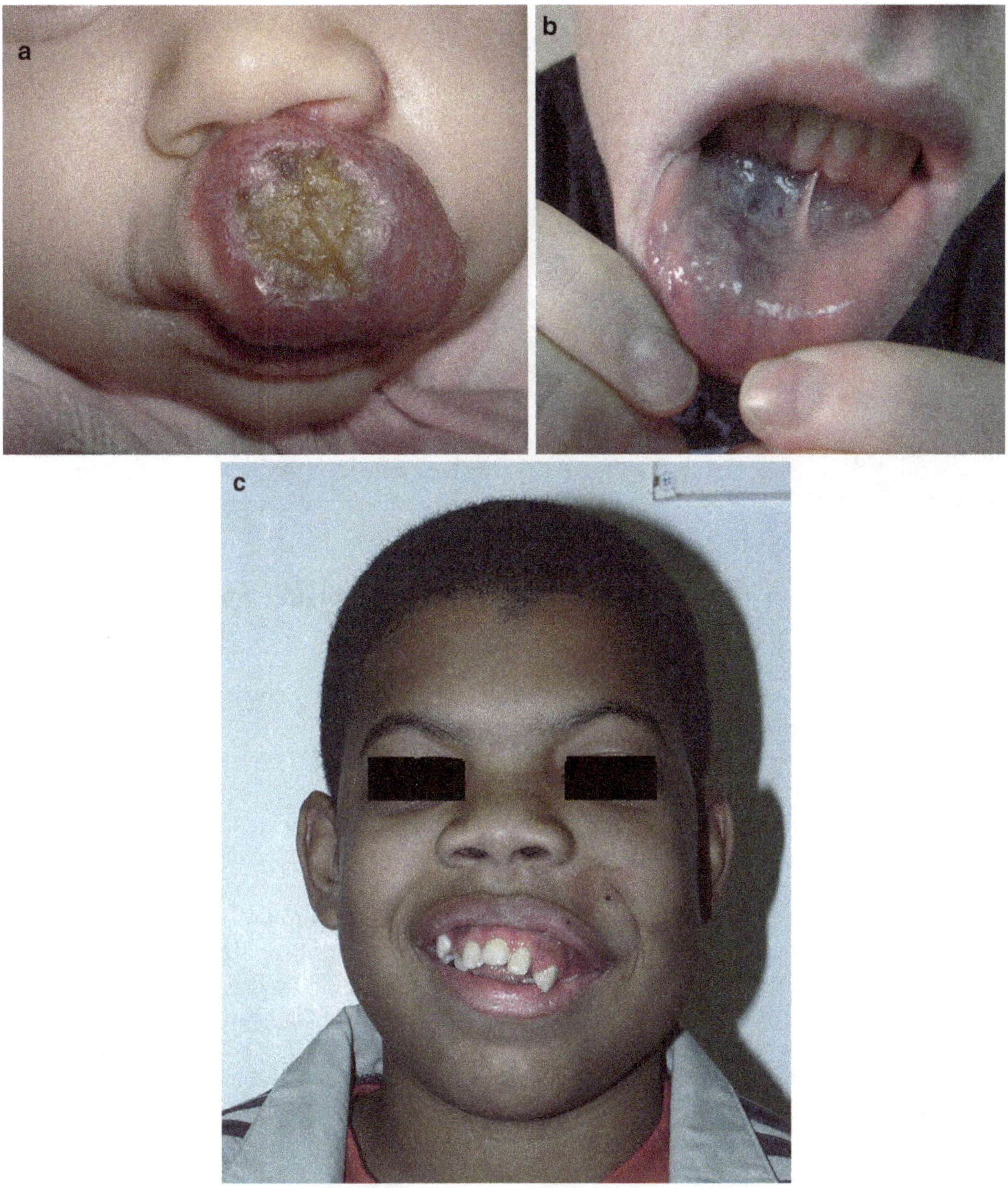

Fig. 4.7 Photographs demonstrating the variation in appearance of facial birthmarks. (**a**) Upper lip ulcerating hemangioma. (**b**) Venous malformation of lower lip. (**c**) Arterial venous malformation distorting left maxilla in young boy (Images courtesy of David W. Low, MD, Attending Surgeon, The Children's Hospital of Philadelphia; Associate Professor, Department of Plastic Surgery, University of Pennsylvania School of Medicine)

Management

Most hemangiomas may simply be observed so long as there are no functional or cosmetic concerns. Pulsed dye laser therapy may be effective for treatment of flat (less than 1 mm) superficial hemangiomas, for healing and pain control of ulcerated hemangiomas, and for the elimination of residual post-involutional telangiectasias. Intralesional corticosteroids may be useful for the suppression of small, localized hemangiomas, but their use should be avoided in the periocular region due to the risk of retinal artery

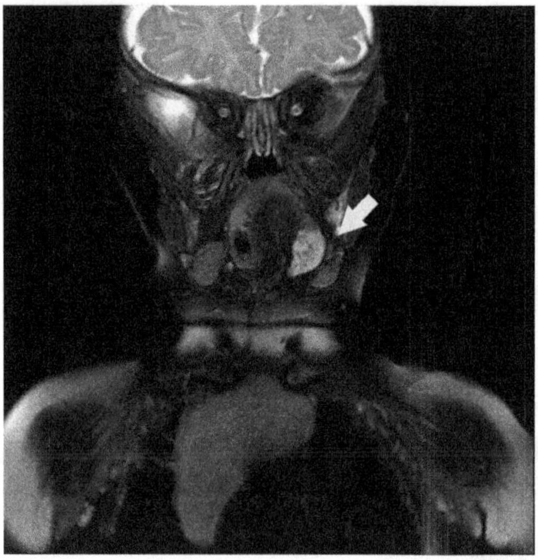

Fig. 4.8 Coronal MRI of head demonstrating left tongue hemangioma

occlusion and blindness. Systemic therapy may be required in patients at risk for functional impairment (e.g., airway obstruction or visual compromise) or for the suppression of lesions in cosmetically sensitive regions. Corticosteroids (2–5 mg/kg/day of oral prednisolone) have been the most commonly used first-line systemic drug for the treatment of proliferative hemangiomas. Adverse effects of corticosteroid administration include irritability, gastritis, immunosuppression, hypertension, adrenal suppression, and growth suppression, all of which are reversible following taper of the medication. Recently, encouraging results have been reported in children treated with propranolol, although the mechanism whereby this nonselective beta-blocker suppresses proliferation of hemangiomas remains uncertain. Potential adverse effects of beta blocker therapy include hypotension, bradycardia, hypoglycemia, bronchospasm, and congestive heart failure. Surgical resection may be indicated in patients who have lesions that may be life-threatening such as may occur when they are located within the oral cavity or airway (especially the subglottis) or for those who fail medical therapy.

Superficial capillary malformations usually respond well to pulsed dye laser therapy. Symptomatic or disfiguring lymphatic, venous, and arteriovenous malformations may require surgical excision, interventional radiologic treatment (sclerotherapy or embolization), or a combination of both).

Malformations of the Tongue

Macroglossia is the most common congenital malformation of the tongue. Aglossia (failure of the tongue to form) and microglossia (small tongue, such as seen with Moebius Syndrome) are extremely rare. Other rare malformations include accessory tongues and bifid tongues (as seen in patients with orodigitofacial syndrome).

Congenital Malformations of the Tongue

Embryology of Tongue

The tongue starts to develop beginning in the fourth week of gestation when the tuberculum impar (median tongue bud) and lateral lingual swellings arising from the first branchial arch mesenchyme form and start to fuse. The lateral lingual swellings grow over the tuberculum impar and form the anterior two-thirds of the tongue. The posterior one-third of the tongue is formed from the third and fourth branchial arch mesenchyme. The mucosa of the anterior two-thirds of the tongue is composed of ectodermal origin, whereas the posterior one-third is of endodermal origin (Fig. 4.9a, b).

Macroglossia

Definition

Macroglossia is defined as a resting tongue that protrudes beyond the teeth/alveolar ridge at rest, with or without enlargement of the tongue tissue. Congenital macroglossia occurs not only when there is enlargement of normal tongue tissue but also when abnormal proportions of tissue types are present. This may be seen when lymphatic

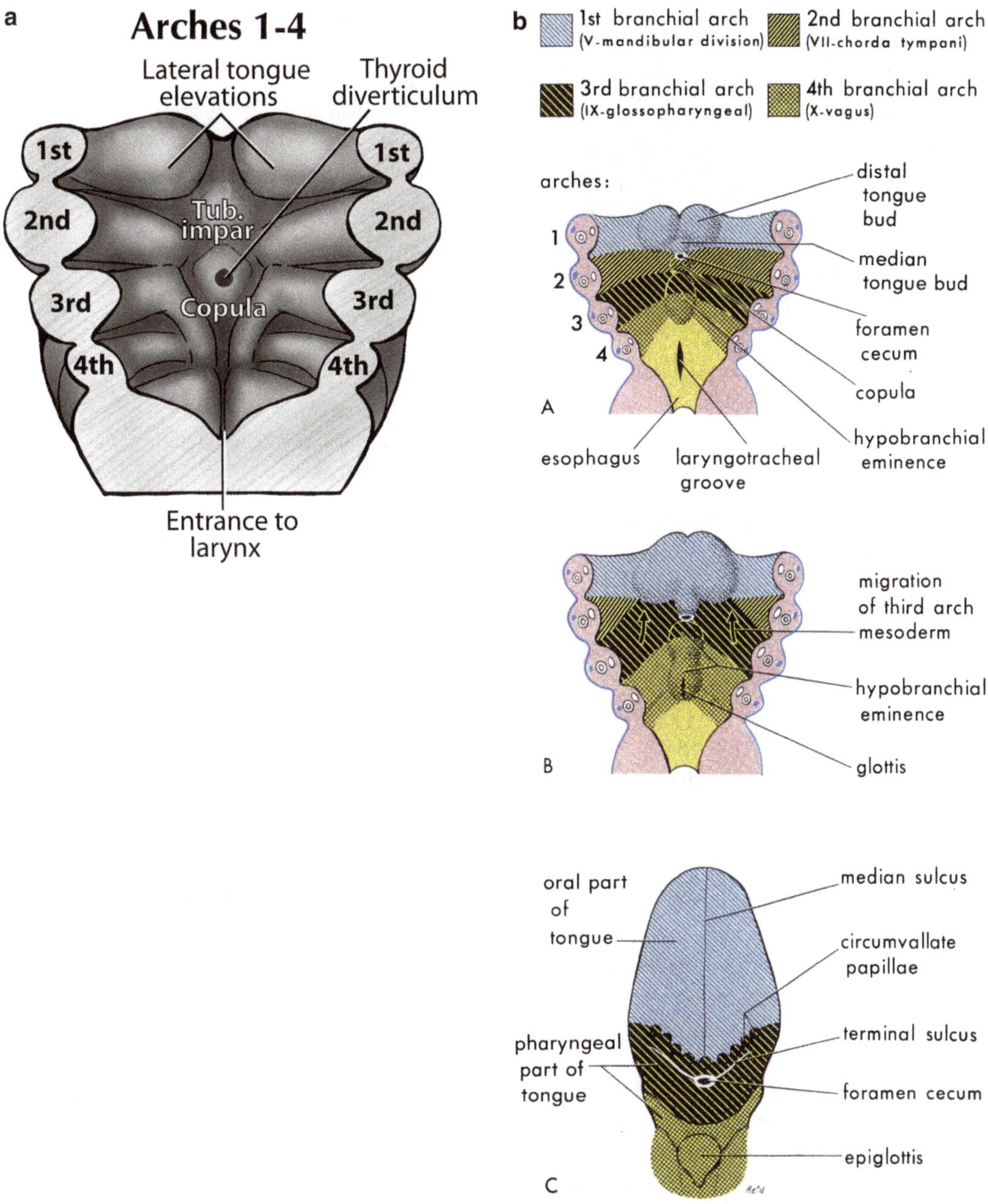

Fig. 4.9 (**a**) Schematic of the embryology of tongue development. (**b**) Schematic demonstrating the origins of various structures from four different branchial arches

malformations, hemangiomas, or other tissue types are found within the tongue, causing enlargement.

Incidence

See associated malformations.

Heredity

The pattern of inheritance depends on the associated condition. However, when isolated it is usually sporadic. An autosomal dominant transmission has been described in two unrelated families [6].

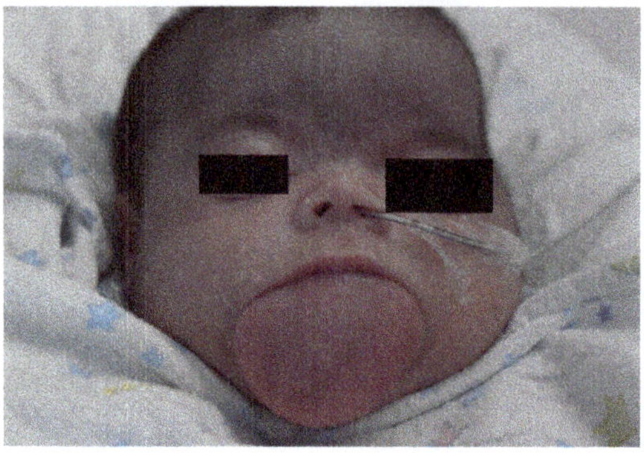

Fig. 4.10 Photograph of infant with macroglossia (Beckwith Wiedemann syndrome)

History

The earliest known written description of tongue lesions such as macroglossia comes from the Egyptian Papyrus Ebers (1150 BC) [7]. Early medical treatments for macroglossia included the use of sclerosing agents (mercury and potassium), leeches, and blood-extracting exercises. Debulking procedures have been described using crusher type instruments, but surgical resection has been the mainstay of treatment since the latter part of the twentieth century.

Etiology

Congenital macroglossia is not common, and when present is frequently associated with specific syndromes that may be characterized by classic physical findings that are obvious at birth. Macroglossia is more common in children who have Beckwith–Weidemann syndrome (Fig. 4.10), Down syndrome (Trisomy 21, relative macroglossia), and congenital hypothyroidism. Idiopathic macroglossia or autosomal dominant macroglossia has also been described. Other more common causes of macroglossia noted at birth include those described elsewhere in this chapter, which relate to masses within the substance of the tongue lymphangioma, hemangioma, vascular lesions, and lingual thyroid. Macroglossia may also be found in children with less common syndromes including Trisomy 22, mucopolysaccharoidosis, gangliosiderosis, Robinow syndrome, and Behmel syndrome (Table 4.2). Some congenital forms of macroglossia that are caused by storage diseases described above may present later in life. In addition, macroglossia may not be noticeable until later in life in those patients with acromegaly or neurofibromatosis.

Table 4.2 Congenital malformations of tongue

Aglossia
Microglossia
Moebius syndrome
Macroglossia
Congenital (observed at birth)
Beckwith–Wiedemann syndrome
Down syndrome (relative macroglossia)
Congenital hypothyroidism
Autosomal dominant
Trisomy 22
Tollner syndrome
Behmel syndrome
Mucopolysaccharidosis
Muscular idiopathic hypertrophy
Observed later in life
Acromegaly
Glycogenosis type IIA
Hypothyroidism
Mucolipidosis
Neurofibromatosis
Amyloidosis

Associated Malformations

Beckwith–Wiedemann Syndrome: Children who have Beckwith–Wiedemann syndrome present with macroglossia in 98 % of cases and the severity of macroglossia varies. The incidence of Beckwith–Wiedemann is 0.73 in 10,000 live births [8]. The mode of inheritance is unknown with both sporadic and familial cases reported in the literature [9]. Most cases are associated with a defect in chromosome number 11. These children have characteristic craniofacial anomalies including maxillary hypoplasia, prominent fontanelle, metopic ridge in forehead caused by premature closure of these bones, and they may also have generalized visceromegaly that may relate to fetal hyperinsulinism. Other features include the presence of hydramnios (caused by poor fetal swallowing in utero), omphalocele, or other abdominal wall defects, nephromegaly, gigantism (sometimes unilateral, hemihypertrophy), hepatomegaly, heart defects, and genital anomalies.

Affected children frequently have perinatal hypoglycemia that may contribute to mental retardation found in some of these patients. These children are also more prone to developing a Wilm's tumor and adrenal tumors.

Down Syndrome: Down syndrome is the most common genetic disorder (Trisomy 21), occurring in about 1 of 700 live births. Many of these children have protruding tongues and chronically opened mouths. However, MRI studies have shown that the tongue size is not large and instead the oral cavity is small resulting in relative macroglossia [10]. These patients also have characteristic facial traits including epicanthus, oblique lid axis, saddle nose, hypotonia, and microgenia.

Congenital Hypothyroidism: Children with congenital hypothyroidism may present similarly to those who have Beckwith–Wiedemann in that these children frequently have macroglossia associated with large fontanelles, hypotonia, and distended abdomens with or without umbilical hernia. Twenty-three percent may also have a lingual thyroid present (refer below).

Clinical Features

The clinical impact of macroglossia depends on the size of the tongue. Severely affected infants frequently present with drooling, swallowing problems, and less often failure to thrive. Many children have symptoms and signs of obstructive sleep apnea and airway problems. Speech problems from dysarthria and excessive saliva may need to be addressed as the child starts to talk. Finally, drying of the mouth, dental hygiene problems, cross-bite, and other malocclusion problems may develop.

Diagnosis

Diagnosis is usually obvious on clinical exam. Given the strong associations with other syndromes, evaluation by a geneticist is frequently warranted. Biopsies or imaging studies such as MRIs or CTs are rarely needed to confirm the diagnosis. A speech therapist may be helpful to ensure the child feeds well and to monitor for speech problems. Sleep studies should be considered in those with Beckwith–Wiedemann and Down syndrome as there is a high rate of undiagnosed sleep apnea.

Management

The mainstay of treatment remains surgical. Orofacial therapy using palate devices to stimulate muscle tone of the tongue and palate have been used with variable success. Surgical therapies depend on the location of the extra tissue. In some instances when sleep apnea is of more concern, the obstructing tissue is in the posterior third of tongue and submucosal reduction using radiofrequency (coblation tools) may be helpful. The coblation instrument dissolves tissue at low temperatures but may cause localized swelling as the tissue heals.

In more severe cases of macroglossia, partial tongue resection is necessary, especially when the tongue protrudes out of the mouth during rest. The anterior wedge resection or keyhole methods have been the most commonly used (Fig. 4.11a, b). The keyhole method, whereby a posterior circle of tissue is excised, allows the anterior and posterior tongue to be reduced (Fig. 4.11c, d, e).

Lymphatic Malformations

Definition

Lymphatic malformations (LMs) consist of abnormal lymphatic channels and cystic spaces that contain clear lymph fluid. These low-flow lesions may be classified as microcystic, macrocystic (formerly known and cystic hygromas), or mixed microcystic and macrocystic.

Incidence

LMs represent less than 5 % of all congenital head and neck masses.

Heredity

Most LMs that occur in the head and neck occur sporadically but are more commonly found in some syndromes.

Etiology

The lymphatic system begins to develop at the end of the fifth week of embryogenesis. LMs are thought to occur when normal lymphatic channels fail to properly form from large central veins during the fifth to sixth week of embryonic life. They represent endothelial outgrowths from

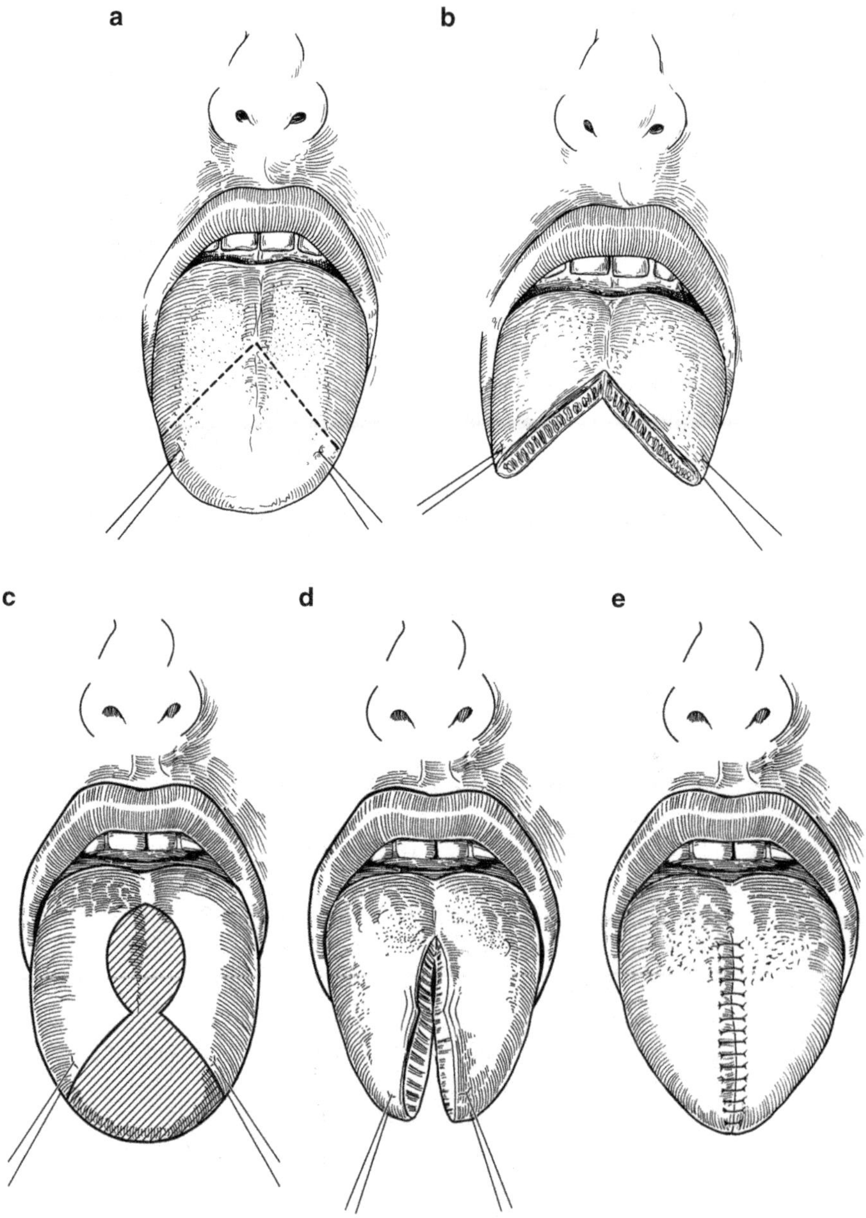

Fig. 4.11 Schematic of two of the types of tongue reduction operations (anterior wedge: **a**, **b** and keyhole: **c**, **d**, **e**)

these veins and they do not have connections with normal lymphatic channels. The cause is unknown, but they may be considered a form of vascular malformation.

Clinical Features

Most LMs present within the first 2 years of birth, but some can appear later in early adulthood or puberty. LMs of the tongue and oropharynx are characterized by the presence of diffuse, often asymmetric soft clear or bluish swellings or masses within the tongue, lip or, less often, within the submucosa of the remaining oral cavity (most often cheek) and oropharynx. These benign lesions may extend to the mucosal surface and may be characterized by the presence of superficial, irregular vesicles. These vesicles may be clear or blood-filled and tend to flare up and

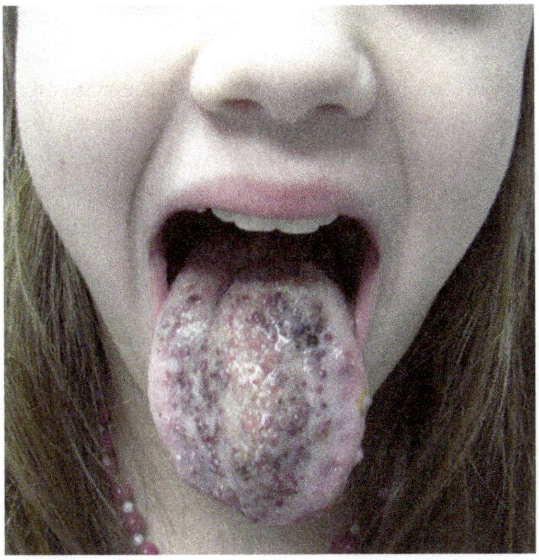

Fig. 4.12 Photograph of child with lymphatic malformation of the tongue (Image courtesy of David W. Low, MD, Attending Surgeon, The Children's Hospital of Philadelphia; Associate Professor, Department of Plastic Surgery, University of Pennsylvania School of Medicine)

bleed in response to trauma or at times when the child has an upper respiratory tract infection (Fig. 4.12). The lesions tend to spread into surrounding tissue and the extent of the lesion may not be apparent on clinical examination. In general, they tend to grow in proportion to the child, but expand and contract depending on the amount of lymph fluid within the channels. Swelling of the tongue, oropharynx, and hypopharynx may result in dysphagia, poor speech, or airway obstruction. Care must be taken to monitor and secure the airway in affected children. The lesions may also be combined with capillary or venous malformations.

Associated Malformations

LMs that are located primarily in the neck may be associated with Turner's syndrome, Trisomy 13, 18, and 21 [11].

Diagnosis

The diagnosis may be made by direct examination and the extent of the lesion confirmed by flexible laryngoscopy, supplemented with contrast MRI or CT. Most LMs do not enhance with contrast unless they are composed of mixed vascular/lymphatic channels.

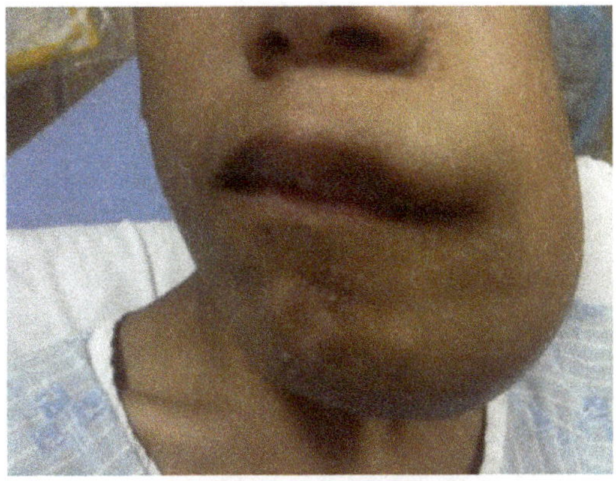

Fig. 4.13 Left facial lymphatic malformation with acute swelling of left cheek and tongue occurring after an upper respiratory tract infection (Image courtesy of David W. Low, MD, Attending Surgeon, The Children's Hospital of Philadelphia; Associate Professor, Department of Plastic Surgery, University of Pennsylvania School of Medicine)

Management

Steroids and antibiotics have been used to reduce acute swelling related to upper respiratory infections or trauma (Fig. 4.13). The options used to treat lesions more definitively depend on the pathological subtype of LM and the location of the mass. Sclerotherapy has been helpful to control macrocystic lesions, but surgical excision/debulking is usually necessary when the lesion is more microcystic in nature. Complete resection is rarely achieved. Those LMs that are microcystic and are located above the suprahyoid muscle are the most difficult to treat and often require multiple surgical procedures to control. It is important to balance the need to preserve normal tissue with resection of LMs that are located within the tongue muscle [12]. Superficial bleeding or lesions that may disfigure the tongue may be controlled with laser or using coblation therapy.

Congenital Ranulas/Mucoceles

Definition

In older children and adults, mucoceles and ranulas are most often caused by trauma to local minor salivary glands in the mucosa or to salivary ducts that run along the floor of the mouth, respectively (Fig. 4.14). However, congenital mucoceles and ranulas have been reported to be

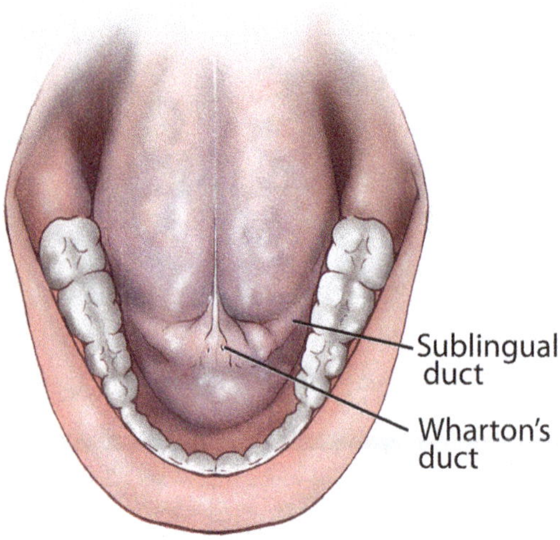

Fig. 4.14 Schematic diagram of floor-of-mouth anatomy

present at or near birth and more likely represent malformation of salivary ducts or glands. Mucoceles tend to be smaller and may be found within the floor of mouth or other mucous membranes in the oral cavity, but ranulas are found exclusively in the floor of mouth and can extend through the myelohyoid muscle into the submandibular space (plunging ranula).

History

The term ranula stems from the Latin word *rana*, meaning frog, because they appear to be similar to the underbelly of a frog.

Incidence

Congenital ranulas and mucoceles are rare without a sex predilection.

Heredity

Sporadic.

Etiology

Mucoceles are usually lined with epithelium, whereas ranulas are pseudocysts that lie adjacent to the sublingual gland in the floor of the mouth. In contrast to older children and adults, congenital mucoceles are thought to result from failure of the normal ducts to open or form properly. Some controversy exists as to the etiology of ranulas because they are not always present at birth and it is difficult to eliminate trauma as a mechanism of their development. Clinical cases have been reported describing children who develop these prior to having teeth, which suggests that they may form because of underdeveloped sublingual gland ducts or because of persistent rests of embryonic tissue.

Clinical Features

Most mucoceles that are present at birth are small 1–2 cm smooth, straw-colored or pale yellow, mucous membrane covered masses found at the orifice of opening of the submandibular duct (Wharton's duct). This duct is located on the under surface of the tongue (on either side of the lingual frenulum) (Fig. 4.15). Other types of mucoceles can also arise from smaller obstructed glands that are located throughout the oral cavity and lip (Fig. 4.16). Ranulas tend to present in older infants and the mass most often is a larger (2–5 cm), pale blue or pink submucosal mass that usually runs along the length of one side of the floor of the mouth (Fig. 4.17a).

Diagnosis

The diagnosis of a mucocele is most often made clinically by examining the mass in the oral cavity, whereas, a ranula usually requires additional studies (such as a contrast MRI or CT of the neck and oral cavity) to determine its extent.

Management

Smaller mucoceles that cause discomfort, feeding or airway problems, or those located at the tip of the submandibular duct can be treated by excision. For those located at the tip of the submandibular duct, the remaining duct should be probed to ensure that it still drains saliva once the mass has been excised. The residual proximal duct may be maintained open with an absorbable suture to reduce the likelihood of recurrence. Larger, floor-of-mouth ranulas (3–6 cm) are prone to infection and require excision or marsupialization. The sublingual gland usually must also be removed to avoid recurrence (Fig. 4.17b).

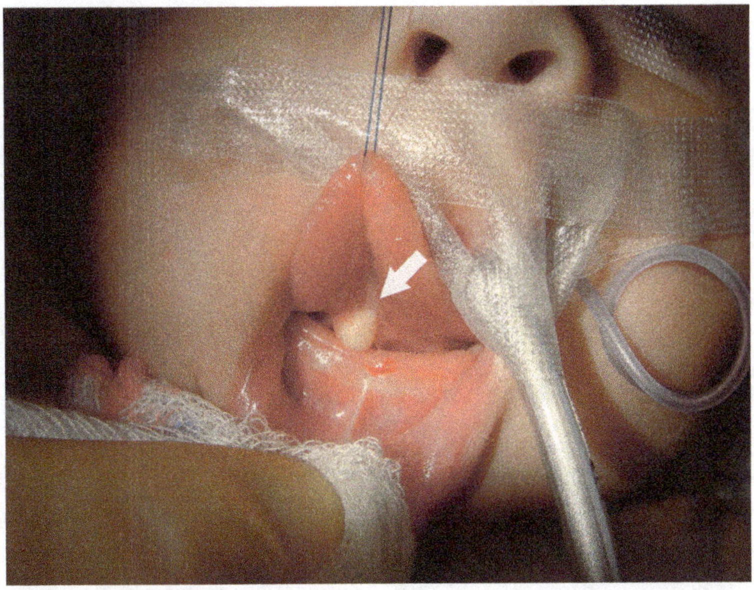

Fig. 4.15 Photograph of salivary cyst (mucocele) at tip of obstructed right submandibular duct

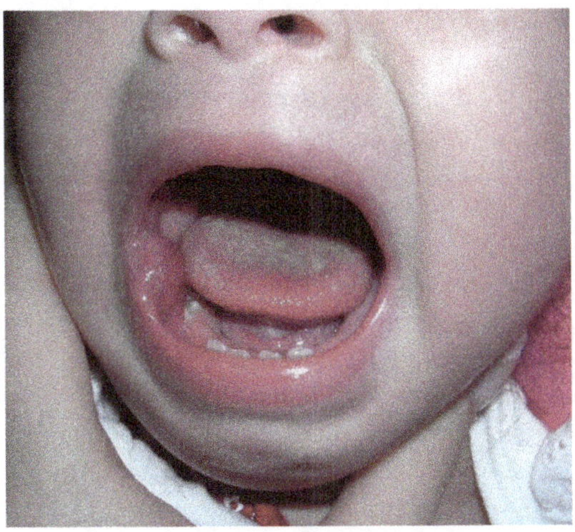

Fig. 4.16 Photograph of child with mucocele of right lower lip (Image courtesy of David W. Low, MD, Attending Surgeon, The Children's Hospital of Philadelphia; Associate Professor, Department of Plastic Surgery, University of Pennsylvania School of Medicine)

Ankyloglossia

Definition

Ankyloglossia "tongue tie" occurs when a persistent frenulum (either epithelium or epithelium and muscle) tethers the under surface of the tip of the tongue to the floor of the mouth (the genioglossus muscle or alveolar ridge). This may cause decreased mobility of the tongue.

Incidence

The prevalence ranges from 0.0.2 to 10 % and occurs more frequently in male than in female infants with a 2.6:1 ratio [13–15].

Heredity

Unknown, but seen more frequently in some families [16].

Clinical Features

In most instances, the tip of the tongue cannot protrude beyond the lower gum line. The tongue may also fail to elevate to touch the palate. The malformation may result in a heart-shaped deformity of the tongue with protrusion (Fig. 4.18).

The more severe the restriction in tongue mobility, the more likely the child will present at birth with poor feeding. Up to 3.2 % of breastfed infants have been found to have poor latch and feeding problems because of ankyloglossia [13–15]. The tightened frenulum prevents the tongue from forming a proper seal for latching so that the jaws must be used to keep the breast in the

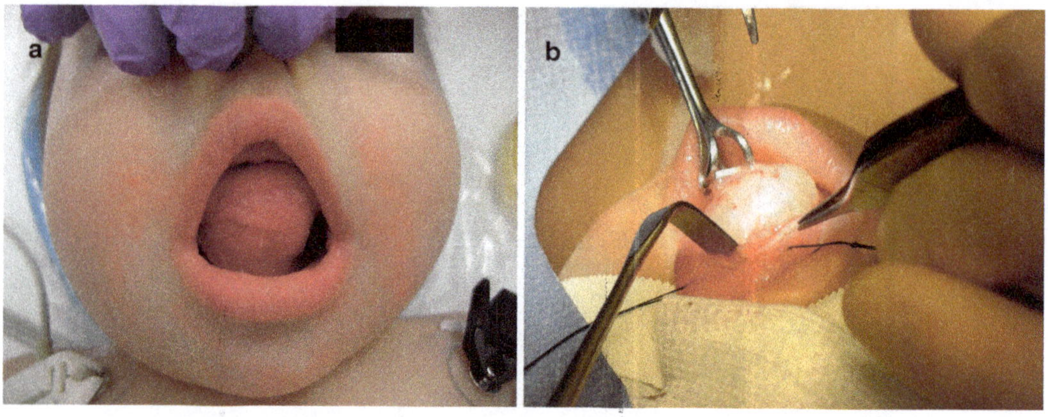

Fig. 4.17 (**a**) Photograph of ranula in the floor of the mouth causing the tongue to elevate superiorly. (**b**) Intraoperative photograph demonstrating ranula being removed from the floor of the mouth

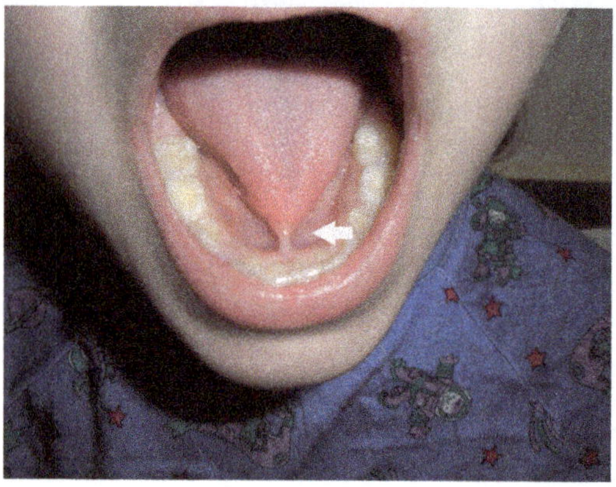

Fig. 4.18 Photograph demonstrating appearance of oral cavity in a child with ankyloglossia restricting tongue elevation

mouth. This results in increased nipple pain and poor weight gain by the infant.

Some children present later as toddlers because they have developed speech articulation problems. Phonemes more likely to be affected include sibilants and lingual sounds (*t*, *d*, *z*, *s*, *n*, and *l*) [16]. Ankyloglossia may also lead to dental problems because the lower teeth cannot be properly cleaned and to anxiety in older children who get teased because they cannot extend their tongues.

Diagnosis

Ankyloglossia is confirmed by passively elevating the tongue tip with a tongue depressor or having the actively move the tongue.

Management

Surgical correction entails division of the band (frenotomy or frenectomy) and, less often, z-plasty (frenuloplasty) may be necessary in more severe cases to prevent recurrence. A tight mucosal band can be incised and released in the physician's office in young infants. In one study, 90 % of the mothers of infants who had this procedure reported marked improvement in comfort of feeding and felt the procedure was helpful [13, 15]. It is difficult to predict which infants will have later problems with speech so preventative surgery is not recommended. General anesthetic is usually required for those with mixed muscular and mucosal bands and in older infants and young children. In those with articulation errors, a trial of speech therapy may be helpful in some instances if the articulation errors are mild. However, if surgery is required, a four flap z-frenuloplasty appears to be most effective in treating the errors (91 % of children had improvement in speech and 64 % of children had complete resolution of articulation errors) [17].

Lingual Thyroid

Embryology

The thyroid gland develops as a midline thickening along the floor of the pharynx during the fourth week of gestation. Thereafter, this thickening grows downward as the thyroid diverticulum and descends anterior to the hyoid bone, reaching its final anatomic position in the lower neck by 7 weeks of gestation. The thyroglossal duct is the tract formed by this migration and usually resorbs when the thyroid has reached the third to fourth tracheal rings. The origin of the gland's descent persists as a small midline pit, the foramen cecum, located at the junction of the anterior tongue and the tongue base (refer to Chap. 8, Fig. 10).

Definition

Lingual thyroid is a rare clinical entity that results from failure of descent of the thyroid anlage during embryogenesis.

Etiology

A lingual thyroid is the most common form of thyroid dysgenesis, a spectrum of disorders describing abnormal formation and migration of thyroid tissue. The spectrum includes failure of thyroid development (athyreosis), thyroid hypoplasia, and ectopic thyroid. Ectopic thyroid tissue may be found anywhere along the normal path of the gland's descent, from the foramen cecum to its usual location superficial to the third to six tracheal cartilages in the neck. Small foci of usually nonfunctioning ectopic tissue may also be found within thyroglossal duct cysts and tracts, which remain when the thyroglossal duct fails to resorb. Of all ectopic thyroids, 70 % are located on the lingual dorsum and are usually diagnosed as part of the evaluation for congenital hypothyroidism [18–20].

Incidence

Primary congenital hypothyroidism occurs in approximately 1 in 2,000–4,254 live births. Eighty-five percent are caused by thyroid dysgenesis, whereby, the thyroid fails to form compared with 15 % that are caused by inborn errors of biosynthesis [18, 19]. Of the infants with thyroid dysgenesis, approximately 23 % have ectopic thyroid, mostly located at the base of the tongue. However, the incidence may be under reported as many individuals develop symptoms later in life. Lingual thyroid has been reported to be two to four times more common in females than in males.

Heredity

Most cases of thyroid dysgenesis are thought to occur sporadically, although, a recent study suggests that 2 % may be inherited, involving dominant genetic predisposition with low penetrance [20].

Clinical Features

A lingual thyroid most often presents as an asymptomatic mass on the midline of the posterior tongue (near the junction of the anterior 2/3 and posterior 1/3). It tends to be smaller than a normal thyroid. The lesion is usually pink or red in color, and its surface contour may be either smooth or irregular. Occasionally, ulceration and bleeding may be present. Rarely, the ectopic gland may be large enough to interfere with swallowing and breathing.

Approximately two-thirds of patients with lingual thyroid lack any additional thyroid tissue, and up to 70 % of patients with lingual thyroid are hypothyroid. Serologic studies usually demonstrate normal or marginal gland function with normal to decreased levels of T3 and T4 and elevated levels of thyroid stimulating hormone (TSH). Hypertrophy of the ectopic gland may occur in response to elevations in TSH levels generated by the increased metabolic demand for thyroid hormone during puberty or during other states of metabolic stress, such as pregnancy, trauma, and infection. Rare cases of thyroid carcinoma arising in the mass have been reported, almost always in males [20, 21].

Diagnosis

Imaging studies are essential for confirmation of the diagnosis. The mass is usually located in the midline of the tongue between the junction of the anterior two-thirds and posterior one-third (near the region of the foramen cecum) (Fig. 4.19a). Technetium or iodine scanning typically shows radionucleide activity within the tongue without activity in the neck. Biopsy is rarely necessary and carries a significant risk of hemorrhage and thyroid storm [20–22].

Management

The clinical management of lingual thyroid remains somewhat controversial. The best initial

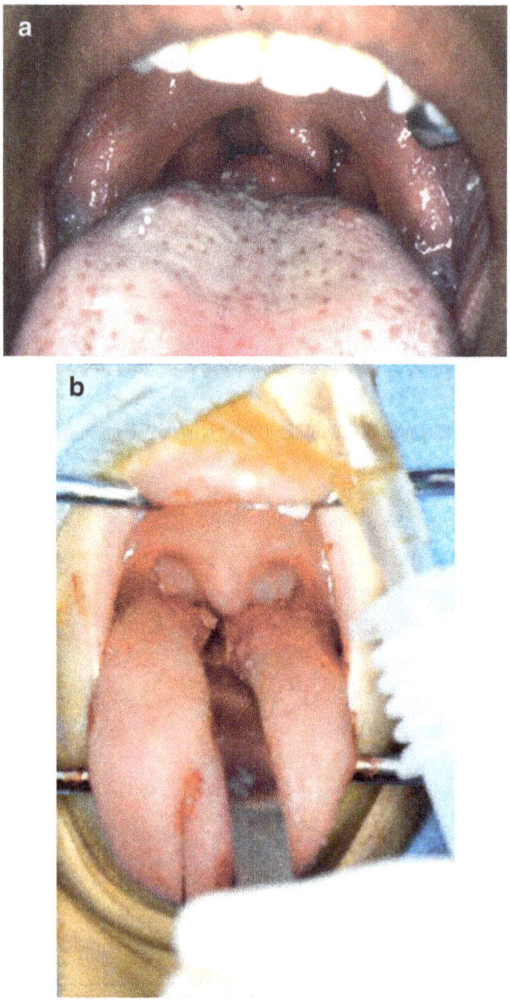

Fig. 4.19 (**a**) Photograph of lingual thyroid in the midline of the tongue (between the junction of the anterior 2/3 and posterior 1/3, in the area of the foramen cecum. (**b**) Intraoperative photograph demonstrating midline division of tongue to access lingual thyroid

guide to treatment is the presence or absence of symptoms. Administration of suppressive exogenous thyroid hormone is currently the mainstay of medical management. The goal of such therapy is to suppress TSH, thereby removing the stimulus for gland enlargement [20].

Most cases of lingual thyroid require no surgical treatment, and excision of the lesion should be reserved for patients who fail to respond to medical therapy or who present with significant dysphagia, airway compromise, or recurrent bleeding. Such treatment should not be attempted until a technetium or iodine radioisotope scan has been performed to determine that there is adequate thyroid tissue in the neck. MRI is useful for evaluation of the extent of the lesion and in determining the best surgical approach for removal. In patients lacking additional thyroid tissue, the lingual thyroid can be excised and autotransplanted to the muscles of the neck (Fig. 4.19b) [23, 24]. Radioactive iodine ablation can be used as an alternative to surgical excision of a symptomatic lingual thyroid in patients who are unfit for surgery or who refuse surgical treatment. Patients treated by radioactive iodine ablation require lifelong thyroid hormone replacement [21–24].

References

1. Kupers AM, Andriessen P, van Kempen MJ, et al. Congenital epulis of the jaw: a series of five cases and review of literature. Pediatr Surg Int. 2009;25(2):207–10.
2. Metry DW. Ten lessons learned from a hemangioma clinic. Semin Plast Surg. 2006;20:157–62.
3. Metry DW, Hawrot A, Altman C, et al. Association of solitary, segmental hemangiomas of the skin with visceral hemangiomatosis. Arch Dermatol. 2004;140(5):591–6.
4. Haggstrom AN, Drolet BA, Baselga E, et al. Prospective study of infantile hemangiomas: clinical characteristics predicting complications and treatment. Pediatrics. 2006;118(3):882–7.
5. Teresa MO, Alexander RE, Lando T, et al. Segmental hemangiomas of the upper airway. Laryngoscope. 2009;119:2242–7.
6. Eeynosos MC, Hearnandez A, Soto F, et al. Autosomal dominant macroglossia in two unrelated families. Hum Genet. 1986;74(2):200–2.
7. Thrasher RD III. Otitis media with effusion differential diagnoses. http://emedicine.medscape.com/article/858990-differential. Accessed 26 Sep 2012.
8. Pettenati MJ, Haines JL, Higgins RR, et al. Wiedemann-Beckwith syndrome: presentation of clinical and cytogenetic data on 22 new cases and review of the literature. Hum Genet. 1986;74:173.
9. Ping AJ, Reeve AE, Law DJ, et al. Genetic linkage of Beckwith-Wiedemann syndrome to 11p15. Am J Hum Genet. 1989;44:720–3.
10. Guimaraes CV, Donnelly LF, Shott SR, et al. Relative rather than absolute macroglossia in patients with Down syndrome: implications for treatment of obstructive sleep apnea. Pediatr Radiol. 2008;38(10):1062–7.

11. Breugem CC, van Der Horst CM, Hennekam RC. Progress toward understanding vascular malformations. Plast Reconstr Surg. 2001;107(6):1509–23.
12. Perkins JA, Manning SC, Tempero RM, et al. Lymphatic malformations: review of current treatment. Otolaryngol Head Neck Surg. 2010;142(6): 795–803.
13. Segal LM, et al. Prevalence, diagnosis, and treatment of ankyloglossia. Can Fam Physician. 2007;53(6): 1027–33.
14. Messner AH, Lalakea MH. Ankyloglossia: controversies in management. Int J Pediatr Otorhinolaryngol. 2000;54:123–31.
15. Ballard J, Auer JC, Khoury J. Ankyloglossia: assessment, incidence, and effect of frenuloplasty on the breastfeeding dyad. Pediatrics. 2002;110(5):1–6.
16. Klockars T. Familial ankyloglossia. Int J Pediatr Otorhinolaryngol. 2007;71(8):1321–9.
17. Heller J, Gabbay J, O'Hara C, Heller M, Bradley JP. Improved ankyloglossia correction with four-flap Z-frenuloplasty. Ann Plast Surg. 2005;54(6):623–8.
18. Fisher D, Dussault J, Foley T, et al. Screening for congenital hypothyroidism: results of screening of one million North American infants. J Pediatr. 1979;94:700–5.
19. Rastogi MV, Lafranchi SH. Congenital hypothyroidism. Orphanet J Rare Dis. 2010;5(1):17.
20. Castanet M, Marinovic D, Polak M, et al. Epidemiology of thyroid dysgenesis: the familial component. Horm Res Paediatr. 2010;73:231–7.
21. Kansal P, Sakati N, Rifai A, Woodhouseet N. Lingual thyroid: diagnosis and treatment. Arch Intern Med. 1987;147:2046–8.
22. Neinas FW, Gorman CA, Devine KD, Woolner LB. Lingual thyroid: clinical characteristics of 15 cases. Ann Intern Med. 1973;79:205–10.
23. Okstad S, Mair IW, Sundsfjord JA, et al. Ectopic thyroid tissue in the head and neck. J Otolaryngol. 1986;15:52–5.
24. Williams JD, Sclafani AP, Slupchinskij O, Douge C. Evaluation and management of the lingual thyroid gland. Ann Otol Rhinol Laryngol. 1996;105:312–6.

Cleft Lip and Palate Malformations

5

Gregory D. Pearson and Richard E. Kirschner

Abstract

This chapter describes the embryology and development of cleft lip and palate deformities in children. Schematic figures and clinical photographs illustrate the more common anomalies and surgeries used to correct these malformations.

Keywords

Cleft lip • Cleft palate • Embryology of oral cavity • Congenital oral malformations

Embryology

The formation of the face begins early in fetal development. The early oral pit, or stoma, is apparent at approximately 4 weeks of age. The facial structures continue to rapidly develop in the ensuing weeks. The nasal placodes are present laterally with the development of medial and lateral nasal prominences during the fifth week of development. During the sixth week, the medial nasal processes join in the midline to form the nasal tip, columella, prolabial segment, and primary palate. The maxillary prominences join with the lateral aspect of each medial nasal process to form the lateral components of the upper lip (Fig. 5.1). During this time, the secondary palate begins to form. Bilateral vertical outgrowths from the maxillary prominences develop during the sixth week. The paired palatal shelves, which initially are vertically oriented, rotate to a transverse position over the following 2 weeks. Once the shelves assume a horizontal orientation (eighth week), they begin to fuse in the midline, a process that is complete by 12 weeks gestation (Fig. 5.2). Thus, by week 8, the lips, primary palate, and secondary palate have all obtained their initial morphology [1]. The classic theory on the formation of a cleft lip holds that during week 6, the medial nasal processes fail to fuse with the maxillary prominences resulting in a cleft of the lip and/or primary palate [2, 3]. Failure of fusion of the palatal shelves during the eighth week

G.D. Pearson, M.D. (✉)
Department of Plastic and Reconstructive Surgery, Center for Complex Craniofacial Disorders, Nationwide Children's Hospital, 700 Children's Drive, Columbus, OH 43205, USA
e-mail: gregory.pearson@nationwidechildrens.org

R.E. Kirschner, M.D., F.A.C.S., F.A.A.P.
Section of Plastic and Reconstructive, Nationwide Children's Hospital, 700 Children's Drive, Columbus, OH 43205, USA
e-mail: richard.kirschner@nationwidechildrens.org

L.M. Elden and K.B. Zur (eds.), *Congenital Malformations of the Head and Neck*,
DOI 10.1007/978-1-4419-1714-0_5, © Springer Science+Business Media New York 2014

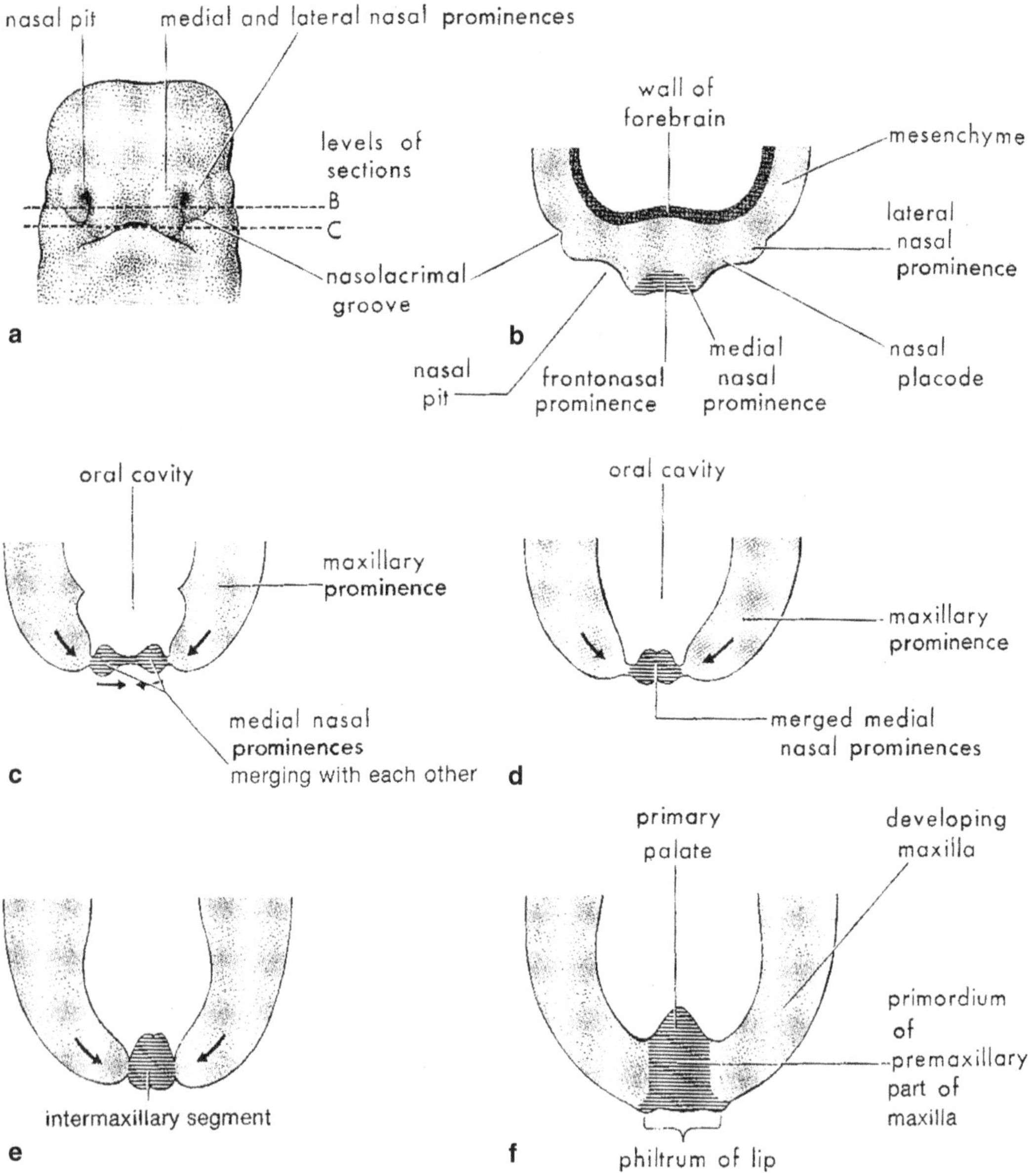

Fig. 5.1 Embryologic development of the lip (from Moore KL, Persaud TVN. *The Developing Human: Clinically Oriented Embryology*, 5th ed. Philadelphia: W.B. Saunders; 1993. Copyright Elsevier 1993)

results in a cleft of the secondary palate. A second theory of cleft pathogenesis invokes a failure of mesodermal penetration. This theory holds that the medial nasal processes and maxillary processes join but, due to a lack of mesoderm within this union, the processes are unable to maintain their fusion, resulting in breakdown and cleft formation [4].

Definition

Due to their differing embryologic development, cleft lip with or without cleft palate (CL/P) is an entity distinct from isolated cleft palate (CP). Clefting of the lip and primary palate results from incomplete fusion of the maxillary and medial

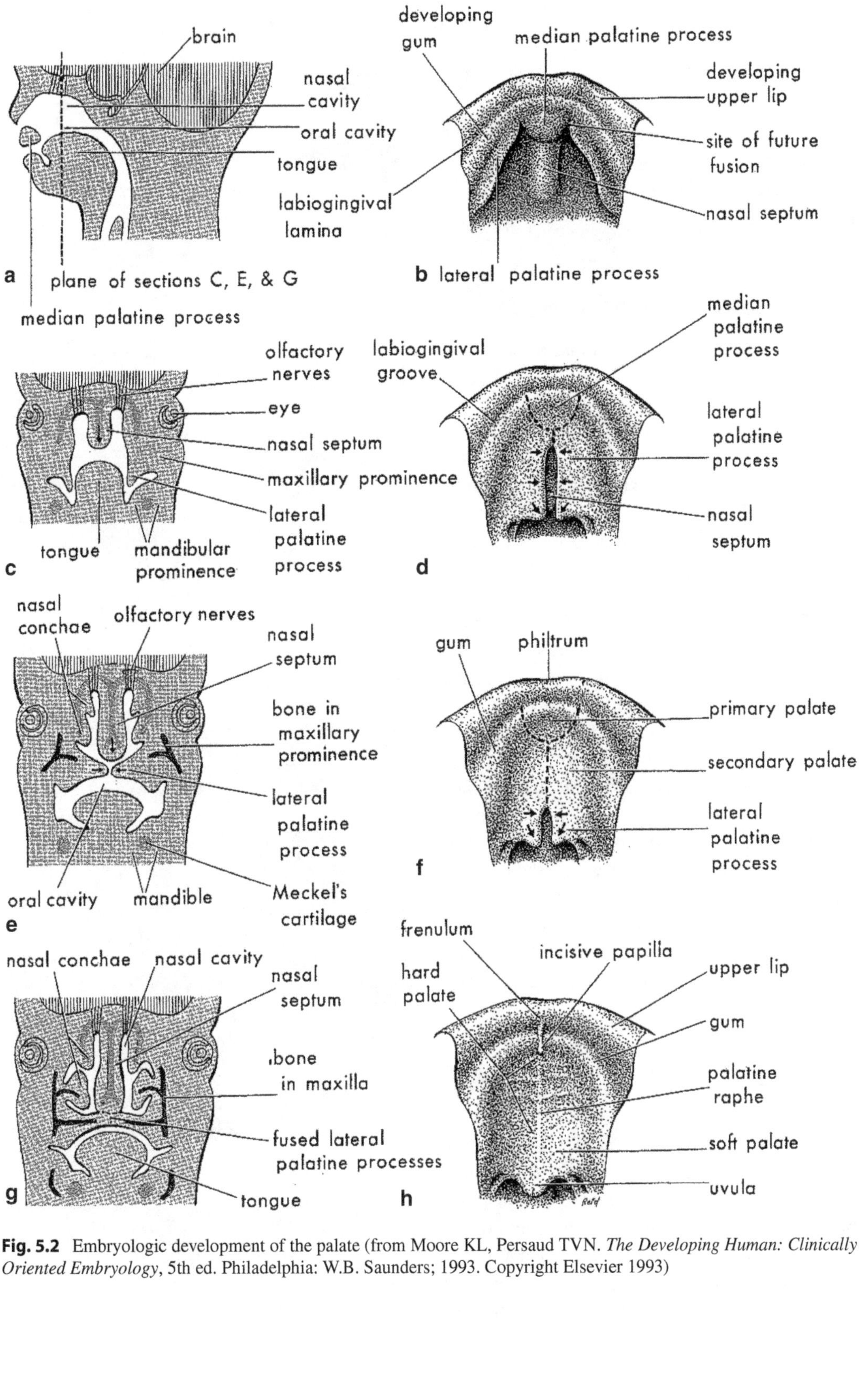

Fig. 5.2 Embryologic development of the palate (from Moore KL, Persaud TVN. *The Developing Human: Clinically Oriented Embryology*, 5th ed. Philadelphia: W.B. Saunders; 1993. Copyright Elsevier 1993)

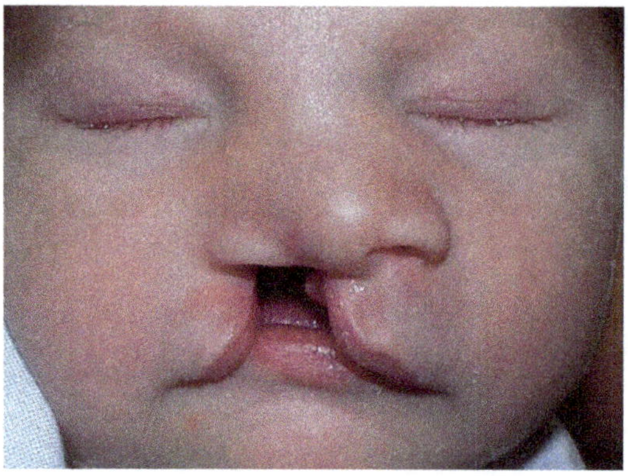

Fig. 5.3 Complete unilateral cleft lip and palate

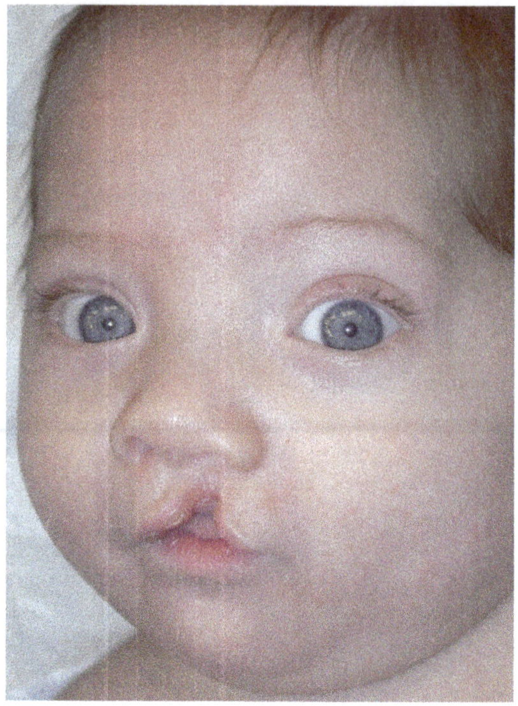

Fig. 5.4 Incomplete unilateral cleft lip and palate

nasal processes, whereas clefting of the secondary palate results from failure of fusion of the palatal shelves. Cleft lip/palate may be defined by the laterality of clefting (left, right, or bilateral) or by whether the cleft is incomplete or complete. In a complete cleft lip, no tissue connects the medial and lateral lip segments (Fig. 5.3). In an incomplete cleft of the lip, a band of tissue of variable width (Simonart's band) connects the medial and lateral lip segments in the superior portion of the lip (Fig. 5.4). Clefting of the secondary palate occurs from the incisive foramen posteriorly and may involve the soft palate alone or both the soft and hard palate (Fig. 5.5). A submucous cleft palate is identified as a bifid uvula, notching of the posterior hard palate, and a zona pellucidum within the soft palate [5] (Fig. 5.6). In a submucous cleft palate, the mucosa of the soft palate is intact but the muscular levator sling is disrupted, with the levator veli palatini aberrantly inserting onto the posterior edge of the hard palate.

Incidence

Cleft lip/palate has variable incidence depending upon race and gender of the patient. The relative occurrence of CL/P is a 6:3:1 ratio of left: right: bilateral. Cleft lip/palate is more common in males compared to females. Race plays a role in the incidence of CL/P as well, with Native Americans and Asians having the highest

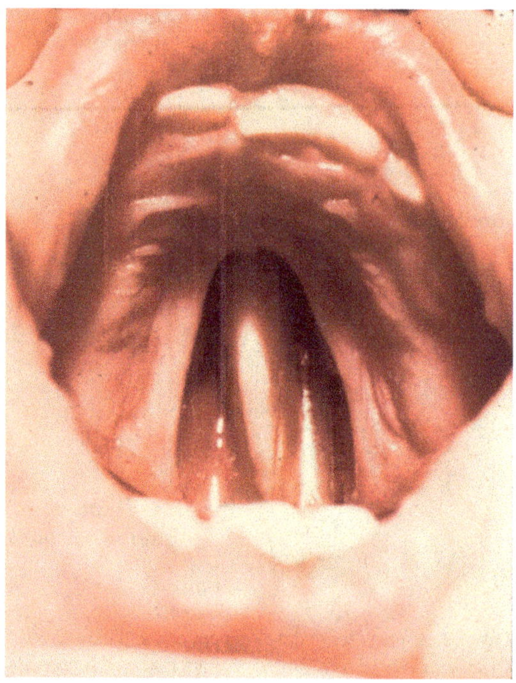

Fig. 5.5 Cleft of the secondary palate

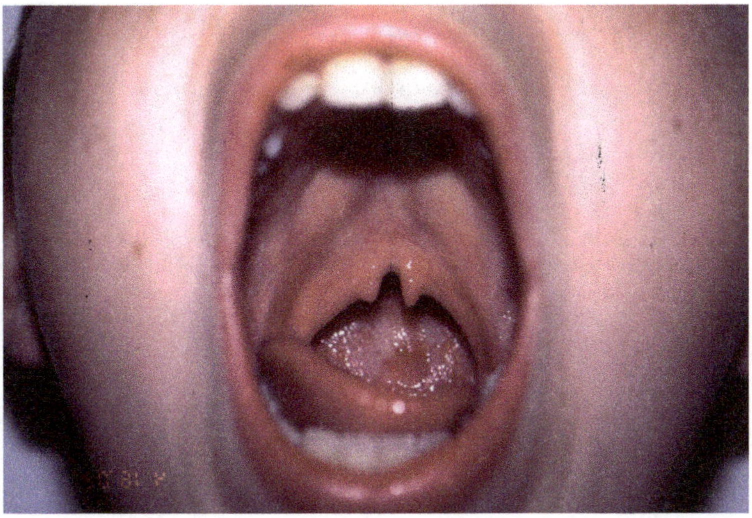

Fig. 5.6 Submucous cleft palate

incidence (3.6 and 2.1 per 1,000 live births, respectively). The incidence of CL/P in Caucasians is 1.0 per 1,000 live births, and that in African Americans is 0.5 per 1,000 live births [6]. Unlike CL/P, isolated cleft palate has a uniform incidence across all races (0.5 per 1,000 live births). CP occurs more frequently in females than in males.

History

The first cleft lip repair to appear in the world's literature was that performed by a Chinese surgeon on a poor farm boy in the fourth century AD. The patient, Wei Yang-Chi, would later become the Governor General of six Chinese provinces, an extraordinary historical testament to the social impact of cleft surgery. For more than a millennium thereafter, cleft lip surgery did not advance much beyond simple cauterization or paring of the cleft edges with simple approximation of the lip segments. Attempts to restore adequate lip length began with the use of curved incisions, as first described by von Graefe and later by Rose and Thompson, and later progressed to the use of rectangular (LeMesurier) and later triangular (Tennison and Randall) flaps from the lateral lip. The rotation-advancement technique, introduced by Millard in 1955, was based on the understanding that the entire Cupid's bow is invariably present on the medial lip segment and is rotated superiorly. Downward rotation of the entire philtral complex, noted Millard, levels the Cupid's bow and opens a gap in the superior lip into which a flap derived from the lateral lip element may be advanced. The rotation-advancement technique has been modified by many cleft surgeons since its introduction and remains widely used throughout the world.

The first anecdotal report of cleft palate repair in 1766 is attributed to LeMonnier, a French dentist. He simply placed several sutures across the cleft, cauterized the mucosa along the cleft margin, and then tied the sutures. In 1819, Dr. Philibert Roux reported repair of the cleft soft palate of a Canadian medical student named John Stephenson. Bernard von Langenbeck is credited with first describing closure of hard palatal clefts by elevating full-thickness mucoperiosteal flaps in 1861. His technique of raising the mucoperiosteum from the posterior edge of the cleft hard palate to the posterior aspect of the alveolus is still commonly used today in the procedure that bears his name (Fig. 5.7a–c). In the early twentieth century, cleft palate surgeons began to focus

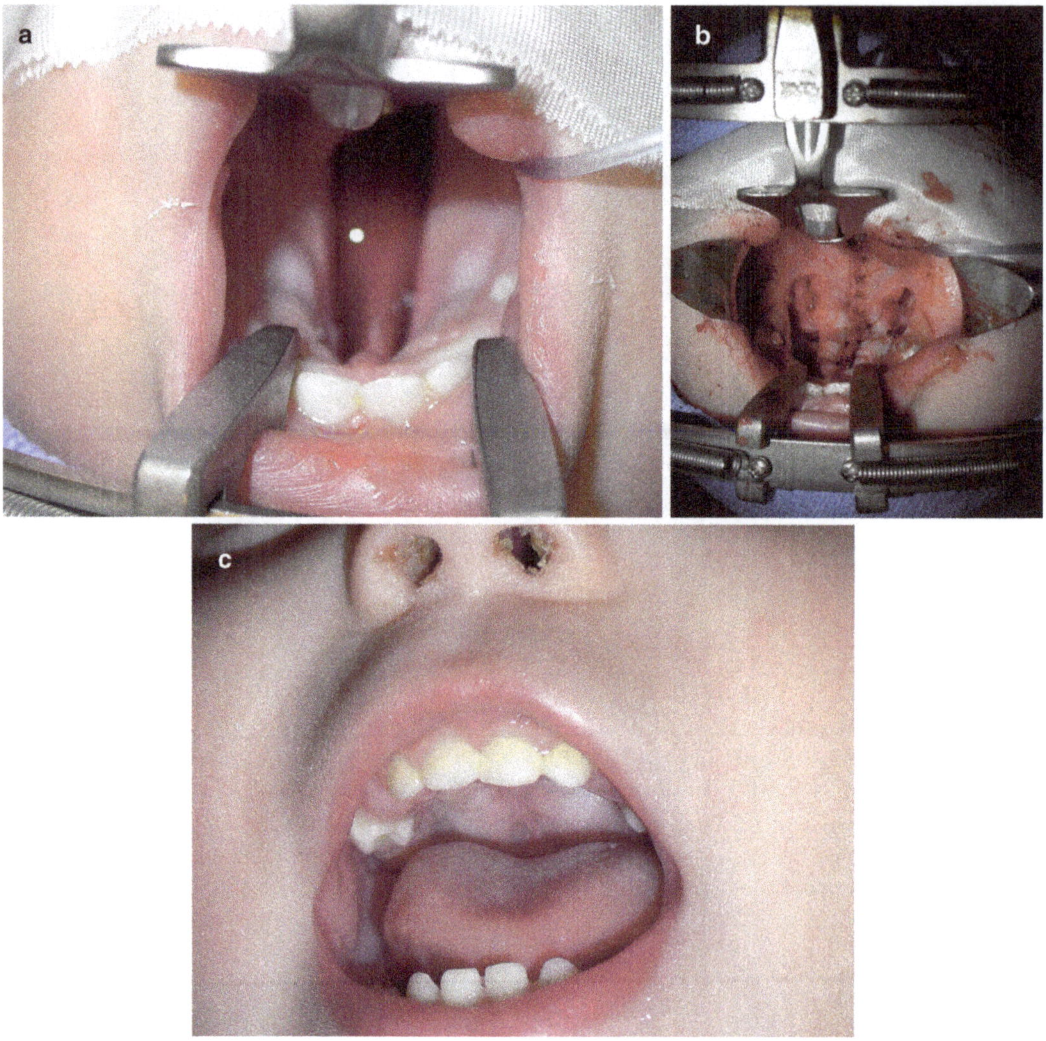

Fig. 5.7 (**a**–**c**) Von Langenbeck cleft palate repair (**a** and **b** demonstrates the surgeon's view from the top of the stretcher with the patient lying supine.)

their attention on means by which to improve speech outcomes by lengthening the palate at the time of repair. The most popular of these techniques, the V–Y pushback technique described by Wardill, and Kilner, remains in widespread use today. In 1978, Leonard Furlow of the University of Florida first described a novel technique of velar repair utilizing opposing mirror-image Z-plasties of the oral and nasal mucosa. The technique offered several advantages over straight-line techniques. Use of Z-plasty closure provided for palatal lengthening without the need for pushback procedures, and transposition of the posteriorly based myomucosal flaps reoriented the levator muscle bundles into anatomical position, reconstructing the levator sling [7] (Fig. 5.8a, b).

Heredity

Genetic analyses have shown that nonsyndromic cleft lip with or without cleft palate has complex inheritance patterns, and there is substantial data to support an etiologic role for genetic factors. Although segregation analysis has provided significant insights, the mode of inheritance for nonsyndromic orofacial clefts remains uncertain.

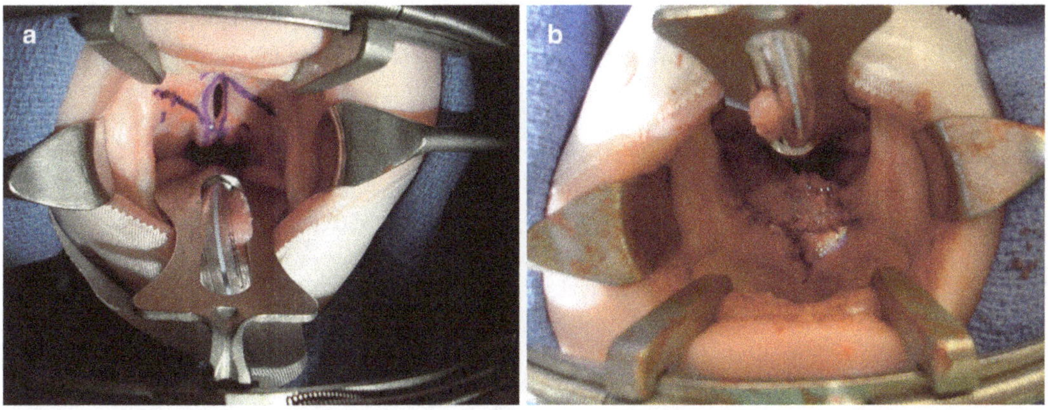

Fig. 5.8 (**a** and **b**) Furlow cleft palate repair (surgeon's view from the top of the stretcher)

It is widely believed that cleft lip with or without cleft palate is a heterogeneous disorder and that 3–20 genes may interact with one another and/or with environmental factors to produce orofacial clefting [8, 9]. Certainly, a family history is one of the strongest risk factors for cleft lip/palate and cleft palate alone. The risk of cleft lip/palate in first-degree relatives is approximately 4 %, increasing to 10 % when two first-degree relatives are affected. For cleft palate alone, the overall risk in first-degree relatives is approximately 2 %, increasing to 8 % when two first-degree relatives are affected [10].

Etiology

As noted above, there is clear evidence for a genetic etiology of nonsyndromic orofacial clefting. In addition, several environmental factors have been implicated, including pharmacologic agents (retinoids, anti-convulsants, folate antagonists, benzodiazepines, and corticosteroids), maternal diseases (diabetes mellitus), and maternal smoking.

Associated Conditions

Understanding the conditions associated with syndromic orofacial clefts are essential to proper clinical management. Over 400 distinct syndromes associated with orofacial clefts, some quite rare, have been described. Associated abnormalities are seen in 25–35 % of clefts of the lip with or without cleft palate in the fetal and newborn period, and yet only 10–15 % of older children with cleft lip with or without cleft palate have associated defects, indicating that many infants with associated severe malformations do not survive infancy [11, 12]. The most common syndrome associated with cleft lip with or without cleft palate is van der Woude syndrome, an autosomal dominant condition most often caused mutations in interferon inhibiting factor 6 (IRF6) [13]. In addition to orofacial clefts, the syndrome often presents with hypodontia and lower lip pits (Fig. 5.9). CHARGE Association (coloboma, heart defect, atresia choanae, retarded growth and development, genital anomalies and hypogonadism, and ear anomalies and deafness), an autosomal dominant condition most often associated with mutations in CHD7, is the second most common syndrome associated with cleft lip with or without cleft palate [14].

In contrast to clefts of the lip with or without cleft palate, the incidence of associated anomalies in infants with cleft palate alone is approximately 50 %. Clefts of the palate alone may be associated with Pierre Robin sequence, a constellation of anomalies including microretrognathia, glossoptosis, and upper airway obstruction (Fig. 5.10). Roughly half of all cases of Robin sequence are syndromic. Of the syndromes associated with cleft palate alone, Stickler syndrome is the most common (5 %), and Stickler syndrome accounts for nearly half of all syndromic cases of Robin sequence. The syndrome is an autosomal dominant disorder caused by mutations in the genes that code for either type 2 or type 11 collagen [15]. Affected patients often present with a flattened midface, myopia, hypotonia, and joint laxity (see Fig. 1 in Chap. 1). The second most common syndrome associated with cleft palate is 22q11.2 deletion syndrome (velocardiofacial syndrome, DiGeorge syndrome), a disorder characterized by short palpebral fissures and hooded eyelids, a broad nasal root, hypoplastic alae, external ear anomalies, conotruncal cardiac defect, immune deficiency, and velopharyngeal dysfunction [16] (see Fig. 3 in Chap. 1).

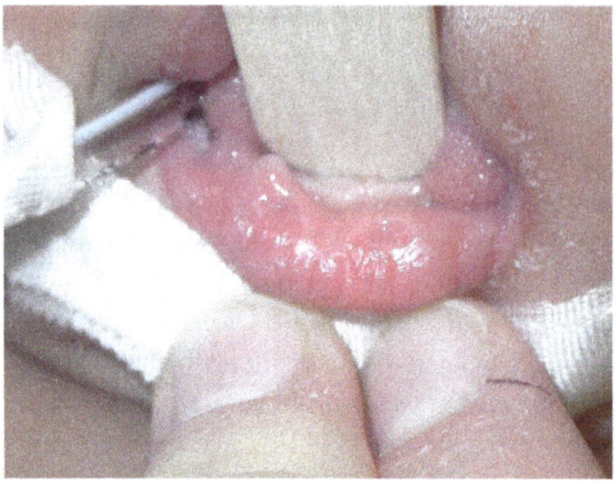

Fig. 5.9 Lip pits in van der Woude syndrome

Clinical Features

There is wide variability in cleft severity (Figs. 5.11, 5.12, 5.13, 5.14, and 5.15) Clefts of the lip with or without cleft palate may be complete (the cleft extends through the entire lip and into the nasal floor) or incomplete (a bridge of tissue remains in the upper portion of the lip). Such clefts may or may not involve the maxillary alveolus and the palate. Incomplete clefts may vary from microform types to more typical patterns. Isolated palatal clefts may involve the levator muscle alone (submucosal clefts), the muscle and mucosa of the velum alone, or the entire thickness of the velum and hard palate.

Some degree of nasal deformity accompanies all clefts of the lip, again varying from minor to severe. In the unilateral cleft, the ala is flattened and posterolaterally displaced. The septum of the nose tends form a C shape with the caudal end

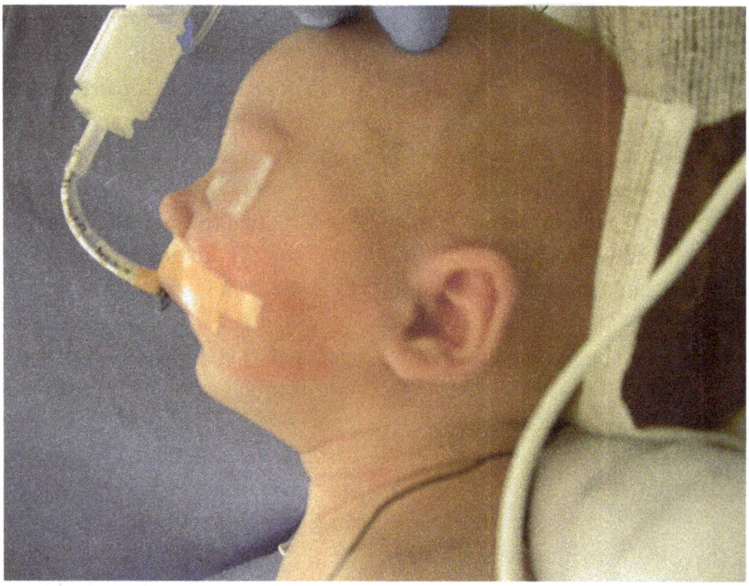

Fig. 5.10 Infant with Pierre-Robin sequence

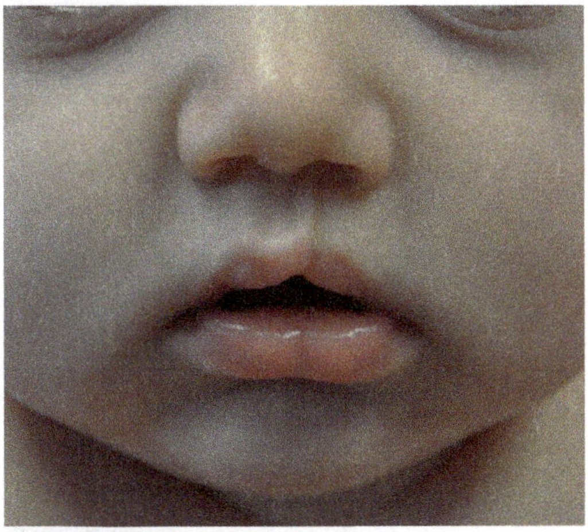

Fig. 5.11 Microform cleft lip

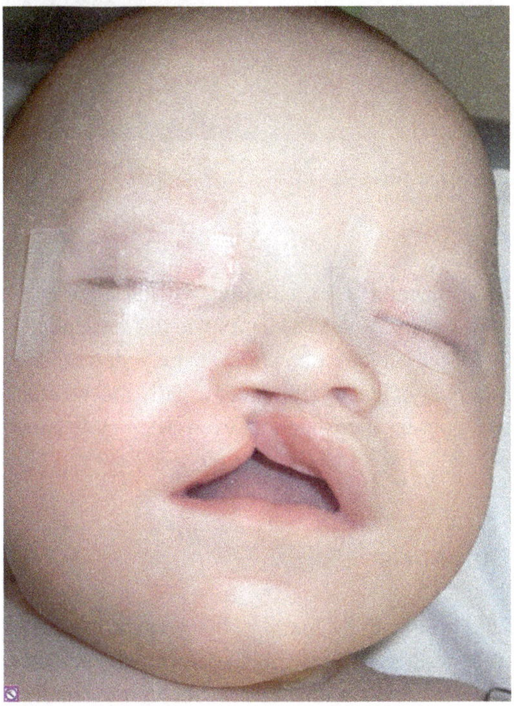

Fig. 5.12 Unilateral incomplete cleft lip

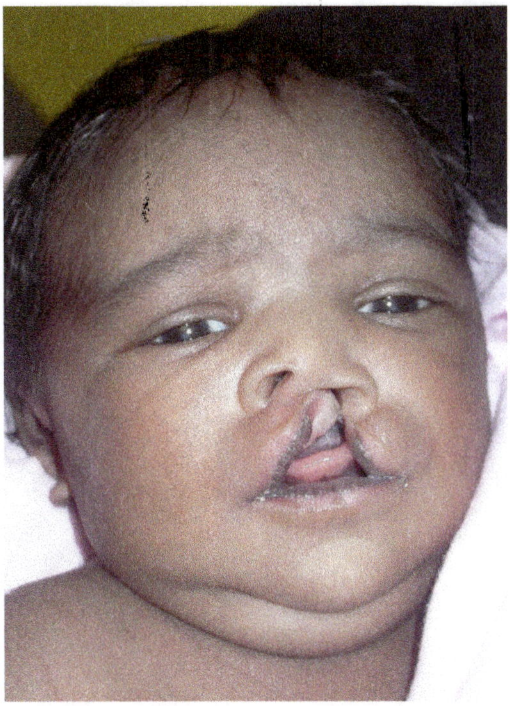

Fig. 5.13 Unilateral complete cleft lip

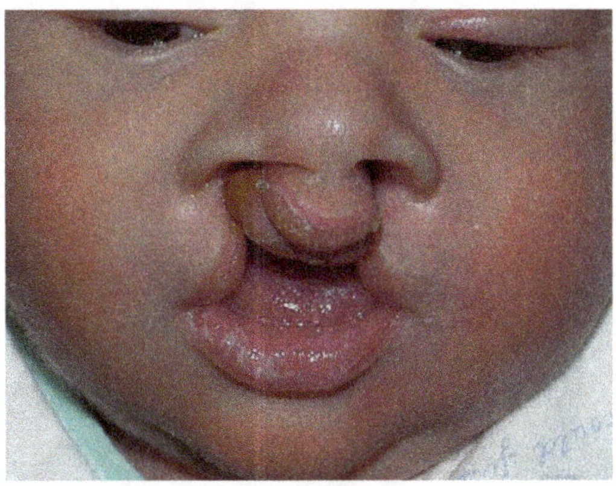

Fig. 5.14 Bilateral complete cleft lip and palate

lying in the normal side of the nares. The premaxilla rotates outward with collapse of the lateral maxillary segment (Fig. 5.16). The lateral incisor and/or canine can be missing in up to 56 % of all cleft patients [17]. In the child with bilateral cleft lip with or without cleft palate child, the nose and premaxilla may be even more severely affected. The premaxilla typically attains a ventral-dorsal alignment since it is not tethered by any soft tissue restraints. The lateral alar cartilages are flattened bilaterally, and the columella is foreshortened (Fig. 5.17).

Children with cleft palate often present with Eustachian tube dysfunction secondary to improper mechanics of the levator and tensor veli palatini muscles. The incidence of tympanostomy

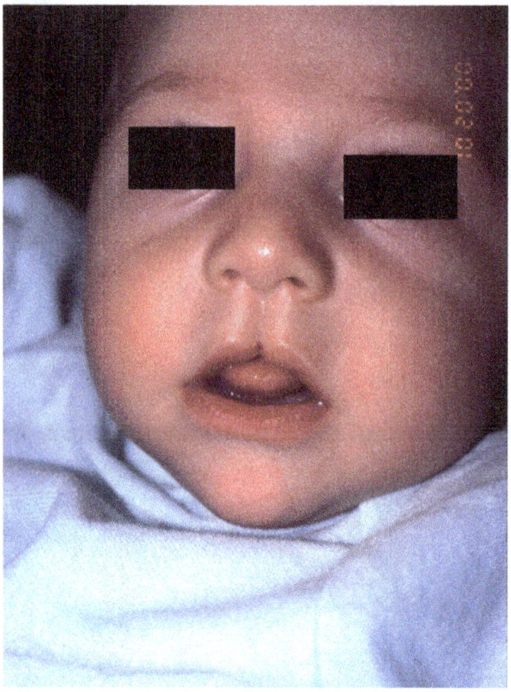

Fig. 5.15 Rare midline cleft lip

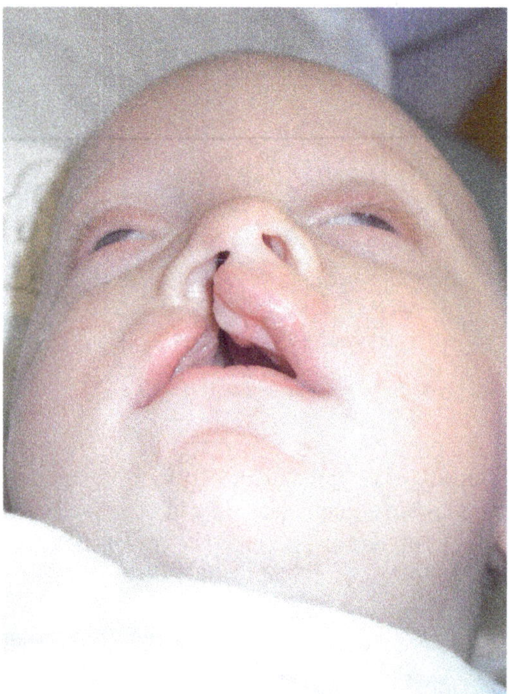

Fig. 5.16 Unilateral cleft nasal deformity

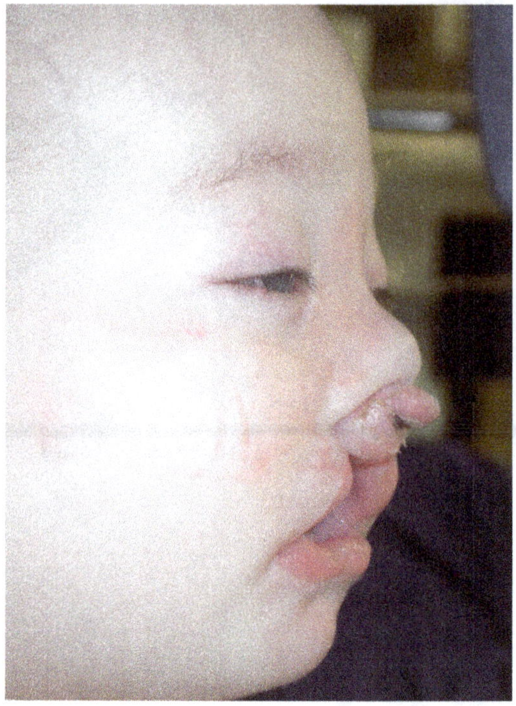

Fig. 5.17 Bilateral cleft nasal deformity

tube placement in children with palatal clefts approaches 90 % [18, 19]. Since the soft palate is an organ of speech, children may demonstrate velopharyngeal dysfunction, usually most evident as hypernasal resonance, even after cleft palate repair.

Diagnosis

Diagnosis can be made in the prenatal period or after delivery. The ability to detect clefts of the lip depends upon many factors including amniotic fluid volume, position of the child, cleft severity, and expertise of the sonographer. Clefts of the palate are more difficult to detect with sonography. Consequently, clefts of the palate alone are rarely identified prenatally. Prenatal MRI has been utilized to delineate clefts of the lip and palate, offering increased sensitivity and specificity when compared to sonography. Upon delivery, clefts of the lip are readily apparent, although microform clefts may elude early diagnosis.

Clefts of the palate can usually be diagnosed with proper intraoral examination, although submucosal clefts may be difficult to diagnose in the neonatal period.

Treatment

No consensus exists for the ideal timing of cleft lip repair. Some centers advocate early repair (within the first few weeks of life), while most centers begin surgery around 3–4 months of life. Presurgical orthopedics have become more popular with lip taping, obturators, nasoalveolar molding (NAM), and the Latham device all having their advocates. Surgical lip adhesion is also a technique for primary orthopedic work. All of these methods seek to improve the lip, nasal, and alveolar form and relationships prior to primary lip repair. The Millard rotation-advancement technique (or some variation thereof) is the most widely utilized technique for repair of the unilateral cleft lip (Figs. 5.18a–5.19b) For the bilateral cleft lip, a modification of the Millard bilateral cleft lip repair modification of this procedure is typically performed (Fig. 5.20a, b).

The approach to repair of alveolar clefts also demonstrates significant variability. Some surgeons advocate repair at the time of the initial cleft lip repair by performing a primary gingivoperiosteoplasty [20]. Other centers have advocated primary alveolar bone grafting in infancy. An abundance of evidence suggests, however, that this approach may result in significant maxillary growth restriction [21]. A more time-honored approach is that of secondary bone grafting performed during the mixed-dentition stage (7–9 years of age), with cancellous iliac bone grafts most commonly employed. More recently, some have advocated the use of bone morphogenic protein (BMP) in conjunction with biodegradable matrix scaffolds as a substitute for autologous bone [22]. While this method offers the advantage

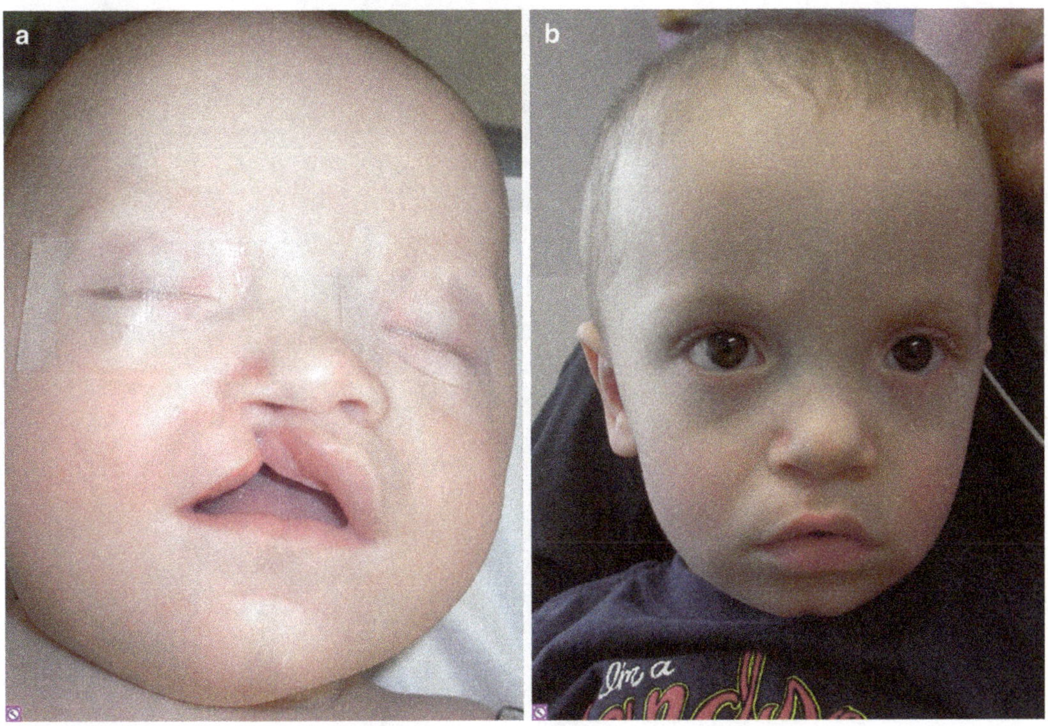

Fig. 5.18 (**a** and **b**) Unilateral incomplete cleft lip repair (Millard)

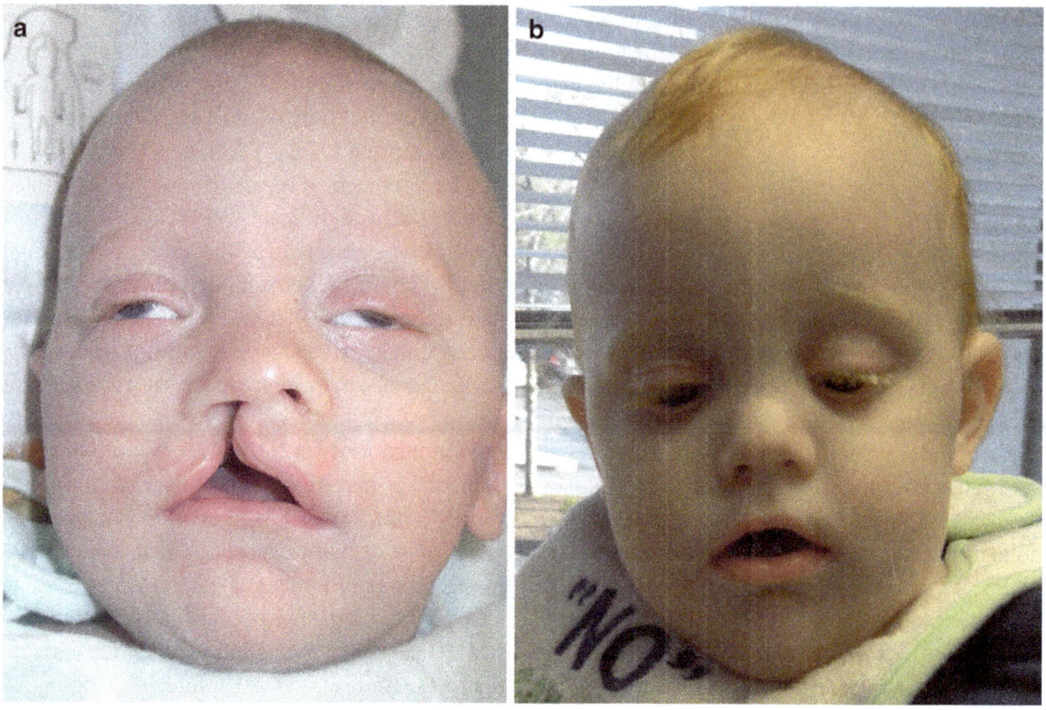

Fig. 5.19 (**a** and **b**) Unilateral complete cleft lip repair (Millard)

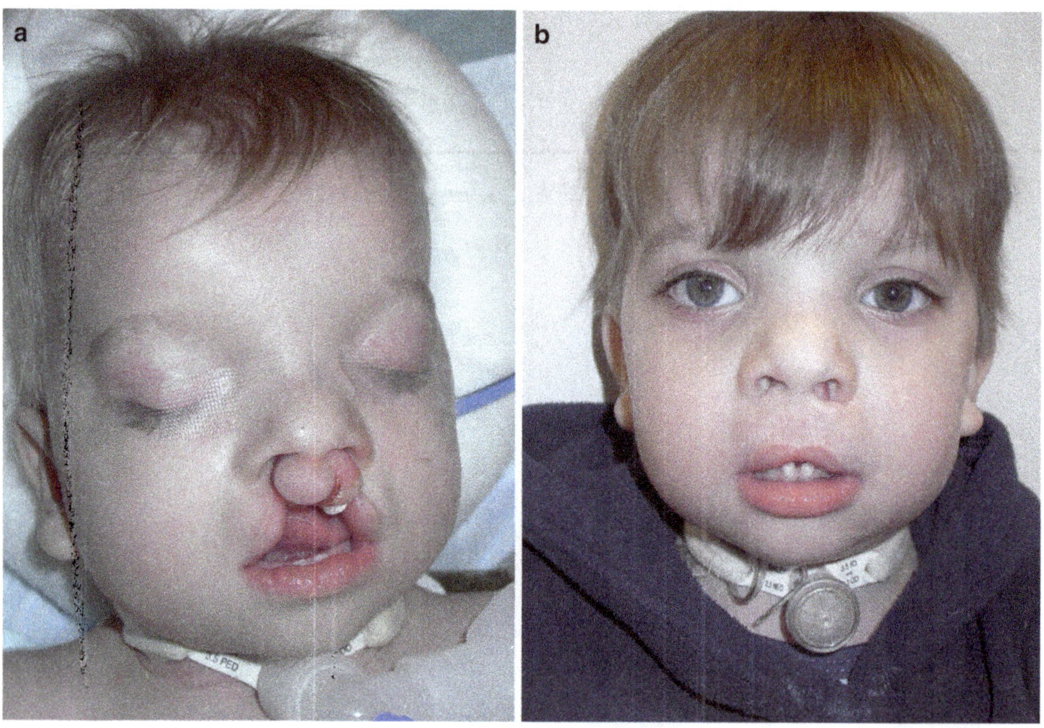

Fig. 5.20 (**a** and **b**) Bilateral complete cleft lip repair

of eliminating donor site morbidity, its long-term efficacy and reliability remain to be established.

Cleft palate repair is typically performed between 9 and12 months of age. Mucoperiosteal flaps from the hard palate are mobilized utilizing lateral releasing incisions and sutured to the midline. The levator veli palatini muscles are detached from the posterior hard palate and reoriented in the posterior velum to reconstruct the levator sling. The soft palate and levator can be repaired by either an intravelar veloplasty or Furlow double opposing z-plasty technique. Submucosal clefts of the palate need only be repaired if they are associated with velopharyngeal dysfunction and are therefore repaired later in childhood. To date, there have been no well-controlled, randomized studies to establish the optimal timing and technique of palate repair (refer to Figs. 5.7 and 5.8 for palatal repairs.)

Secondary surgical procedures are commonly required in children with cleft lip and/or cleft palate. Lip revision and tip rhinoplasty are commonly performed in the school-aged child. Operations to improve velopharyngeal function (posterior pharyngeal flap or sphincter pharyngoplasty) may be necessary in 10–25 % of cleft palate patients and can be completed once the child has achieved sufficient phonologic development and diagnostic studies can be performed (typically 4–6 years of age). Orthognathic surgery can be accomplished upon the completion of facial growth if jaw and occlusal discrepancies exist, and septorhinoplasty can be carried out upon in the teenage years for cleft patients with persistent cleft nasal deformities.

References

1. Sperber GH, Sperber SM. Embryology of orofacial clefting. In: Losee JE, Kirschner RE, editors. Comprehensive cleft care. 1st ed. New York, NY: McGraw Hill; 2009. p. 7–19.
2. Dursey E. Zur Entwicklungsgeschichte des Kopfes des Menschen und der Hohren Wirbeltheire. Tubingen: H Lauppschen; 1869.
3. His W. Unsere Koerperform und des physiologische Problem ihrer Entstohung. Leipzig: Verlag von Vogel; 1874.
4. Jones MC. Facial clefting. Etiology and developmental pathogenesis. Clin Plast Surg. 1993;20:599–606.
5. Calnan JS. Submucous cleft palate. Br J Plast Surg. 1954;6:264.
6. Jones MC. Etiology of facial clefts: prospective evaluation of 428 patients. Cleft Palate J. 1988;25:16.
7. Randall P, Jackson O. A short history of cleft lip and cleft palate. In: Losee JE, Kirschner RE, editors. Comprehensive cleft care. 1st ed. New York, NY: McGraw Hill; 2009. p. 187–207.
8. Marazita ML, Murray JC, Lidral AC, et al. Meta-analysis of 13 genome scans reveals multiple cleft lip/palate genes with novel loci on 9q21 and 2q32-35. Am J Hum Genet. 2004;75:161–73.
9. Vieira AR, Avila JR, Daack-Hirsch S, Dragan E, Félix TM, Rahimov F, et al. Medical sequencing of candidate genes for nonsyndromic cleft lip and palate. PLoS Genet. 2005;1:e64.
10. McDonald-McGinn DM, Driscoll D, Matthews M. Prenatal and genetic counseling. In: Losee JE, Kirschner RE, editors. Comprehensive cleft care. 1st ed. New York, NY: McGraw Hill; 2009. p. 81.
11. Croen LA, Gm S, Wasserman CR, Tolarove MM. Racial and ethnic variations in the prevalence of orofacial clefts in California, 1983–1992. Am J Med Genet. 1988;79:42–7.
12. Stoll C, Alembik Y, Dott B, Roth MP. Associated malformations in cases with oral clefts. Cleft Palate J. 2000;37:41–7.
13. Zucchero T, Cooper ME, Maher BS, et al. Interferon regulatory factor 6 (IRF6) gene variants and the risk of isolated cleft lip or palate. N Engl J Med. 2004;351:769–80.
14. Kniffin CL, et al. Mendelian Inheritance in Man. CHARGE Syndrome (#214800). http://omim.org/entry/214800. Accessed 24 Jan 2011.
15. Kniffin CL, et al. Mendelian Inheritance in Man. Stickler Syndrome; type I; STL1 (#108300). http://omim.org/entry/108300. Accessed 24 Jan 2011.
16. Kniffin CL, et al. Mendelian Inheritance in Man. Velocardiofacial syndrome (#192430). http://omim.org/entry/192430. Accessed 24 Jan 2011.
17. Suzuki A, Watabane M, Nakano M, et al. Maxillary lateral incisors of subjects with cleft lip and/or palate, part 2. Cleft Palate Craniofac J. 1992;29:380–4.
18. Bluestone C. Eustachian tube obstruction in the infant with cleft palate. Ann Otol Rhinol Laryngol. 1971;80:1–30.
19. Cole R, Cole J, Intaraprason S. Eustachian tube function in cleft lip and palate patients. Arch Otolaryngol. 1974;99:3337–41.
20. Santiago P, Grayson B, Cutting C, et al. Reduced need for alveolar bone grafting by presurgical orthopedics and primary gingivoperiosteoplasty. Cleft Palate Craniofac J. 1998;35:77–80.
21. Trotman C-A, Long Jr RE, Sheldon W, et al. Comparison of facial form in primary alveolar bone-grafted and nongrafted unilateral cleft lip and palate patients: Intercenter Retrospective Study. Cleft Palate Craniofac J. 1996;33:91–5.
22. Herford AS, Boyne PJ, Rawson R, et al. Bone morphogenetic protein-induced repair of the premaxillary cleft. J Oral Maxillofac Surg. 2007;65:2136–42.

Congenital Malformations of the Larynx

6

Michael J. Rutter and J. Matthew Dickson

Abstract

Congenital laryngeal anomalies comprise a spectrum of malformations that may present at birth or later in childhood. This chapter will focus on laryngomalacia, laryngeal cysts, webs, and atresia, vocal cord paralysis, laryngotracheoesophageal clefts, vascular anomalies, and subglottic stenosis.

Keywords

Laryngomalacia • Laryngocele • Saccular cyst • Vallecular cysts • Vocal cord paralysis • Laryngotracheoesophageal clefts • Congenital subglottic stenosis • Laryngeal webs • Subglottic hemangioma

Embryology of the Larynx

The respiratory system begins its development during the fourth week of gestation as an outgrowth of the ventral wall of the foregut (respiratory diverticulum). The endodermal lining gives rise to the epithelial lining of the larynx, tracheal, bronchi, and alveoli. The larynx develops from this endodermal tissue and adjacent mesenchyme of the foregut located between the fourth and sixth branchial arches. The ventral laryngotracheal groove forms at 20 days of gestation and differentiates into the primitive laryngeal sulcus and the respiratory primordium. The laryngotracheal groove continues to deepen until its lateral edges fuse. By day 26, this tube descends caudally, where the trachea becomes separated from the esophagus by the tracheoesophageal septum, which has a persistent thin vertical opening into the pharynx. Fusion occurs in the caudal-to-cranial direction. Incomplete fusion results in development of persistent communication (or clefting) between the larynx or trachea and the esophagus (Fig. 6.1).

The primitive larynx is first evident at 32 days of gestation when the mesenchymal arytenoid swellings derived from the sixth branchial arch

M.J. Rutter, M.D., F.R.A.C.S. (✉)
Department of Otolaryngology,
Cincinnati Children's Hospital Medical Center,
3333 Burnet Avenue, MLC 2018, Cincinnati,
OH 45229, USA
e-mail: mike.rutter@cchmc.org

J.M. Dickson, B.Sc., M.D., F.R.C.S(C)
Division of Otolaryngology, Department of Surgery,
Surrey Memorial Hospital, University of British
Columbia, #303, 9808 King George Boulevard,
Surrey, BC, Canada, V3T 2V6
e-mail: mc.dickson@mac.com

L.M. Elden and K.B. Zur (eds.), *Congenital Malformations of the Head and Neck*,
DOI 10.1007/978-1-4419-1714-0_6, © Springer Science+Business Media New York 2014

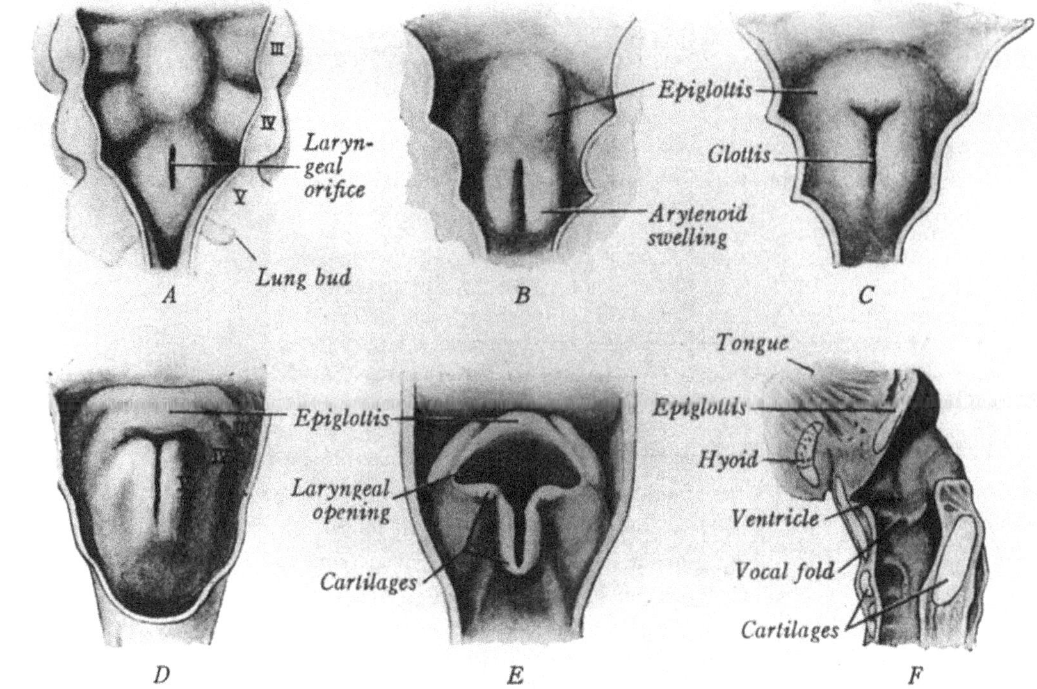

Fig. 6.1 Embryology of the larynx

form on either side of the laryngeal orifice and abut the tissue superiorly (hypobranchial eminence), creating a T-shaped aditus. The hypobranchial eminence gives rise to the epiglottis, cuneiform cartilages, and supraglottic structures. The arytenoid swellings fuse in the midline, and then grow cranially to differentiate into the arytenoid and corniculate cartilages and aryepiglottic folds. The thyroid cartilage develops from surrounding tissue from the fourth branchial arch. During this time, the laryngeal epithelium proliferates causing a temporary occlusion of the laryngeal lumen, which then recanalizes allowing the glottis to be patent and for the laryngeal ventricles to form. Failure of recanalization may lead to webs or atresia of the supraglottis, glottis, or subglottis (refer to below).

Endoscopic Anatomy of the Larynx

The larynx consists of a cartilaginous skeleton, intrinsic and extrinsic muscles, and mucosal lining. The larynx can be divided into three sections: the supraglottis (including superior to the ventrical, the epiglottis, aryepiglottic folds, and false cords), the glottis (the vocal folds), and the subglottis. The saccule is a small diverticulum lined by mucous glands extending upward from the anterior ventricle of the larynx and the inside surface of the thyroid cartilage lamina. The piriform sinus is located within the hypopharynx and is lateral to the laryngeal orifice, bounded medially by the aryepiglottic fold and laterally by the thyroid cartilage and hypothyroid membrane. The vallecula is a space bounded by the lingual surface of the epiglottis and base of the tongue. The postcricoid space is posterior to the arytenoid cartilages (Fig. 6.2). Figure 6.3a, b depict the normal larynx and vocal cords as viewed during direct laryngoscopy.

Laryngomalacia

Definition

Laryngomalacia is a condition in which laryngeal tone is weak, resulting in dynamic prolapse of supraglottic tissue into the airway [1]. This condition is characterized by inspiratory stridor and is associated with varying degrees of airway obstruction.

History

Laryngomalacia was first described by Jackson and Jackson in 1942 in relation to a flaccid larynx and the collapse of supraglottic tissue onto the glottis during inspiration [2]. Historically, severe cases of laryngomalacia required placement of a tracheotomy. In the 1970s, supraglottoplasty was introduced. This currently remains the operative procedure of choice [3].

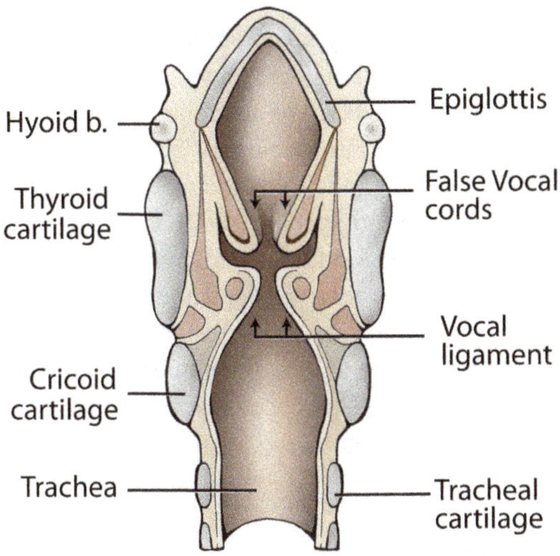

Fig. 6.2 Illustration demonstrating the anatomy of the larynx

Incidence

The true incidence of laryngomalacia is not known; however, this condition is the most common cause of stridor in the newborn [4–7], accounting for 60–75 % of cases [6, 8].

Heredity

The mode of inheritance has not been defined.

Etiology

Although there is no consensus as to the etiology of laryngomalacia, several theories have been proposed. The anatomic theory suggests that characteristic stridor and airway obstruction are caused by the abnormal anatomic location of flaccid laryngeal tissue. The cartilaginous theory proposes that the disease is caused by immaturity and pliability of the laryngeal cartilages. The neurologic theory includes multiple mechanisms including neuromuscular hypotonia, disrupted cortical function, and abnormal neural pathways. The etiology is likely multifactorial, with contributions from all three theories [1].

Associated Malformations

Laryngomalacia is seen in otherwise healthy children and in those with a wide range of

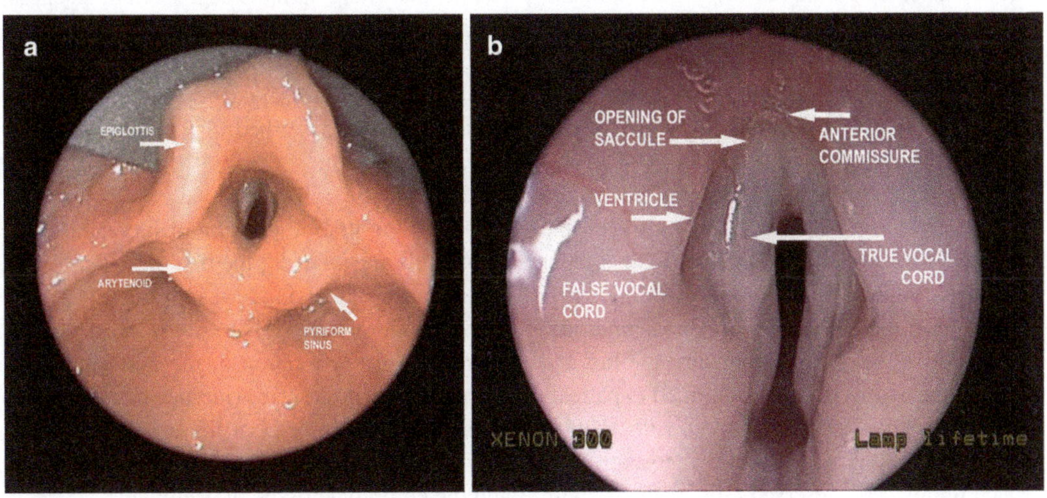

Fig. 6.3 Endoscopic photographs demonstrating the surface anatomy of a normal larynx

comorbidities, including neurologic disease, cardiopulmonary disease, congenital anomalies, and syndromes. Up to 80 % of children with laryngomalacia have gastroesophageal reflux disease (GERD). Synchronous airway lesions have been reported in 12–64 % of children with laryngomalacia [8, 9]. Of these lesions, subglottic stenosis, tracheomalacia, and vocal cord paralysis are the most common [5, 8–10].

Clinical Features

Laryngomalacia is characterized by the onset of high-pitched inspiratory stridor within the first two weeks of life. Stridor is exacerbated by feeding, crying, and lying in a supine position. Symptoms typically peak around 6 months of age, and spontaneously resolve by 12–24 months. Symptoms range from mild inspiratory stridor and feeding difficulties to life-threatening airway obstruction, and cardiopulmonary complications. In severe cases, apneic spells, cyanosis, and failure to thrive may result [3]. Classification of laryngomalacia is described based on the site of supraglottic obstruction [8] or symptoms and clinical findings [1]. We currently classify laryngomalacia based on clinical findings.

Diagnosis

Transnasal flexible fiberoptic laryngoscopy is the gold standard for diagnosis of laryngomalacia. Characteristic findings include short aryepiglottic folds (100 %), floppy cuneiforms (60 %), and an omega-shaped epiglottis (20 %). Figure 6.4 demonstrates schematic illustrations and endoscopic photographs of airways of infants who have laryngomalacia. Figure 6.4a, c represents the more common finding of anterior prolapse of the epiglottis and aryepiglottic folds. Figures 6.4b, d represent the less common form, whereby the mucosa over the arytenoid and cuneiform cartilages and aryepiglottic folds are redundant. In the latter case, the children may present with a lower-pitched purring or rattling stridor on inspiration.

Adjunctive studies, including airway films and airway fluoroscopy, may be performed in patients whose symptoms are inconsistent with flexible laryngoscopy findings. Microlaryngoscopy and bronchoscopy are reserved for patients with suspected synchronous airway lesions or for those requiring surgical intervention for laryngomalacia.

Management

The management of laryngomalacia depends on individual clinical findings and disease progression. Most patients are monitored closely and do not require surgical intervention. Patients are managed medically with anti-reflux therapy. Parental reassurance should also be given. Surgical intervention is required in up to 20 % of patients with laryngomalacia [1]. Indications for operative management of severe cases include failure to thrive, hypoxia, pulmonary hypertension, and cor pulmonale. Supraglottoplasty is performed with laser or microlaryngeal instruments, with the aim of surgery being to release the tight aryepiglottic folds and reduce redundant supra-arytenoid tissue (Fig. 6.5). This approach can be tailored to individual laryngeal pathology. Tracheotomy is reserved for children in whom supraglottoplasty has failed, usually those with significant comorbidities. In children with severe neurologic deficits, tracheotomy may be an alternative to supraglottoplasty.

Laryngeal Cysts

Definition

Congenital laryngeal cysts are fluid- or air-filled lesions that cause variable degrees of hoarseness, dysphagia, stridor, and airway obstruction. Saccular cysts, laryngoceles, vallecular cysts, and lingual thyroglossal duct cysts are the lesions most commonly described.

History

Although the first description of laryngeal cysts is not well documented, the first classification of cystic laryngeal lesions was proposed by De Santo et al. in 1970 [11]. Arens et al. subsequently used the location of the cyst and histomorphology to describe laryngeal cysts [12]. More recently, Forte et al. have classified congenital laryngeal cysts by the extent of the lesion and the embryonic tissue of origin [13].

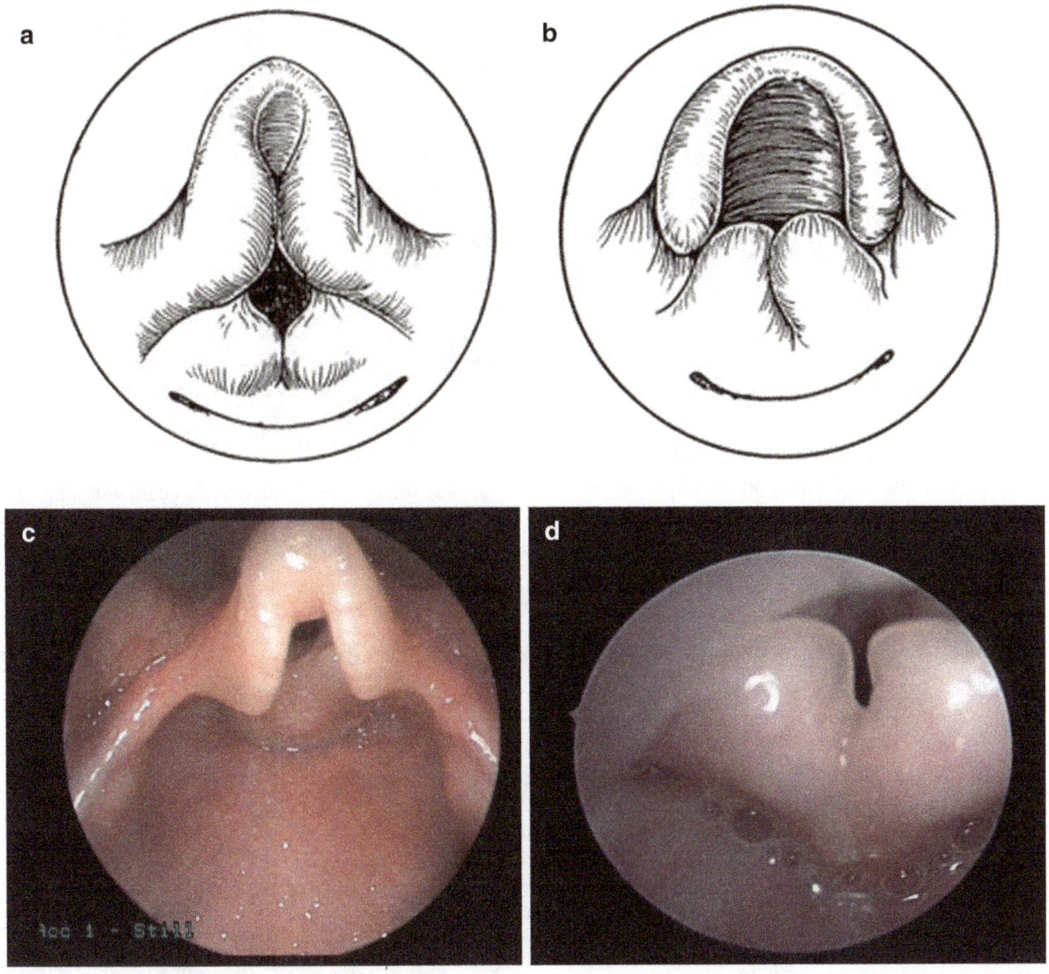

Fig. 6.4 (**a** and **c**) Illustration and endoscopic photograph demonstrating the most common form of laryngomalacia (anterior prolapse). (**b** and **d**) Illustration and endoscopic photograph demonstrating less common posterior prolapse

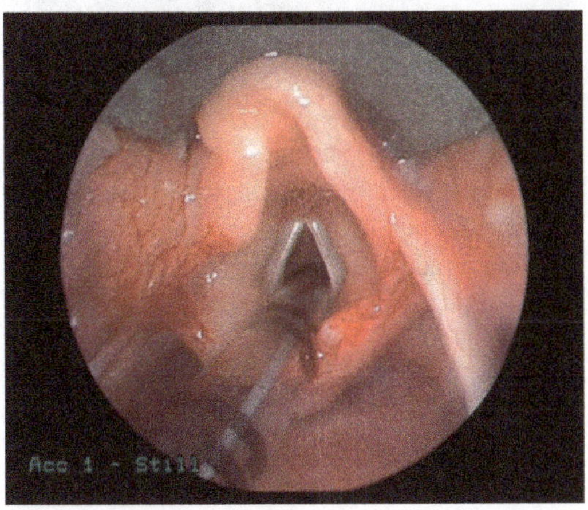

Fig. 6.5 Endoscopic photograph demonstrating postoperative results following supraglottoplasty performed to treat severe laryngomalacia

Incidence

The incidence of congenital laryngeal cysts has not been reported; however, these lesions are considered rare causes of airway and swallowing symptoms in the newborn.

Heredity

The mode of inheritance is unknown.

Etiology

The etiology of laryngeal cysts varies, depending on the type of cyst. Saccular cysts and laryngoceles arise from the saccule, a vestigial laryngeal structure. The saccule contains mucous glands thought to help lubricate the vocal cords. Congenital obstruction of the saccular orifice results in the development of a mucous-filled cyst. A laryngocele is an abnormal dilation of the saccule that maintains patency with the laryngeal lumen. This communication with the laryngeal lumen leads to an intermittent air-filled sac that causes variable airway symptoms. Vallecular cysts are thought to arise from obstruction of mucosal glands in the vallecula or base of tongue. The etiology of lingual thyroglossal duct cysts relates to the embryology of the thyroid. The thyroglossal duct is an epithelial-lined structure connecting the foramen cecum to the thyroid as it descends in the neck. Failure of this duct to obliterate between the fifth and tenth weeks of gestation can lead to the formation of a cyst anywhere along its tract; this can include the base of tongue, larynx, or neck.

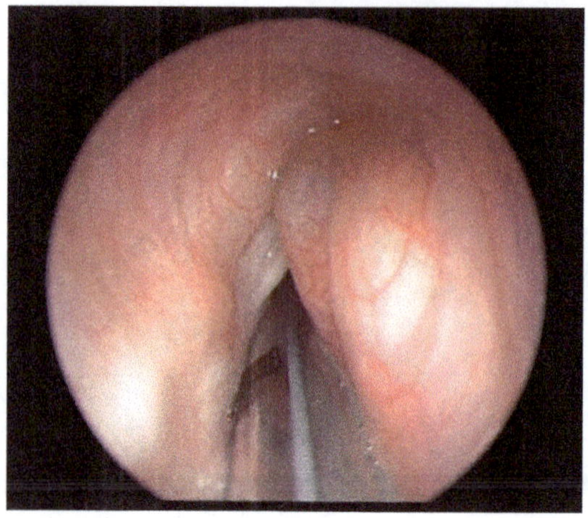

Fig. 6.6 Endoscopic photograph demonstrating an obstructing anterior-based saccular cyst

Associated Malformations

There is no evidence that laryngeal cysts are associated with other anomalies or are more common in specific syndromes or conditions.

Clinical Features

Congenital laryngeal cysts present with airway symptoms and feeding difficulties. In neonates, any of these cysts may be life-threatening. Saccular cysts may present with life-threatening airway obstruction or gradual onset of stridor, depending on the size of the lesion at birth (Fig. 6.6). Laryngoceles typically cause intermittent symptoms including hoarseness and dyspnea made worse by crying (Fig. 6.7). Vallecular cysts often cause early onset of stridor associated with cough and cyanotic episodes (Fig. 6.8). Swallowing difficulties and failure to thrive may also occur. Symptoms related to thyroglossal duct cysts depend on cyst location and can include all of the above.

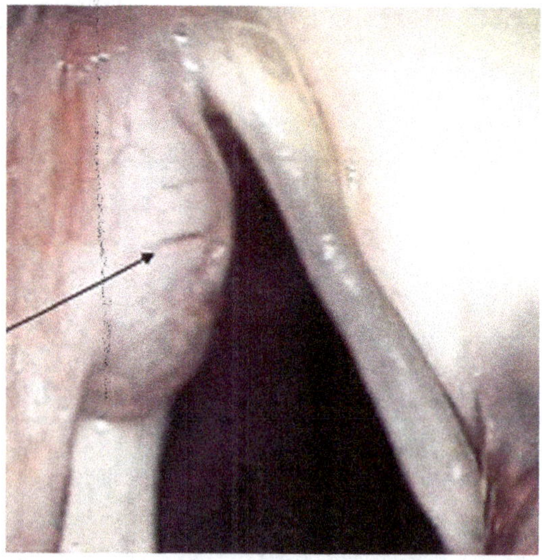

Fig. 6.7 Endoscopic photograph demonstrating a laryngocele of the larynx

Diagnosis

The gold standard for diagnosing laryngeal cysts is the use of transnasal flexible fiberoptic laryngoscopy. A soft-tissue lateral radiograph may be part of the initial evaluation prior to otolaryngology referral. Computed tomography (CT) can be useful in confirming the diagnosis and determining the extent of the lesion. Microlaryngoscopy and bronchoscopy are used at the time of surgery to evaluate the possible presence of secondary airway lesions and to secure the airway. Biopsy helps differentiate thyroglossal duct cysts from vallecular cysts by the presence of thyroid follicles.

Diagnostic investigations help to classify these lesions, allowing for appropriate treatment. Saccular cysts are classified as lateral (involving the false cord and aryepiglottic fold posterosuperiorly) or as anterior (protruding from the ventricle into the laryngeal lumen). Laryngoceles are

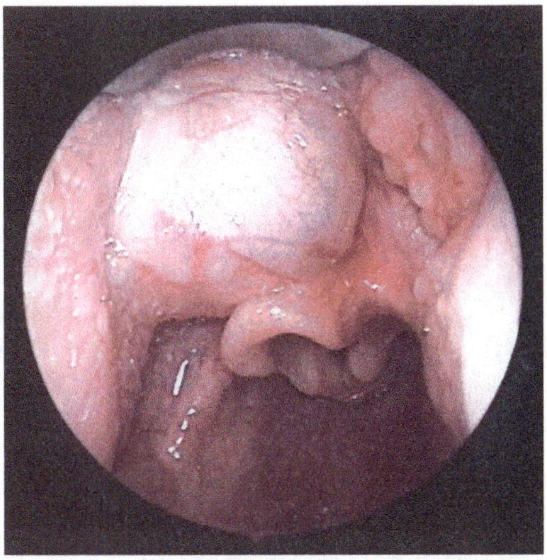

Fig. 6.8 Endoscopic photograph demonstrating a vallecular cyst

considered internal if they are confined to the larynx and involve the false vocal cord and aryepiglottic fold (Fig. 6.9). External lesions extend beyond the thyrohyoid membrane.

Management

Treatment of laryngeal cysts is surgical. The diagnosis of saccular cysts is often confirmed with aspiration at the time of surgery. We advocate a lateral cervical approach as the primary surgical intervention. Temporary tracheotomy placement may be required for large life-threatening cysts. Laryngoceles may be treated endoscopically or through an external approach. Vallecular cysts are managed definitively with endoscopic marsupialization, or excision. We recommend that lingual thyroglossal duct cysts be endoscopically excised. Recurrences may require an external approach.

Laryngeal Webs and Atresia

Definition

Laryngeal webs are malformations in which abnormal tissue forms between two structures in the larynx [14]. True anterior glottic webs are a gossamer-thin membrane that connects the anterior true vocal cords; however, most laryngeal webs are actually thick, and involve not only the vocal cords but also the subglottis. These webs should be considered a milder version within the spectrum of laryngeal atresia.

History

The first classification of laryngeal webs was proposed by Benjamin in 1983. This system defined four degrees of laryngeal atresia by their anatomic location [14]. In 1985, Cohen classified webs according to their thickness and degree of glottic narrowing [15].

Incidence

Although the incidence of laryngeal webs is unknown, anterior glottic webs account for 5 % of congenital laryngeal anomalies. More than 90 % of congenital laryngeal webs are anterior glottic webs; less than 2 % are found in the supraglottis; and 7 % are found in the subglottis. Complete laryngeal atresia is extremely rare.

Heredity

More than 50 % of children with partial laryngeal atresia have chromosome 22q11.2 deletion, an autosomal dominant heritable condition that usually presents as velocardiofacial syndrome (VCFS) or Di George syndrome. As the clinical manifestation of VCFS may be subtle, we recommend that all children with partial laryngeal atresia undergo genetic testing for chromosome 22q11.2 deletion [16]. It should, however, be noted that the incidence of partial laryngeal atresia in children with VCFS is low.

Etiology

Laryngeal webbing or atresia results from a failure in embryogenesis. The primitive laryngeal aditus becomes a t-shaped opening by the growth of three masses that later form the epiglottis and two arytenoid cartilages. As they develop during the fifth to seventh weeks of gestation, the lumen obliterates. Failure of the lumen to recanalize by week 10 of gestation leads to varying degrees of obstruction in the form of webs or atresia.

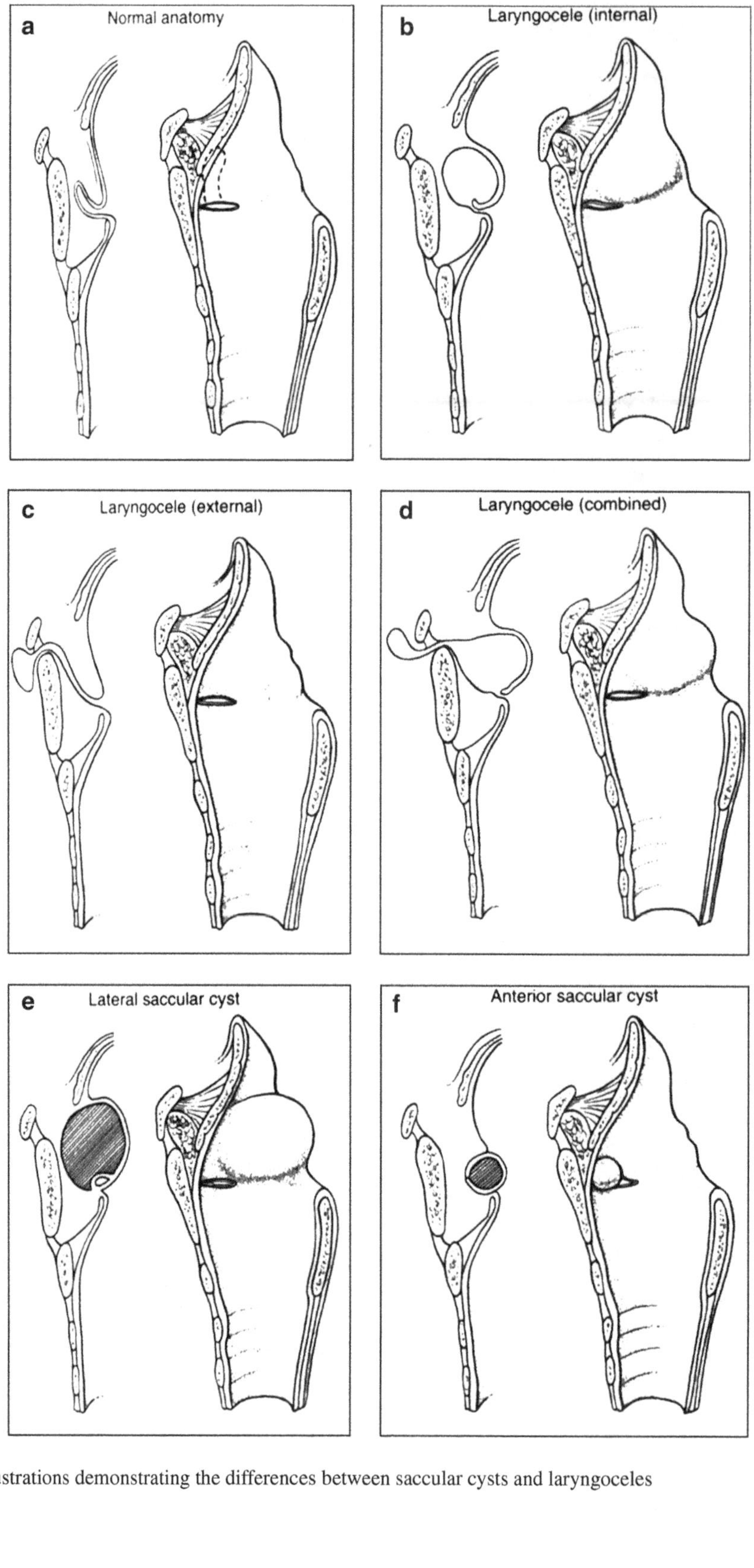

Fig. 6.9 Illustrations demonstrating the differences between saccular cysts and laryngoceles

Associated Malformations

The most common conditions associated with laryngeal atresia are VCFS and DiGeorge syndrome [16]. Glottic and supraglottic atresia are also associated with other foregut and non-foregut anomalies. These include esophageal atresia, tracheoesophageal fistula (TEF), limb defects, and urinary tract abnormalities [17].

Clinical Features

Thin anterior glottic webs may be asymptomatic or present with mild voice dysfunction and hoarseness. Severe webs that are thick and involve the anterior and posterior glottis are more likely to present with biphasic stridor (particularly when infants are feeding or upset), life-threatening airway compromise, and aphonia. Infants are, nevertheless, remarkably tolerant of congenital airway compromise. They may present with subtle airway symptoms and yet have moderate to severe webbing [18]. Complete laryngeal atresia is not compatible with life unless ventilation through a TEF is achieved or the pathology is noted prior to birth and an EXIT (ex utero intrapartum treatment) procedure is performed to allow tracheotomy to be performed while maternal-fetal circulation is maintained.

Diagnosis

Initial evaluation is made by awake transnasal flexible fiberoptic laryngoscopy. This may suggest the need for rigid microlaryngoscopy or bronchoscopy in the operating room to confirm the diagnosis. The degree of webbing is noted and categorized according to the classification described by Cohen [15]. Type 1 webs are anterior and thin, occupying 35 % or less of the glottis. Type 2 webs involve 35–50 % of the glottis and have a thicker anterior component (Fig. 6.10). Type 3 webs are again anterior and occlude 50–75 % of the glottis. The thick anterior component may be associated with cricoid cartilage involvement and the vocal cords may not be seen. Type 4 webs are thick anteriorly and posteriorly, compromising 75–90 % of the glottis; there is a subglottic component and the vocal cords are not discernible (Fig. 6.11). Isolated posterior glottic webs are typically thin, but may have interarytenoid involvement with resultant vocal cord fixation. Vocal cord mobility should be documented during microlaryngoscopy and bronchoscopy. Imaging studies, including high-voltage lateral radiographs and CT are useful to help diagnose cricoid involvement or other airway anomalies.

Laryngeal atresia can be diagnosed prenatally by ultrasound. Obstruction of the laryngeal lumen can result in congenital high airway obstruction syndrome (CHAOS). Signs of CHAOS are seen on ultrasound and include a flattened diaphragm, a fluid-filled, dilated airway distal to the obstruction, fetal hydrops, and enlarged hyperechogenic lungs. These signs indicate the need for color-flow Doppler to localize the level of obstruction [19, 20].

Management

Treatment for laryngeal webs involves either endoscopic or open surgical techniques that are typically delayed until 3–4 years of age. Thin anterior webs can be treated endoscopically with microlaryngeal instruments. Silastic sheeting or keels can be placed endoscopically or with open techniques to prevent stenosis. In this setting, a tracheotomy is usually placed to ensure a safe airway.

Webbing that involves the subglottis and cricoid plate requires a formal laryngotracheoplasty with laryngofissure. The CO_2 laser is not recommended because it can cause scarring. The web is divided and the cricoid is addressed by submucosal resection of the cricoid cartilage, the use of anterior cartilage grafting, or partial cricotracheal resection. This can be performed with the use of a keel and a temporary tracheotomy or in a single-stage fashion with intubation for up to 2 weeks. Revision surgery is often required. Alternatively, open reconstruction of the anterior commissure can be performed when at least 25 % of the laryngeal lumen is patent. Immediate surgical intervention with a tracheotomy at birth may be necessary for type 3 and type 4 webs. Posterior glottic webs often can be addressed by endoscopic division, but may require open placement of a posterior costal cartilage graft for interarytenoid involvement.

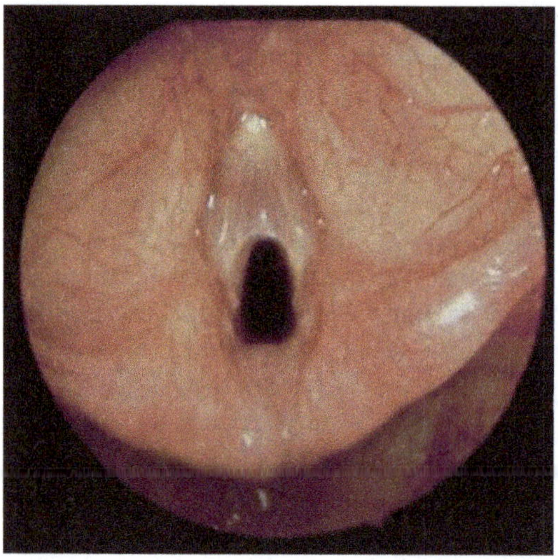

Fig. 6.10 Endoscopic photograph of a Cohen type 2 anterior glottis web

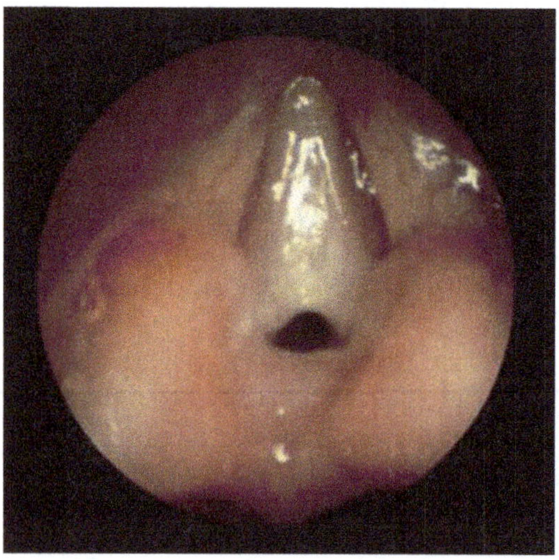

Fig. 6.11 Endoscopic photograph of a Cohen type 4 glottic web

In patients with a complete congenital laryngeal web and a TEF, esophageal intubation may permit oxygenation prior to placement of a tracheotomy; however, congenital laryngeal atresia without a TEF results in CHAOS. This is usually diagnosed prenatally, allowing for a subsequent EXIT procedure to secure the infant's airway. In either case, once the airway is secured, definitive repair is delayed until the child is 4 years of age [20].

Vocal Cord Paralysis

Definition

Vocal cord paralysis is defined as the inability of one or both vocal cords to move. The paralysis is generally caused by abnormal nerve input to the laryngeal muscles, either from the central nervous system or of peripheral nerve origin. Symptoms vary from voice dysfunction to airway and swallowing problems.

History

In 1882, Guy's Hospital Reports first published evidence of vocal cord paralysis in a child. Chevalier Jackson later attributed asphyxiation in infants to bilateral abductor paralysis. In 1970, Goff classified vocal cord paralysis according to whether the etiology was congenital or acquired [21]. These classifications are further subdivided into unilateral and bilateral paralysis. In infants, bilateral paralysis is generally congenital, whereas unilateral paralysis is typically an acquired condition caused by damage to the recurrent laryngeal nerve.

Incidence

Although the incidence of congenital vocal cord paralysis is unknown, it is the second most common cause of stridor in the newborn, and accounts for 10 % of congenital laryngeal anomalies [22].

Heredity

Autosomal dominant inheritance has been described in some cases of bilateral vocal cord paralysis [23]. Rarely, hereditary motor and sensory neuropathy (Charcot-Marie-Tooth Disease), may cause bilateral paralysis [24]. In unilateral cases, there is no known genetic link.

Etiology

Although the majority of cases of congenital vocal cord paralysis are idiopathic, a number of conditions may lead to this pathology. In rare cases, birth trauma may cause stretching of the recurrent laryngeal nerve. Central nervous system disorders such as Arnold-Chiari malformation (ACM) and hydrocephalus typically cause bilateral paralysis, as can peripheral nervous

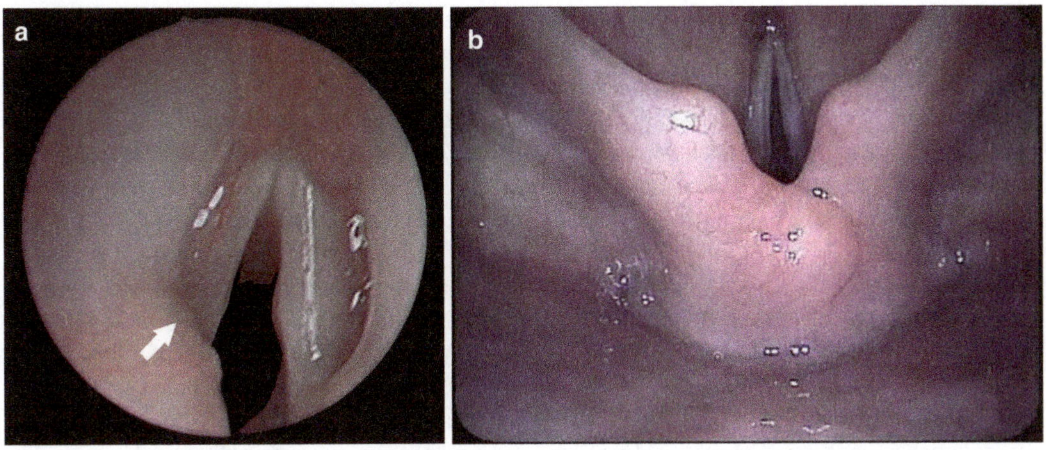

Fig. 6.12 (**a**) Endoscopic photograph demonstrating the findings in a patient with unilateral vocal cord paralysis. The paralyzed cord is positioned just off the midline in the paramedian position (see *arrow*). (**b**) Endoscopic photograph demonstrating the findings in a patient with bilateral vocal cord paralysis resulting in narrowing of the opening of the glottis

system disorders such as spinal muscle atrophy and myasthenia gravis. In both central nervous system and peripheral nervous system disorders, unilateral paralysis is observed only rarely. Other peripheral causes of unilateral paralysis include cardiovascular and mediastinal anomalies.

Clinical Features

Symptoms of unilateral paralysis include a weak, breathy cry and difficulty with feeding. Recurrent aspiration can result from an inability to approximate the vocal cords and protect the airway because the paralyzed cord sits within the paramedian position (just off the midline) (Fig. 6.12a). Bilateral paralysis usually presents with high-pitched inspiratory stridor associated with a normal cry (Fig. 6.12b). The paralyzed vocal cords are situated so they rest close to midline on either side, reducing the glottis airway size. Respiratory distress and acute airway obstruction may require emergent airway management.

Diagnosis

The diagnosis is established with awake transnasal flexible fiberoptic laryngoscopy. Microlaryngoscopy and bronchoscopy under anesthesia are performed to check the mobility of the cricoarytenoid joints and evaluate for other laryngeal pathology. All patients should undergo a detailed neck exam and imaging of the chest. A video swallow study (VSS) is performed to assess swallowing function in patients with feeding difficulties and to help delineate mediastinal pathology. All patients with bilateral paralysis require central nervous system imaging to rule out ACM or other brainstem abnormalities. In most cases of vocal cord paralysis with an unknown etiology, the entire course of the vagus nerve is imaged, including the head, neck, and chest.

Management

In some children, treatment of the underlying cause of paralysis may be sufficient to restore vocal cord mobility. In children with stridor and retractions caused by bilateral paralysis, tracheotomy placement is generally (90 %) required. Approximately 50 % of patients with congenital bilateral vocal cord paralysis experience spontaneous recovery by 1 year of age [25]. When vocal cord function is not restored, other procedures can be performed to achieve decannulation. These procedures include vocal cord lateralization, cordotomy, partial or complete arytenoidectomy, and posterior cricoid cartilage grafting. Both open and endoscopic techniques are used.

In most children with unilateral vocal cord paralysis, surgical intervention is not needed. In infants with significant aspiration, a gastrostomy tube may be required for nutritional support, and occasionally, a tracheotomy is needed for pulmonary toilet. With growth of the airway, medialization procedures can be used to help achieve better voice quality. Injection medialization and type 1 thyroplasty have been performed, though little is known about their effects on the developing larynx.

Laryngotracheoesophageal Clefts

Definition

Laryngotracheoesophageal clefts (LTECs) are posterior, midline airway defects that represent a fusion defect during embryogenesis. These clefts may be minor and short, or may extend to the carina or beyond. They are classified according to their anatomic extent.

History

The first documented case of LTEC was described by Richter in 1792 in a child with multiple anomalies. Finlay established the modern diagnosis in 1949, and Pettersson was the first to report a successful repair in 1955 [26, 27].

Incidence

Owing to diagnostic advancements, the reported incidence of LTECs has increased significantly over the last 20 years. The incidence is currently estimated at 1 in 2,000 live births [28].

Heredity

Opitz-Frias syndrome and Pallister-Hall syndrome, both of which are associated with LTECs, are autosomal dominant conditions. Opitz-Frias syndrome may be associated with an X-linked recessive inheritance pattern.

Etiology

LTECs result from a fusion failure during embryogenesis. The larynx and trachea develop from a groove in the foregut floor posterior to the hyobranchial eminence, which deepens until the lung buds form. In the fourth week of gestation, this tracheoesophageal groove fuses in a caudal to cephalad direction to form the tracheoesophageal septum. Fusion failure results in varying degrees of posterior clefting.

Associated Malformations

LTECs are associated with many other congenital anomalies. Airway anomalies include tracheomalacia (greater than 80 %) and TEF (20–37 %) [3, 29]. Defects of the gastrointestinal tract (e.g., esophageal atresia, anal defects, malrotation, or intestinal fixation) are the most common non-airway findings. Gastroesophageal reflux disease (GERD) is a near universal finding. Genitourinary anomalies (e.g., hypospadias, inguinal hernias, and renal agenesis) and cardiovascular anomalies (e.g., ventricular septal defects, coarctation, and transposition of the great vessels) have also been described.

Clinical Features

Symptoms of LTEC depend on the severity of disease. The hallmark feature of the disorder is aspiration. This represents a continuum from silent microaspiration to gross aspiration with apnea, cyanosis, and pneumonia. Minor clefts may be asymptomatic or present with hoarseness, coughing, choking, brief cyanotic episodes, and recurrent respiratory infections. Major clefts typically present with feeding difficulties, respiratory distress, and severe airway obstruction. Severe clefts may be associated with polyhydramnios and prematurity.

Diagnosis

Diagnosing a LTEC can be challenging, and requires a high index of suspicion. Although the gold standard for evaluation is airway endoscopy, minor clefts often appear normal on repeated endoscopies, and thus can go undiagnosed for years. Suspension microlaryngoscopy with distraction and probing of the interarytenoid area most reliably excludes or confirms a laryngeal cleft. A multidisciplinary approach including evaluations by the pulmonary and gastroenterology services helps determine the degree of pulmonary dysfunction and GERD; this is especially valuable in the older child. Adjunctive tests include a VSS and a functional endoscopic evaluation of swallowing (FEES) to assess for aspiration.

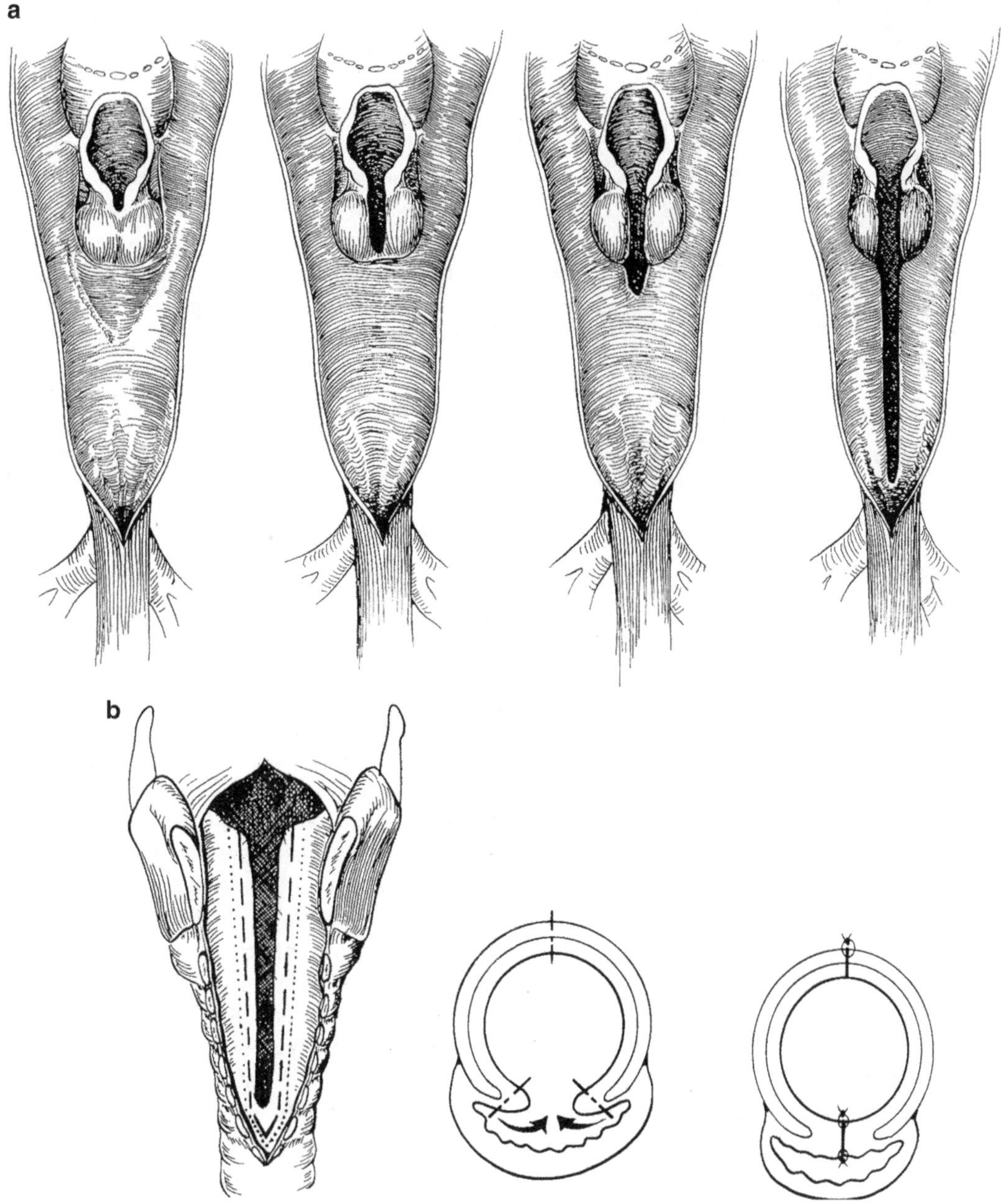

Fig. 6.13 Illustration of the four types of laryngeal clefts (Reprinted with permission from Cotton RT, Myer CM III, eds. *Practical Pediatric Otolaryngology*. Philadelphia, PA: Lippincott-Raven; 1999: 506)

Radiographs of the chest and lateral neck can aid in diagnosing aspiration pneumonia or allow visualization of a posteriorly displaced endotracheal tube or anteriorly displaced nasogastric tube.

The most commonly used classification of LTECs is described by Benjamin and Inglis [30] (Fig. 6.13). Type I clefts are interarytenoid defects that do not extend inferior to the vocal cords. Type II clefts are partial cricoid defects,

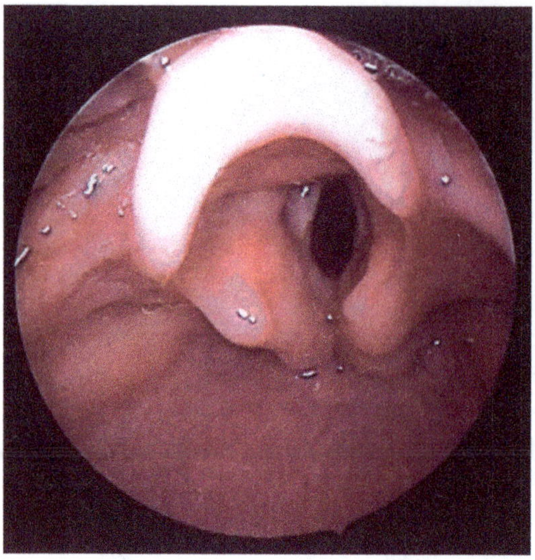

Fig. 6.14 Endoscopic photograph demonstrating a posterior laryngeal cleft causing separation of the arytenoid cartilages

whereas type III clefts are total cricoid clefts with or without cervical tracheal involvement. Type IV clefts involve the intrathoracic trachea. Rutter has proposed a modification of this classification, which differentiates intrathoracic defects by carinal involvement [31]. Type IV long clefts comprise defects that involve the carina. These defects are often seen in infants with multiple congenital anomalies. They are associated with anastomotic dehiscence and mortality rates greater than 90 % [3, 29].

Management

Treatment varies according to clinical findings and the severity of the cleft. Early intervention is important to prevent permanent pulmonary dysfunction. Type I clefts with minimal symptoms can be managed nonoperatively with anti-reflux therapy, a thickened diet, and supraglottic swallowing strategies. Symptomatic clefts are treated surgically with either endoscopic or open techniques. Endoscopic management is usually reserved for type I and type II clefts (Fig. 6.14). Open procedural techniques include anterior laryngofissure and lateral pharyngotomy. Our preference is an anterior approach with a two or three layer closure. A three layer closure involves an interposition graft of periosteum, fascia, or cartilage. Complete LTEC usually requires a thoracotomy or sternotomy; this is often performed on cardiopulmonary bypass or with extracorporeal membrane oxygenation (ECMO).

When possible and practical, airway protection should be addressed prior to definitive repair. A tracheotomy may be required; however, it is best to avoid this if possible because decannulation is often delayed in the setting of tracheomalacia. All patients should be managed with anti-reflux therapy or surgical interventions, which may include gastrojejunostomy tube placement or Nissen fundoplication and gastrostomy tube placement.

Vascular Anomalies

Definitions

Hemangiomas and vascular malformations are the two major types of pediatric vascular lesions. Hemangiomas are benign vascular tumors of infancy. They are characterized by endothelial cell hyperplasia and mast cell proliferation. These tumors generally undergo a phase of rapid postnatal proliferation, followed by a phase of gradual spontaneous regression that occurs over several years. Hemangiomas typically present cutaneously, though they can present anywhere within the tracheobronchial tree, with the subglottis being the most common site.

Vascular malformations arise from errors in vascular morphogenesis. Unlike hemangiomas, they have normal endothelial turnover, normal numbers of mast cells, and do not resolve spontaneously. Malformations encompass a wide spectrum of anomalies (capillary, venous, arterial, lymphatic, and combined lesions) having varying presentations. Lymphatic malformations and lymphatic-venous malformations can affect the larynx, though these cases are rare.

History

In 1982, Mulliken and Glowacki proposed a classification system to differentiate vascular tumors from vascular malformations [32]. The classification was subsequently modified in 1996, with consensus from the International Society for the Study of Vascular Anomalies.

Sharp reported the first excision of a subglottic hemangioma in 1949 [33].

Incidence

Hemangiomas are the most common tumors of infancy, affecting 1–10 % of infants. These lesions occur most commonly in the head and neck (60 %), though they account for only about 1 % of congenital laryngeal anomalies. The actual incidence of airway hemangiomas and vascular malformations is unknown.

Heredity

The mode of inheritance of these lesions has not been defined.

Associated Malformations

More than 50 % of patients with subglottic hemangiomas also have cutaneous lesions, which may indicate a possible coexisting airway lesion [3]. As well, many infants (65 %) with cutaneous hemangiomas in a cervicofacial or "beard" distribution have airway involvement [34].

Clinical Features

Presentation of vascular airway anomalies depends on the location and severity of the lesion. Only 30 % of airway hemangiomas are evident at birth. Infants typically become symptomatic within the first few months of life. Characteristic symptoms include progressive biphasic stridor and retractions. A barking cough, hoarseness, dysphagia, cyanosis, and even hemoptysis can be a part of the clinical picture. Patients may have been seen and treated repeatedly for croup. Hemangiomas follow a predetermined course, involving a proliferative phase followed by an involutive phase. This process is typically shorter with subglottic hemangiomas. Lymphatic malformations typically have more extensive head and neck involvement and are categorized as microcytic, macrocystic, or mixed disease. They can enlarge suddenly due to infection or trauma.

Diagnosis

The diagnosis of both hemangiomas and vascular malformations is based on history, physical exam, endoscopic findings, and imaging. Transnasal flexible fiberoptic laryngoscopy is performed to rule out other causes of neonatal stridor, including laryngomalacia and vocal cord paralysis.

Microlaryngoscopy and bronchoscopy under anesthesia are the gold standard for evaluation of airway hemangiomas. A sessile, compressible mass is typically seen in the posterolateral aspect of the subglottis (Fig. 6.14). These masses are more common on the left side, are usually submucosal, and often have a bluish or reddish hue. Biopsy is usually not necessary or recommended. Figure 6.15 demonstrates a less common hemangioma because it is located in the supraglottis. Contrast-enhanced magnetic resonance imaging (MRI) and CT are used to ensure there is no extension of the hemangioma beyond the trachea.

Management

The treatment of subglottic hemangiomas is based on clinical symptoms and the degree of airway obstruction. In older children, observation is appropriate if there are minimal airway symptoms and less than 50 % of the airway is compromised. In children with mild to moderate symptoms, treatment with high-dose systemic corticosteroids can hasten involution, though long-term treatment is strongly discouraged. Propranalol, a nonselective beta-blocker, has been found to be effective in promoting involution during the rapid growth phase of infantile hemangiomas. However, patients may develop side effects including hypotension, bradycardia, exacerbation of reactive airway disease and hypoglycemia so should be monitored closely throughout the treatment course (usually given over a 6 month period if found to be effective) [35]. Most patients require endoscopic or open procedures for definitive treatment. The endoscopic use of CO_2 and potassium titanyl phosphate (KTP) lasers has been advocated but can lead to postoperative subglottic stenosis in up to 20 % of patients [36]. Intralesional steroid injection and microdebrider submucosal resection also have been performed endoscopically. Open excision through a vertical laryngofissure for large and rapidly growing subglottic hemangiomas is a promising alternative to tracheotomy [37]. This procedure involves submucosal resection allowing for airway augmentation with

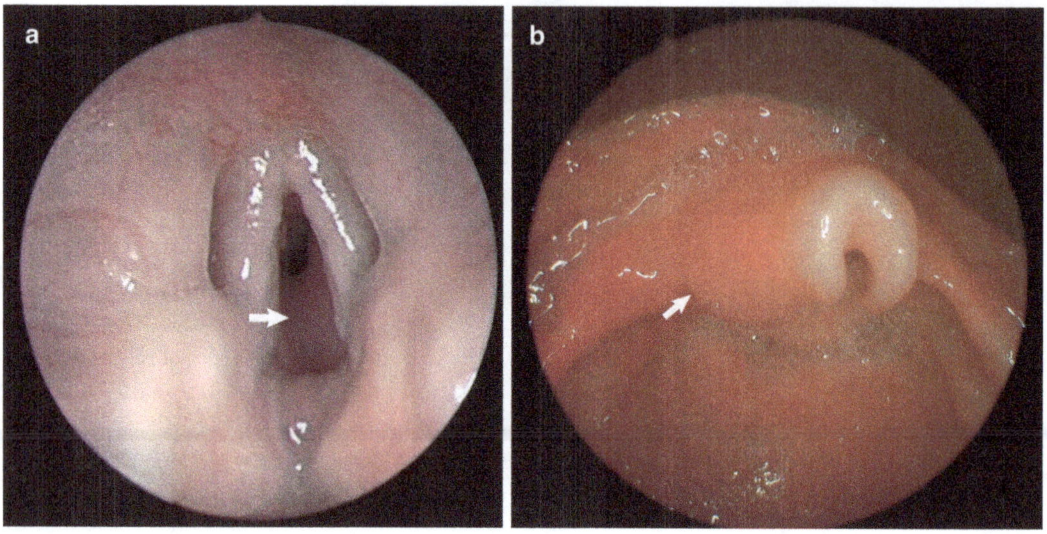

Fig. 6.15 (**a**) Endoscopic photograph of a subglottic hemangioma (arrow). (**b**) Endoscopic photograph of a supraglottic hemangioma (arrow)

a thyroid ala cartilage graft when a coexisting subglottic stenosis is present. In selected cases, the hemangioma may be removed through an anterior approach without performing a complete laryngofissure. Alternatively, tracheotomy can provide a safe and stable airway during the natural history of the disease. Decannulation is achieved when involution is sufficient.

The management of vascular malformations depends on the extent of disease. When large and extensive lesions are present, complete surgical excision is often not possible. Multiple procedures may thus be necessary. A tracheotomy may be required.

Subglottic Stenosis

Definition

Subglottic stenosis (SGS) in the neonate is defined as a narrowing in the cricoid region of less than 4 mm in a full-term infant and less than 3 mm in a premature infant. The greatest area of narrowing is typically 2–3 mm below the vocal cords. Congenital SGS can be classified as membranous or cartilaginous and occurs when there is no history of intubation or surgical trauma [38].

History

In 1954, Holinger first described congenital SGS manifesting as an abnormally shaped cricoid cartilage [39].

Incidence

Although the incidence of congenital SGS is unknown, it is rare when compared to the incidence of acquired SGS. Congenital SGS is considered the third most common cause of stridor in the newborn.

Heredity

The mode of inheritance has not been defined.

Etiology

The etiology of congenital SGS is attributed to failure of the laryngeal lumen to fully recanalize by the tenth week of embryogenesis. The condition is part of the continuum encompassing laryngeal webbing, stenosis, and atresia discussed earlier. Membranous SGS is caused by hyperplastic mucous glands with increased fibrous connective tissue in the subglottis, and is typically circumferential. Cartilaginous SGS is caused by a thickening or deformity of the cricoid cartilage, which typically presents as a small

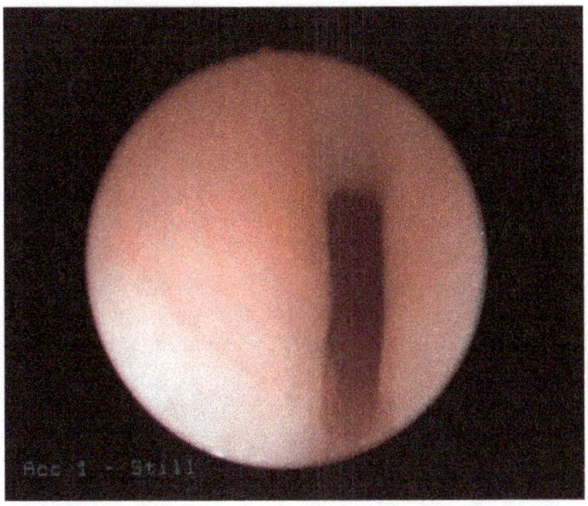

Fig. 6.16 Endoscopic photograph of congenital subglottic stenosis which is elliptical in nature causing narrowing in the lateral dimensions of the subglottis

posterior or elliptical opening. A trapped first tracheal ring can also lead to stenosis.

Associated Malformations

Congenital SGS is sometimes associated with a number of other congenital head and neck anomalies (e.g., vocal cord paralysis, laryngeal webs, posterior laryngeal clefts). It may also be associated with a number of syndromes (e.g., infants with Down syndrome typically have a small larynx and subglottis). GERD can potentiate the condition, and intubation or instrumentation increases the risk of an acquired stenosis in addition to the underlying congenital pathology.

Clinical Features

Presentation depends on the degree of stenosis and can range from minimal dyspnea to acute airway obstruction at birth. Symptoms include biphasic stridor, dyspnea, tachypnea, and cyanosis. Nevertheless, infants are often surprisingly asymptomatic. Congenital SGS can also present during intubation for a surgical procedure or can manifest later in childhood as exercise intolerance. Congenital SGS is typically less severe than acquired stenosis (Fig. 6.16).

Diagnosis

The diagnosis is based on endoscopic findings during rigid microlaryngoscopy and bronchoscopy. SGS is suspected when upper respiratory infections or recurrent croup cause significant airway compromise. The severity of the stenosis is determined by the Myer-Cotton grading system, using the diameter of endotracheal tubes to size the airway [40]. This classification divides SGS into four categories. Grade I represents less than 50 % stenosis; grade II includes 51–70 % stenosis; grade III includes 71–99 % stenosis; and grade IV includes lesions with no detectable lumen. Flexible, transnasal fiberoptic laryngoscopy should also be performed to rule out other glottic and supraglottic causes of stridor, such as laryngomalacia or vocal cord paralysis.

Radiographic evaluation of a patient who is not intubated can aid in the diagnosis prior to endoscopy, and can help define the characteristics of the stenosis.

Management

Treatment of congenital SGS depends on the severity of the symptoms and grade of stenosis. In mild to moderate cases, observation alone may be appropriate. Children commonly outgrow the condition within the first few years of life, and less than 50 % will require a tracheotomy [22, 41]. Decannulation is achieved in most infants by 24–36 months of age [42]. Dilation plays a limited role in cartilaginous SGS. Endoscopic laser procedures can be useful for grade I and grade II lesions. Other surgical interventions are also used to try to avoid tracheotomy placement. Cotton first described the anterior cricoid split procedure in 1980 [43]. For more severe SGS, open techniques such as laryngotracheal reconstruction with cartilage grafting and cricotracheal resection are performed.

Acknowledgement We would like to thank Aliza Cohen for assistance in writing this chapter.

References

1. Thompson DM. Abnormal sensorimotor integrative function of the larynx in congenital laryngomalacia: a new theory of etiology. Laryngoscope. 2007;117(6 Pt 2 Suppl 114):1–33.
2. Jackson C, Jackson CL, editors. Diseases and injuries of the larynx. New York: Macmillan; 1942.

3. Rutter MJ. Evaluation and management of upper airway disorders in children. Semin Pediatr Surg. 2006;15(2):116–23.
4. Cotton R, Prescott AJ. Congenital anomalies of the larynx. In: Cotton RT, Meyer III CM, editors. Practical pediatric otolaryngology. Philadelphia, PA: Lippincott-Raven; 1999. p. 497–514.
5. Friedman EM, Vastola AP, McGill TJ, Healy GB. Chronic pediatric stridor: etiology and outcome. Laryngoscope. 1990;100(3):277–80.
6. Holinger LD. Etiology of stridor in the neonate, infant and child. Ann Otol Rhinol Laryngol. 1980;89(5 Pt 1):397–400.
7. Zoumalan R, Maddalozzo J, Holinger LD. Etiology of stridor in infants. Ann Otol Rhinol Laryngol. 2007;116(5):329–34.
8. Olney DR, Greinwald Jr JH, Smith RJ, Bauman NM. Laryngomalacia and its treatment. Laryngoscope. 1999;109(11):1770–5.
9. Mancuso RF, Choi SS, Zalzal GH, Grundfast KM. Laryngomalacia. The search for the second lesion. Arch Otolaryngol Head Neck Surg. 1996;122(3): 302–6.
10. Gonzalez C, Reilly JS, Bluestone CD. Synchronous airway lesions in infancy. Ann Otol Rhinol Laryngol. 1987;96(1 Pt 1):77–80.
11. DeSanto LW, Devine KD, Weiland LH. Cysts of the larynx—classification. Laryngoscope. 1970;80(1):145–76.
12. Arens C, Glanz H, Kleinsasser O. Clinical and morphological aspects of laryngeal cysts. Eur Arch Otorhinolaryngol. 1997;254(9–10):430–6.
13. Forte V, Fuoco G, James A. A new classification system for congenital laryngeal cysts. Laryngoscope. 2004;114(6):1123–7.
14. Nicollas R, Triglia JM. The anterior laryngeal webs. Otolaryngol Clin North Am. 2008;41(5):877–88, viii.
15. Cohen SR. Congenital glottic webs in children. A retrospective review of 51 patients. Ann Otol Rhinol Laryngol Suppl. 1985;121:2–16.
16. Miyamoto RC, Cotton RT, Rope AF, et al. Association of anterior glottic webs with velocardiofacial syndrome (chromosome 22q11.2 deletion). Otolaryngol Head Neck Surg. 2004;130(4):415–7.
17. Hartnick CJ, Cotton RT. Congenital laryngeal anomalies. Laryngeal atresia, stenosis, webs, and clefts. Otolaryngol Clin North Am. 2000;33(6):1293–308.
18. Rutter M. Laryngeal webs and subglottic hemangioma. In: Graham JS, Scadding GK, Bull PD, editors. Pediatric ENT. New York, NY: Springer; 2007. p. 211–22.
19. DeCou JM, Jones DC, Jacobs HD, Touloukian RJ. Successful ex utero intrapartum treatment (EXIT) procedure for congenital high airway obstruction syndrome (CHAOS) owing to laryngeal atresia. J Pediatr Surg. 1998;33(10):1563–5.
20. Hartnick CJ, Rutter M, Lang F, Willging JP, Cotton RT. Congenital high airway obstruction syndrome and airway reconstruction: an evolving paradigm. Arch Otolaryngol Head Neck Surg. 2002;128(5):567–70.
21. Goff WF. Vocal cord paralysis analysis of 229 cases. JAMA. 1970;212(8):1378–9.
22. Wiatrak BJ. Congenital anomalies of the larynx and trachea. Otolaryngol Clin North Am. 2000;33(1): 91–110.
23. Manaligod JM, Skaggs J, Smith RJ. Localization of the gene for familial laryngeal abductor paralysis to chromosome 6q16. Arch Otolaryngol Head Neck Surg. 2001;127(8):913–7.
24. Lacy PD, Hartley BE, Rutter MJ, Cotton RT. Familial bilateral vocal cord paralysis and Charcot-Marie-tooth disease type II-C. Arch Otolaryngol Head Neck Surg. 2001;127(3):322–4.
25. Miyamoto RC, Parikh SR, Gellad W, Licameli GR. Bilateral congenital vocal cord paralysis: a 16-year institutional review. Otolaryngol Head Neck Surg. 2005;133(2):241–5.
26. Finlay HV. Familial congenital stridor. Arch Dis Child. 1949;24(119):219–23.
27. Pettersson G. Inhibited separation of larynx and the upper part of trachea from oesophagus in a newborn; report of a case successfully operated upon. Acta Chir Scand. 1955;110(3):250–4.
28. Sandu K, Monnier P. Congenital tracheal anomalies. Otolaryngol Clin North Am. 2007;40(1):193–217, viii.
29. Chitkara AE, Tadros M, Kim HJ, Harley EH. Complete laryngotracheoesophageal cleft: complicated management issues. Laryngoscope. 2003;113(8):1314–20.
30. Benjamin B, Inglis A. Minor congenital laryngeal clefts: diagnosis and classification. Ann Otol Rhinol Laryngol. 1989;98(6):417–20.
31. Rutter M, Azizkhan RG, Cotton RT. Posterior laryngeal cleft. In: Ziegler M, Azizkhan RG, Weber TR, editors. Operative pediatric surgery. New York: McGraw-Hill Companies; 2003. p. 313–20.
32. Mulliken JB, Glowacki J. Hemangiomas and vascular malformations in infants and children: a classification based on endothelial characteristics. Plast Reconstr Surg. 1982;69(3):412–22.
33. Sharp HS. Haemangioma of the trachea in an infant; successful removal. J Laryngol Otol. 1949; 63(7):413.
34. Orlow SJ, Isakoff MS, Blei F. Increased risk of symptomatic hemangiomas of the airway in association with cutaneous hemangiomas in a "beard" distribution. J Pediatr. 1997;131(4):643–6.
35. Leaute-Labreze C, Taieb A. Efficacy of beta-blockers in infantile capillary haemangiomas: the pysiopahtological significance and therapeutic consequences. Ann Dermatol Venereol. 2008;135:860–2.
36. Sie KC, McGill T, Healy GB. Subglottic hemangioma: ten years' experience with the carbon dioxide laser. Ann Otol Rhinol Laryngol. 1994;103(3): 167–72.
37. Vijayasekaran S, White DR, Hartley BE, Rutter MJ, Elluru RG, Cotton RT. Open excision of subglottic hemangiomas to avoid tracheostomy. Arch Otolaryngol Head Neck Surg. 2006;132(2):159–63.

38. Tucker GF, Ossoff RH, Newman AN, Holinger LD. Histopathology of congenital subglottic stenosis. Laryngoscope. 1979;89(6 Pt 1):866–77.
39. Holinger PH, Johnson KC, Schiller F. Congenital anomalies of the larynx. Ann Otol Rhinol Laryngol. 1954;63(3):581–606.
40. Myer 3rd CM, O'Connor DM, Cotton RT. Proposed grading system for subglottic stenosis based on endotracheal tube sizes. Ann Otol Rhinol Laryngol. 1994;103(4 Pt 1):319–23.
41. Hartnick C, Cotton RT. Syndromic and other congenital anomalies of the head and neck. Otolaryngol Clin North Am. 2003;33(6):1293–308.
42. Holinger PH, Kutnick SL, Schild JA, Holinger LD. Subglottic stenosis in infants and children. Ann Otol Rhinol Laryngol. 1976;85(5 Pt.1):591–9.
43. Cotton RT, Seid AB. Management of the extubation problem in the premature child. Anterior cricoid split as an alternative to tracheotomy. Ann Otol Rhinol Laryngol. 1980;89(6 Pt 1):508–11.

Congenital Malformations of the Trachea

7

Karen B. Zur

Abstract

Tracheal malformations consist of a variety of anomalies related to abnormal development of the tracheobronchial tree. The most common clinical findings associated with tracheal narrowing include biphasic stridor with a prolonged expiratory component and cough that can be wet or bronchial in nature (from retained secretions). This chapter focuses on tracheomalacia, tracheal stenosis, tracheoesophageal fistula, tracheal bronchus, and bronchogenic cysts.

Keywords

Tracheomalacia • Tracheal stenosis • Tracheoesophageal fistula • Tracheal bronchus and bronchogenic cysts

Embryology of the Trachea

The lower aerodigestive tract begins its development during the embryonic phase of development (first 8 weeks post conception). This time period is divided into 23 stages according to the Carnegie system, and each is characterized by morphologically distinct structural development [1].

The laryngotracheal diverticulum (respiratory diverticulum) appears between the fourth and sixth branchial arches [2]. On the 20th day of embryonic development (stage 4), the foregut begins to appear and the respiratory diverticulum appears medially. There is no respiratory system development during the first eight stages of the Carnegie system.

The primitive pharynx appears between the arches and pouches as the respiratory diverticulum continues to grow, and around 24 days (stage 11), the respiratory diverticulum splits into the two lung buds (Fig. 7.1a). These buds, marking the tracheal bifurcation, continue to descend while the tracheoesophageal separation

K.B. Zur, M.D. (✉)
Division of Pediatric Otolaryngology, Center for Pediatric Airway Disorders, The Children's Hospital of Philadelphia, 3400 Civic Center Boulevard, 1 Wood ENT, Philadelphia, PA 19104, USA

Department of Otolaryngology: Head and Neck Surgery, Perelman School of Medicine at the University of Pennsylvania, Philadelphia, PA, USA
e-mail: zur@email.chop.edu

L.M. Elden and K.B. Zur (eds.), *Congenital Malformations of the Head and Neck*,
DOI 10.1007/978-1-4419-1714-0_7, © Springer Science+Business Media New York 2014

remains intact. During this stage, the respiratory and digestive systems develop separately, demarkated by the tracheoesophageal septum (Fig. 7.1b).

Early in the fetal stage (30 mm Crown Rump [C-R] stage), the primordium of the circular muscles of the trachealis are visible as are the epiglottis, thyroid cartilage, and the hyaline tracheal cartilage rings. As the fetal stage progresses, the circular muscles of the trachea continue to develop and mature. At 100 mm CR stage both muscular layers are developed.

Anatomy of the Trachea

The trachea begins immediately caudal to the cricoid cartilage at the level of the sixth cervical vertebra (C6) and extends to the carina, where it bifurcates between thoracic vertebrae 4 and 5 (T4-5). In the adult, it measures about 11 cm and is composed of 15–20 rings of U-shaped hyaline cartilages (Fig. 7.2). In males, the trachea grows until about 20 years of age, while in females the growth halts at about 14 years of age.

The fibers of the trachea are innervated by the recurrent laryngeal nerve, and the sympathetic nerve supply is from the middle cervical ganglion. The blood supply is divided into lateral tracheal wall and lateral-anterior tracheal walls. The lateral supply is from the longitudinal vessels of the inferior thyroid artery, subclavian artery, supreme intercostal artery, internal thoracic artery, brachiocephalic trunk, and bronchial arteries at the bifurcation of the trachea. The anterior supply is via transverse segmental vessels that run in the soft tissue between the cartilages. These vessels originate in the longitudinal vessels mentioned above, and then arborize to supply the submucosal capillaries.

The venous drainage is into the left inferior thyroid vein or the laryngeal vein. The inferior thyroid veins originate on the thyroid isthmus.

Lymphatic drainage is into the pretracheal, paratracheal, and tracheobronchial nodal groups.

Tracheomalacia

Definition

This anomaly refers to laxity in the tracheal cartilage rings with resultant airway compression either due to problems related to the intrinsic strength of the cartilage or due to extrinsic compression by vasculature or masses.

History

Tracheomalacia was first described by Sprague et al. in 1933 [3] in relation to vascular compression.

Incidence

The true incidence of tracheomalacia is difficult to report as many cases of mild tracheomalacia are undiagnosed. One report estimates tracheomalacia to be present in 1 in 1,445 infants. Tracheomalacia associated with various syndromes has an incidence that parallels that of the syndrome and is, therefore, much lower [4].

Heredity

The mode of inheritance has not been defined in isolated cases. It is variable when associated with the syndromes that will be described below.

Etiology

Tracheomalacia can be a result of an intrinsic cartilaginous weakness or caused by extrinsic compression of the C-shaped tracheal rings. The intrinsic, or primary tracheomalacia, is due to a weakness and abnormality in the tracheal wall (Fig. 7.3). Secondary tracheomalacia could be due to external forces applied to the tracheal wall such as vascular compression (aberrant innominate artery, double aortic arch, or pulmonary artery sling), tracheoesophageal fistula (TEF) repair, a mediastinal mass leading to localized compression, or due to the presence of a laryngotracheal cleft [5] (Fig. 7.4). Finally, the presence of a tracheostomy tube can cause localized tracheal wall trauma and weakness (Fig. 7.5).

Associated Malformations

As mentioned in the previous section, patients who have cardiac anomalies with vascular aber-

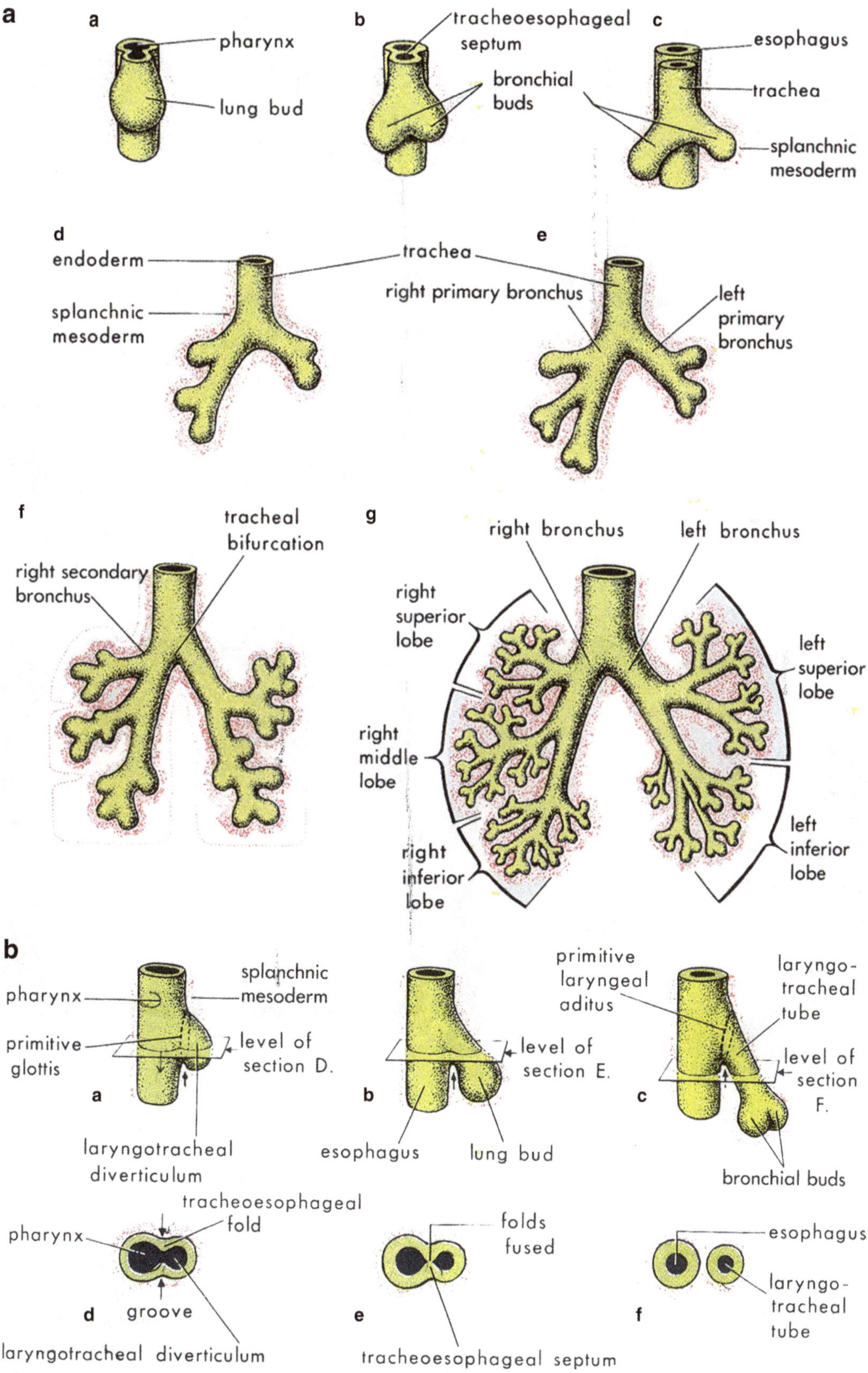

Fig. 7.1 (**a**, **b**) Schematics of embryologic development of trachea and lungs. (From Moore KL, Persaud TVN. *The Developing Human*: *Clinically Oriented Embryology*, 5th ed. Philadelphia: W.B. Saunders; 1993:228. Copyright Elsevier 1993)

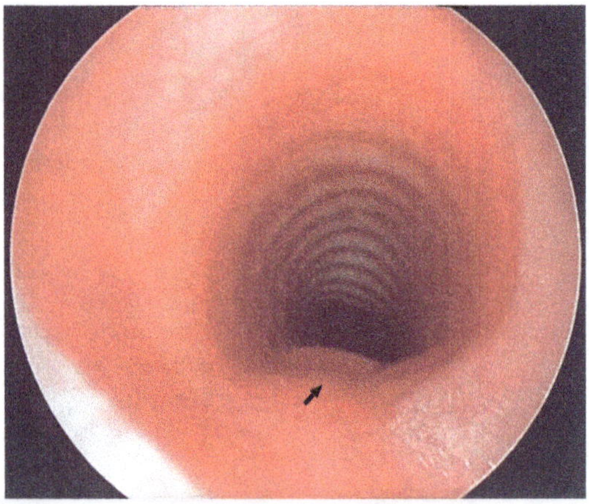

Fig. 7.2 Endoscopic photograph of normal trachea taken just above carina demonstrating horseshoe-shaped cartilages anteriorly and posterior strip of longitudinal muscle which contains no cartilage (*arrow*). (From Moore KL, Persaud TVN. *The Developing Human: Clinically Oriented Embryology*, 5th ed. Philadelphia: W.B. Saunders; 1993:227. Copyright Elsevier 1993)

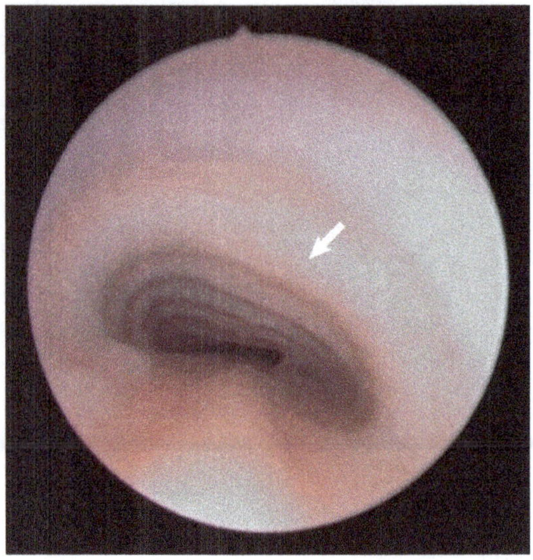

Fig. 7.4 Endoscopic photograph of tracheomalacia caused by external compression from innominate artery. On dynamic endoscopy, pulsations were seen near the arrow

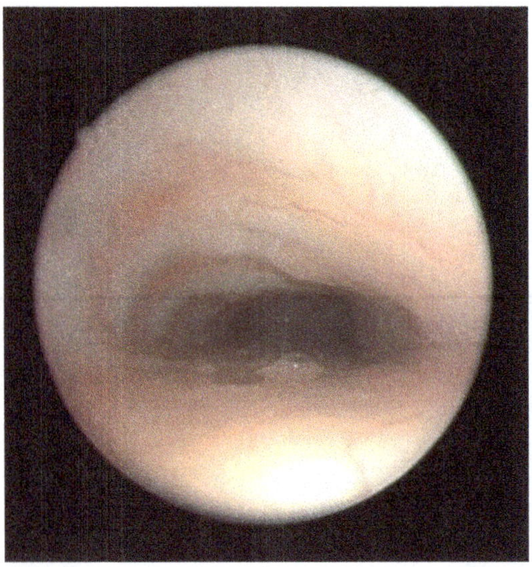

Fig. 7.3 Endoscopic photograph of trachea with intrinsic tracheomalacia. Dynamic endoscopy revealed no pulsations

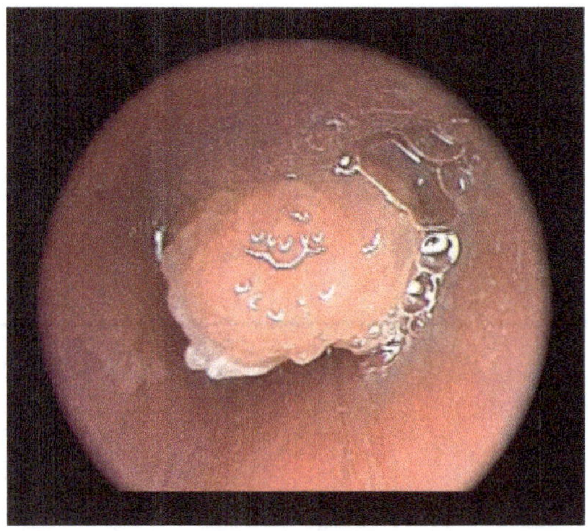

Fig. 7.5 Endoscopic photograph of suprastomal fibroma

rancies and those who have had tracheoesophageal fistula repair are predisposed to tracheomalacia. The resultant extrinsic vascular compression may at times compromise the tracheal wall to such an extent that it intermittently closes off the airway causing severe cough and intermittent life-threatening events may ensue. Patients who have undergone repair of a TEF rarely (1.85 %) continue to have symptoms of tracheomalacia [6].

Clinical Features

Tracheomalacia should be considered in a child presenting with a history of expiratory stridor and/or chronic cough. The symptoms are episodic, and the child may seem healthy with no signs of airway compromise between events. In the neonate, unexplained episodes of cyanosis related to severe agitation, crying or feeding (dying spells) should lead to an investigation that includes tracheomalacia in the differential diagnosis. Cough and grunting are symptoms associated with but not exclusive of tracheomalacia. Grunting leads to an auto-positive end expiratory pressure (PEEP) that effectively stents the tracheal airway open as a compensatory mechanism. In cases of vascular anomalies, dysphagia may be a presenting feature (27 %) as well [7].

Diagnosis

The gold standard used to diagnose tracheomalacia is bronchoscopy [8]. A high index of suspicion is important, however, as tracheomalacia may be misdiagnosed as asthma especially in the older patient. Flexible and rigid bronchoscopy are employed to perform the airway evaluation. Rigid bronchoscopy provides high-definition detailed information to evaluate for laryngotracheal clefting and subglottic stenosis that can often be missed on flexible exam. However, the rigid bronchoscope can stent the trachea during the evaluation, thus under-estimating the tracheomalacia severity or missing more subtle findings. The endoscopic findings of tracheomalacia will include flattening of the tracheal rings with a "fish mouth" appearance of the distal airway (Fig. 7.3). In cases of extrinsic vascular compression, the following three characteristic findings are identified: (1) oblique flattening of the right anterior wall above carina (aberrant innominate artery) (Fig. 7.4), (2) triangular compression above the carina (double aortic arch), and (3) flattened lower tracheal wall with a collapsed right mainstem bronchus (pulmonary artery sling).

Several adjunct studies may also be helpful depending on the severity of findings or symptoms. These include barium swallow, magnetic resonance imaging or computed tomography with or without angiography to evaluate extrinsic compression/vasculature, and echocardiography in cases of suspected cardiac/vascular anomalies.

Management

In the majority of cases, in which symptoms are mild, conservative observation with parental reassurance suffices, as the disease is self-limiting. Usually, the symptoms resolve by 1–2 years of age without surgical intervention [9]. If significant tracheomalacia is identified, with worrisome symptoms including oxygen desaturations, bradycardias, and apnea, several approaches have been utilized, depending on the etiology. For intrinsic tracheomalacia, tracheostomy tube with or without continuous positive airway pressure (CPAP) is recommended. Vascular surgery for those patients with identified vascular anomalies that cause significant airway obstruction can lead to resolution of the symptoms without the need for a tracheostomy tube. Some patient will require the placement of temporary artificial airway until future growth if symptoms persist despite vascular reimplantation. Distal carinal tracheomalacia and bronchomalacia can be managed with CPAP. In some cases, airway reconstruction can remove localized segments of tracheomalacia. This option is reserved for the older child with short segments of collapse, or in cases where an indwelling tracheostomy tube led to suprastomal collapse.

Tracheal Cartilaginous Sleeve

Definition

Tracheal cartilaginous sleeve (TCS) is a congenital malformation characterized by fusion of the tracheal rings that may be isolated to a few tracheal arches, include the entire trachea, or extend beyond the carina into the bronchi. In this condition, distinct tracheal rings cannot be identified [10]. TCS has been reported only in children with craniosynostosis syndromes [11].

Incidence

No data are available on the prevalence of TCS in cartilaginous sleeve (CS) syndromes [12].

Heredity

TCSs are associated with the craniosynostosis syndromes. In a report by Hockstein et al., five of six patients with Pfeiffer syndrome had TCS [10]. All patients had mutations in the Fibroblast

Growth Factor Receptor 2 (FGFR2), transmitted in an autosomal dominant pattern.

Etiology

TCSs are associated with the craniosynostosis syndromes. Pathologic evaluation of postmortem tracheal specimen showed cartilaginous sleeves with posterior interruption but lacking a normal pars membranacea. Davis et al. [12] demonstrated that the stained and cleared tracheas all demonstrate variable ring formation, usually limited to the posterolateral aspect. The functional significance of TCS, if any, is unknown. The formation of TCS implies a common mesenchymal defect in which normally discrete structures fuse and is probably analogous to other mesenchymal abnormalities seen in these patients.

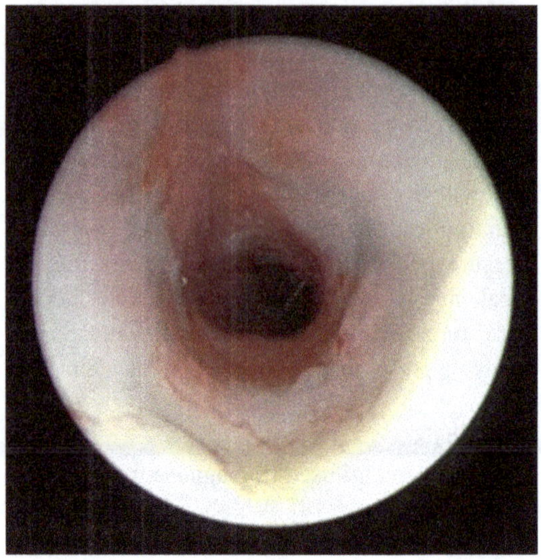

Fig. 7.6 Endoscopic view of tracheal cartilaginous sleeve that consists of a segment of fused cartilages. Note lack of discrete tracheal cartilage

Associated Malformations

TCSs are exclusively associated with the craniosynostosis syndromes and have been described in: Pfeiffer, Crouzon, and Goldenhar's syndromes.

Clinical Features

The presence of TCS may be clinically subtle, as many craniosynostosis patients with this finding are asymptomatic until later in age. In a 1992 report by Inglis et al., four newborn patients developed recurrent lower respiratory tract infections, reactive airway disease, and chronically retained secretions attributable to this anomaly. Neither tracheal stenosis nor stridor was encountered [13]. Many of the tracheal anomalies in these patients are detected later when the patient undergoes evaluation of other upper airway anomalies such as obstructive sleep apnea from midface obstruction or from adeontonsillar hypertrophy.

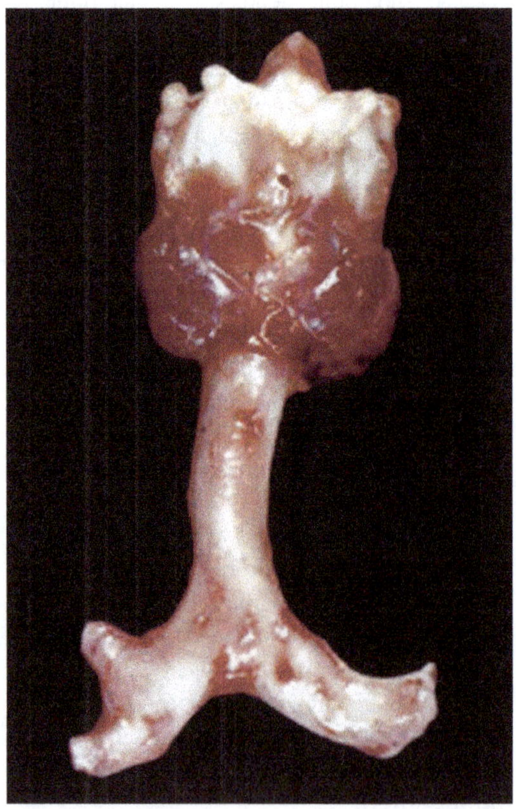

Fig. 7.7 Postmortem photograph of an airway with tracheal sleeve

Diagnosis

A high index of suspicion in patients with the craniosynostosis syndromes is of paramount importance, as TCS has only been described in this select group of patients. Bronchoscopy will delineate the degree of subglottic, tracheal, and bronchial involvement (Figs. 7.6 and 7.7). Due to the rigid nature of the trachea minimal to no respiratory movement is observed during endoscopy.

Management

Therapy is patient directed. In select patients with significant airway compromise or deteriorating pulmonary disease due to toilet issues, a tracheostomy is advisable and may extend the life expectancy [14]. Noorily et al. reported that 45 % of children with Crouzon's syndrome required tracheostomy tube placement [15]. However, many of these children also had inherent obstructive sleep apnea related to the maxillofacial deformities (choanal stenosis, adenotonsillar enlargement, midface hypoplasia). Close monitoring of the airway in the tracheotomized patient is essential, as granulation tissue and tube obstruction have frequently been encountered in these patients [10]. This is thought to be related to the lack of pliability of the trachea, leading to difficulty fitting an appropriately shaped tracheostomy tube, localized trauma, and fibrosis [16]. Tracheal resection or slide tracheoplasty have been reported when less than 40 % of the length of the trachea is involved; however, these may be risky procedures due to the tendency for poor healing noted in this condition [17].

Complete Tracheal Rings

Definition

Complete tracheal rings refer to the most common congenital malformation leading to tracheal stenosis. This condition is characterized by circumferential cartilaginous tracheal ring with no posterior pars membranacea. The pars membranacea is the muscular posterior wall of the trachea which normally lacks tracheal rings.

History

Cohen and Landing were the first to describe the association between pulmonary artery sling and tracheal stenosis [18]. In 1982, the first surgical repair of complete tracheal ring in an infant was reported [19]. and 2 years later, the first successful procedure was accomplished [20].

Incidence

Symptomatic tracheal stenosis due to complete tracheal rings is rare and the incidence of undiagnosed complete tracheal rings is unknown [21].

Heredity

Unknown.

Etiology

Unknown.

Associated Malformations

Complete tracheal rings have been reported to be associated with an aberrant left pulmonary artery (pulmonary artery sling) in 35 % of cases [18, 22]. In a separate review, 50–60 % of patients with pulmonary artery slings had complete tracheal rings and long segment tracheal stenosis. Associated intracardiac anomalies have been reported to occur in 24 % of patients with complete tracheal rings [22]. In addition, patients with trisomy 21 have been shown to have an a higher risk of having complete tracheal rings. A recent report showed that 17.5 % of patients with complete tracheal rings (7/40) had Downs syndrome [23].

Clinical Features

Episodic or progressive respiratory distress, biphasic stridor, "washing machine" breathing sounds [24], cyanosis or a difficult intubation have all been reported as the clinical presentation of complete tracheal rings. Symptoms may often get exacerbated by an upper respiratory infection. Due to the distal trapped secretions, recurrent pulmonary infections can be seen.

Diagnosis

Bronchoscopy is the standard for diagnosis of complete tracheal rings (Fig. 7.8a, b). The endoscopy allows direct visualization of the trachea, ruling-out any other synchronous lesion of the upper airway. Other diagnostic modalities in the stable patient include magnetic resonance imaging (MRI) or computed tomography (CT) imaging to evaluate the pulmonary vasculature (Fig. 7.9a–c). An echocardiogram should be performed in all patients to rule-out pulmonary artery sling.

Management

In a recent report, it had been shown that 10 % of patients with complete tracheal rings will not require any surgical reconstruction or intervention [21]. The remainder will require a tracheal

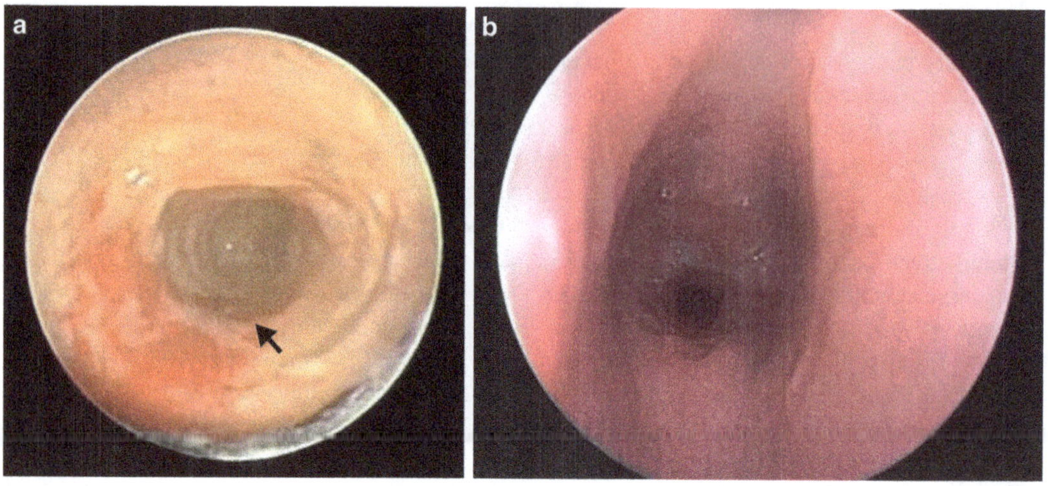

Fig. 7.8 Endoscopic view of complete tracheal ring in two patients which demonstrates (**a**) lack of normal pars membranacea (*arrow*). (**b**) More severe midtracheal stenosis (*arrowhead*)

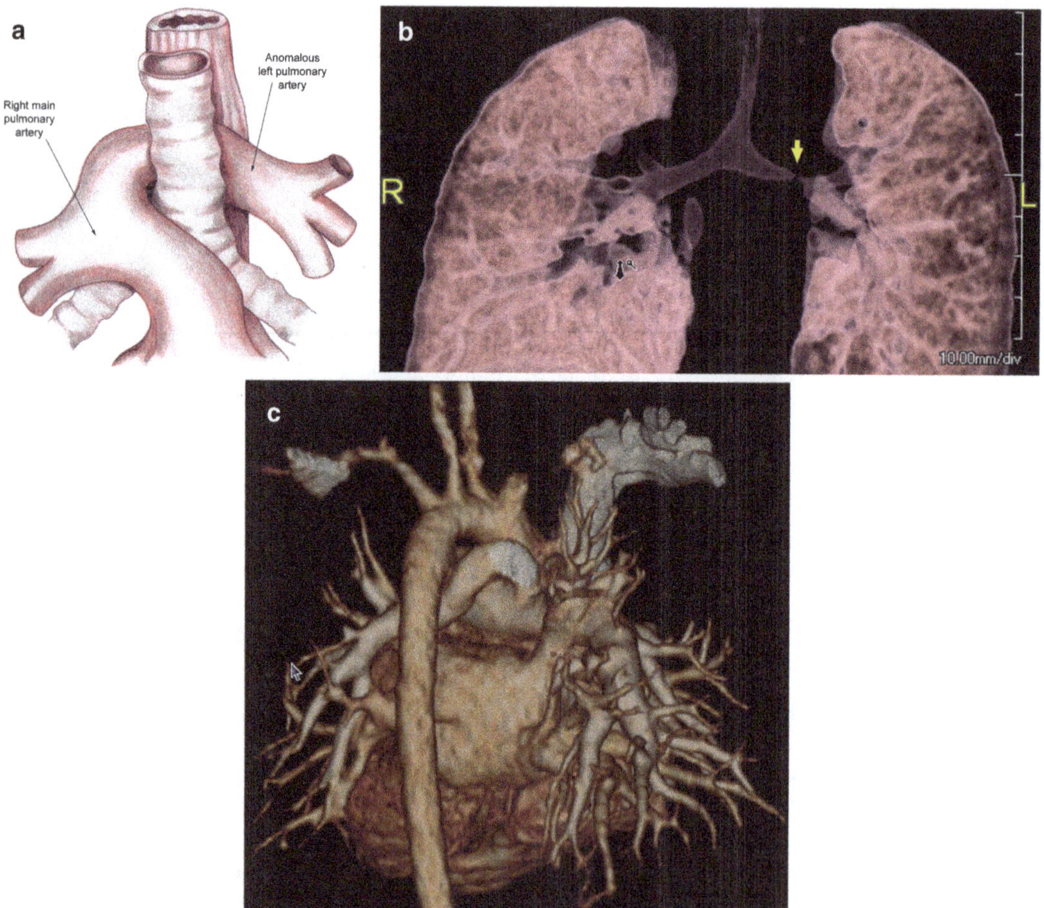

Fig. 7.9 (**a**) Schematic image; (**b**, **c**) 3D rendered volume CT angiogram images demonstrating pulmonary artery sling (*arrow* on **b**)

reconstruction with either a slide tracheoplasty or a patch tracheoplasty [24].

Tracheoesophageal Fistula (TEF)

Definition

Tracheoesophageal fistula (TEF) refers to a communication between the trachea and esophagus. A TEF may be congenital or acquired.

History

The first description of a TEF dates to 1697, Thomas Gibson described a neonate with an esophageal atresia and TEF. The first surgical reconstruction of this lesion was described in 1941 and was associated with a 70 % mortality rate [25].

Incidence

Congenital esophageal atresia and/or TEF have an incidence of 1 in 3,000–4,500 live births [26]. Acquired TEFs are rare and the incidence is not known.

Heredity

VATER/VACTERL (Vertebral, Anal, Cardiac, Tracheo-Esophageal Fistula, Esophageal atresia, Renal, Radial dysplasia) association is a relatively common, nonrandom multiple-malformation condition. The incidence is reported to be 1.6 in 10,000 [27]. No consistent or recurring etiology has been established for the VATER/VACTERL association, but it has been more frequently reported in the offspring of diabetic mothers. Most cases occur as sporadic events with low recurrence risk. The pattern of malformation has generally been a sporadic occurrence; thus, there is probably a low recurrence risk (<1 %) [27].

Etiology

The trachea and esophagus both originate from the primitive foregut. During the fourth to sixth weeks of gestation, the caudal foregut forms a ventral diverticulum that later develops into the trachea. The common membrane between the esophagus and trachea, the tracheoesophageal fold, creates a septum between the two, and if it deviates posteriorly, a communication between both tubes will form. The exact cause is unknown, but it is thought to result from a developmental disorder in formation and separation of the primitive foregut into trachea and esophagus. It is generally felt to be a heterogeneous disorder with the various yet-to-be established etiologies working through a common embryological pathway [27].

Acquired TEF can result from localized trauma after ingestion of toxic foreign bodies such as a battery, localized infection which devascularizes the wall of the esophagus, malignancy or from traumatic or prolonged intubation of the esophagus or trachea (either with an endotracheal tube or a tracheostomy tube). Cuff pressures exceeding 30 cm H_2O can promote trachealis necrosis and a consequent acquired TEF.

Associated Malformations

Nearly 50 % of patient with a congenital esophageal atresia/TEF have one or more anomalies, with cardiac anomalies being the most commonly recognized [26]. Other recognized associations are chromosomal abnormalities (Trisomy 21 and 18, 8 %), and gastrointestinal malformations as seen in VATER/VACTREL and CHARGE: imperforate anus, esophageal atresia, pyloric stenosis, duodenal atresia, and annular pancreas (38 %) [26]. The association between TEF, vertebral anomalies, anal atresia, and radial dysplasia was first described by Quan and Smith in 1972 [28].

Clinical Features

The diagnosis of a congenital TEF is usually made in the early postnatal period as it is often associated with life-threatening pulmonary events, cough related to feeds and copious frothy secretions in the early neonatal period. It should be suspected with a history of recurrent aspiration pneumonias or aspiration.

Diagnosis

Prenatal ultrasonography has facilitated the diagnosis of esophageal atresia and early diagnosis of TEF as it reveals lack of gastric air bubble and is a cause of maternal polyhydramnios. Barium swallow investigation as well as a bronchoscopy are supplemental in the investigation of a potential communication between the tracheal and

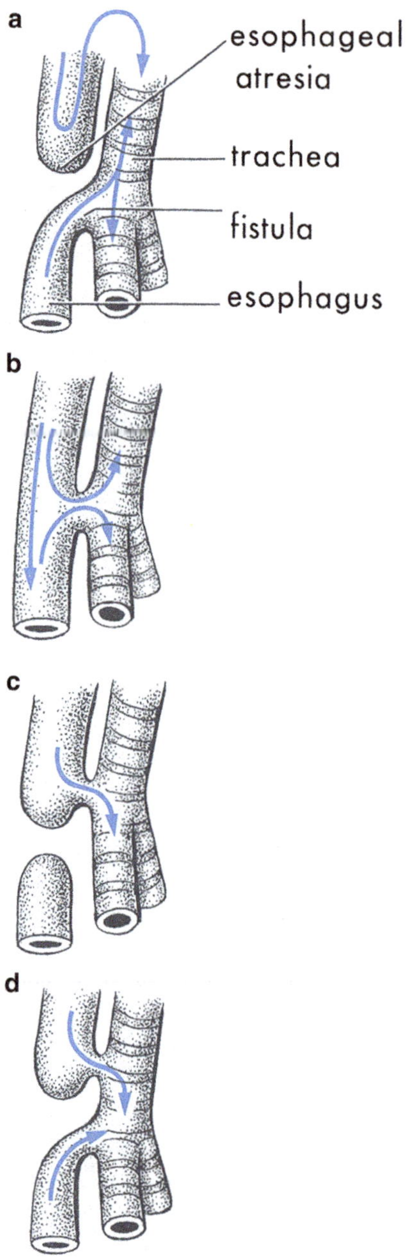

Fig. 7.10 Schematic of more common variations of tracheoesophageal atresia with and without fistula (From Moore KL, Persaud TVN. *The Developing Human: Clinically Oriented Embryology*, 5th ed. Philadelphia: W.B. Saunders; 1993:229. Copyright Elsevier 1993)

esophagus. Although there are several varieties of TEF, the most common association between an esophageal atresia (EA) and TEF is a proximal esophageal atresia and distal TEF (86.5 %) (Figs. 7.10–7.11b).

Management

Surgical management is the mainstay of treatment. Closure of the communication between the trachea and esophagus can be performed transthoracically or trans-tracheally (Fig. 7.12).

Tracheal Agenesis

Definition

Tracheal agenesis is a rare condition in which the trachea intervening between the subglottic cricoid and carina is absent or severely narrowed (atretic) [29].

History

Tracheal agenesis was first described in 1900 by Payne [30].

Incidence

Tracheal agenesis is extremely rare, only 116 reported cases have been found in the literature [29].

Heredity

Unknown.

Etiology

According to the theories described in the TEF section regarding the tracheal and esophageal development, tracheal atresia occurs when there is failure of the distal elongation of the caudal diverticulum which normally forms the trachea [29]. More recent reports purport that hedgehog signaling is involved in this process and that exogenous factors like adriamycin might cause tracheoesophageal malformations by interfering with this signaling pathway [31].

Associated Malformations

Evans reviewed 100 cases of tracheal agenesis and categorized this finding into four groups based on associated malformations. Tracheal agenesis, complex congenital cardiac anomalies, radial ray defects, and duodenal atresia (TACRD) describes an association separate from VATER/VACTREL [32]. This latter group includes either tracheal stenosis or atresia in a group of associated malformations: vertebral, anal atresia,

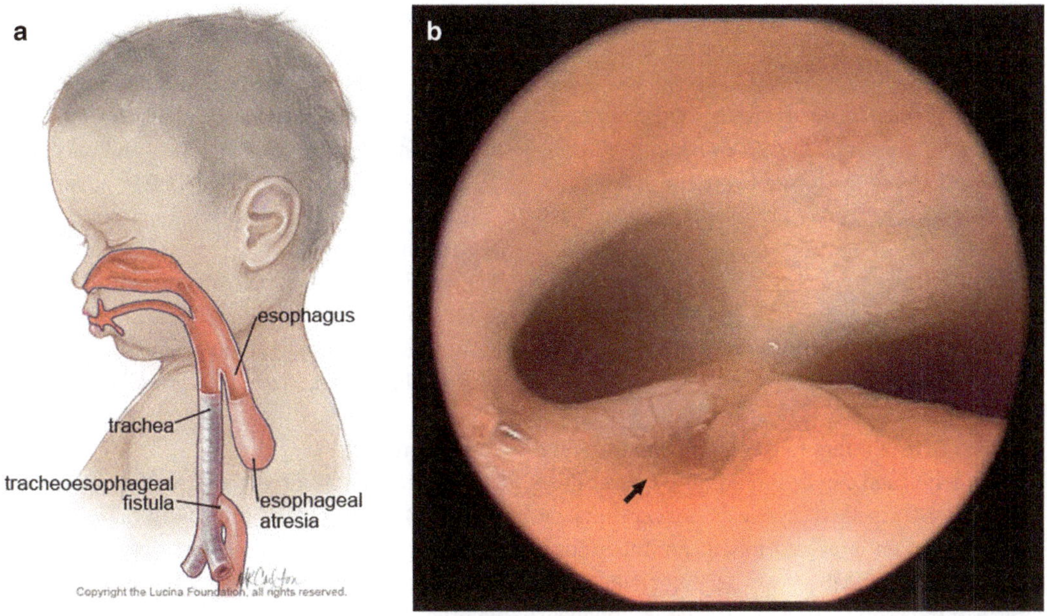

Fig. 7.11 (**a**) Schematic of most common type of tracheoesophageal atresia with distal fistula (Image courtesy of the Lucina Foundation). (**b**) Endoscopic view of fistula in posterior distal trachea

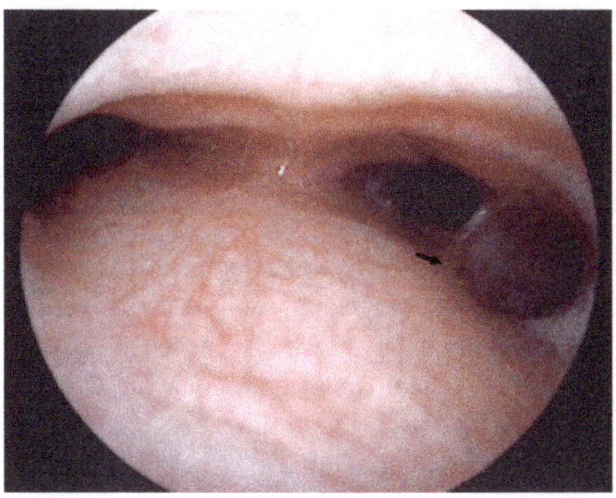

Fig. 7.12 Endoscopic photograph of a pig bronchus (*arrow*)

esophageal esophageal atresia, radial dysplasia, renal defects plus cardiovascular, and limb defects [33]. The underlying mechanisms responsible for these associations remains unclear, but is likely a result of abnormal epithelial mesenchymal interactions or a disruption of early blastogenesis [32].

Clinical Features

Tracheal agenesis is a devastating condition that leads to airway obstruction and absent cry. Some infants are able to survive the first few hours of life, relying on a bronchoesophageal fistula. Intubation is not possible, but mask ventilation can maintain oxygenation through the fistula. To maintain ventilation, pharyngeal intubation has been shown to prolong life in a few report cases.

Diagnosis

Diagnosis is made at birth. Bronchoscopy and esophagoscopy confirm the findings of a blind or severely compromised tracheal pouch and a distal esophago-bronchial communication.

Management

Immediate mask ventilation and pharyngeal intubation are done on an emergent basis as a tracheostomy tube may not be possible due to lack of intervening tracheal cartilages between the larynx and carina. Once the patient is stabilized, a formal cervical pharyngotomy through which the patient remains ventilated has been shown in two case reports to prolong life. Further esophageal reconstruction is necessary to band the lower esophagus, place a gastrostomy, and eventually reconstruct the esophagus. Devastating complications related to the unstable airway and significant morbidity from the esophageal surgery portend a poor prognosis [29].

Tracheal Atresia

Definition

Tracheal atresia refers to a congenital narrowing of the trachea and can be thought of as part of the spectrum of tracheal agenesis, except that a small lumen is present, albeit nonfunctional. Most often, tracheal atresia is associated with atresia of the esophagus and a tracheoesophageal fistula [34].

History

The first reported case of tracheal atresia with an associated esophageal atresia was in 1972.

Incidence

This condition is extremely rare. Only a few reports of tracheal atresia have been found in the literature [31, 34].

Heredity

Unknown. There is a reported male:female ratio of 2:1.

Etiology

During embryonal stages 12 and 13 the trachea starts to form when the lung buds protrude from the foregut and move into a caudal direction. Mesenchymal cells subsequently constitute the tracheoesophageal septum. If this process fails, different forms of esophageal and tracheal atresia and fistulas can develop [31].

Associated Malformations

Ninety percent (90 %) of the cases of tracheal atresia have other associated conditions, mostly affecting the cardiovascular, gastrointestinal, or genitor–urinary systems [35].

Clinical Features

At birth, a constellation of respiratory distress, failure to pass an endotracheal tube below the level of the vocal folds, lack of a cry, ability to bag-mask ventilate are suggestive of a tracheal anomaly such as atresia with a possible distal TEF.

Diagnosis

Prenatal diagnosis of tracheal atresia may be suggested based on ultrasound findings of polyhydramnios, large echogenic lungs, dilated airways, inverted diaphragm, and massive ascites [31].

Management

If congenital high airway obstruction syndrome (CHAOS) is diagnosed prenatally based on the above ultrasonic telltale signs, a procedure to secure the airway while the fetus is still receiving maternal oxygenation can be performed. This surgical intervention, termed EXIT procedure, for ex utero intra partum treatment, allows placement of a tracheostomy tube in these patients via a maternal hysterotomy. Later surgical intervention to reconstruct the airway is possible but not feasible in all cases if the atresia segment is long.

Tracheal Stenosis

Definition

Tracheal stenosis refers to a narrowing of the trachea due to any of the conditions described above in detail (tracheal atresia, agenesis, TCS, and complete tracheal rings). Iatrogenic or acquired tracheal stenosis could result, most commonly, secondary to trauma, intubation injury or burn.

History

Congenital tracheal stenosis was first described in 1899 by Gregor [36]. Postintubation tracheal stenosis was first described by Cooper and Grillo in 1969 [37].

Incidence

The incidence of tracheal stenosis is dependent on the type of stenosis as described in the previous sections. Acquired tracheal stenosis, either due to intubation or an indwelling tracheostomy tube, has been reported to be in the range of 6–20 % and 0.6–20 %, respectively.

Heredity

Not applicable to the acquired tracheal stenosis. See other sections for diagnosis-specific heredity information.

Etiology

Trauma, intubation, and burn injuries, which most commonly afflict the pediatric trachea, can lead to injury due to localized inflammation and devascularization of the tracheal wall/perichondrium. This leads to chondritis (inflammation of the cartilage) and scarring of the trachea which consequently may lead to stenosis.

Associated Malformations

A rare condition recently described in the literature is associated with diffuse tracheal calcification and stenosis. The X-linked recessive form of chondrodysplasia punctata has been reported to have an association with chondrodysplasia and punctate calcification of cartilage, and is believed to result from a defect in the vitamin K-dependent enzyme arylsulfatase E [38].

Clinical Features

Patients with tracheal stenosis may present with shortness of breath (with or without exertion), stridor, and retractions. Dependent on the degree of narrowing, these symptoms may be more or less subtle.

Diagnosis

Bronchoscopy is the gold standard of visualization and diagnosis of tracheal abnormalities, such as tracheal stenosis (Fig. 7.13). Adjunctive studies such as the CT scan or MRI may reveal associated anomalies in cases of congenital tracheal stenosis (see previous sections). Plain airway films or fluoroscopy may allow visualization of gross tracheal stenosis.

Management

The management of tracheal stenosis is dependent on the degree of symptomatology. In mild cases, observation is often possible. In patients with more concerning airway symptoms, tracheal reconstruction either by resection or augmentation has been shown to be successful [24]. Tracheostomy placement is another method to bypass the level of tracheal narrowing either in lieu of or in preparation for future reconstruction. Some surgeons advocate placement of tracheal stents following dilation of the trachea in cases of mild stenosis [39].

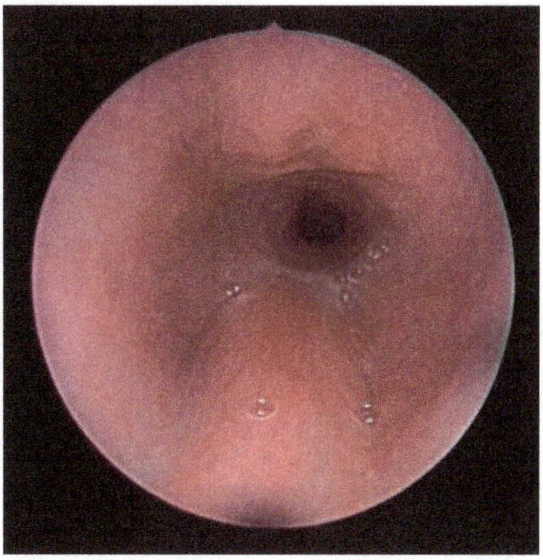

Fig. 7.13 Endoscopic view of tracheal stenosis

Tracheal Bronchus (Pig Bronchus, Tracheal Diverticula, Tracheal Lobe)

Definition

Congenital tracheal bronchus refers to a pouch formation in the distal trachea, between 2 and 6 mm above the bifurcation into the right and left mainstem bronchi. It is often referred to as a Pig Bronchus when the entire right upper lobe bronchus is displaced on the trachea [40].

History

The first report of a right upper lobe tracheal bronchus was by Sandifort in 1785 [40].

Incidence

The incidence of tracheal diverticula has been reported to be about 0.3 % in bronchoscopies

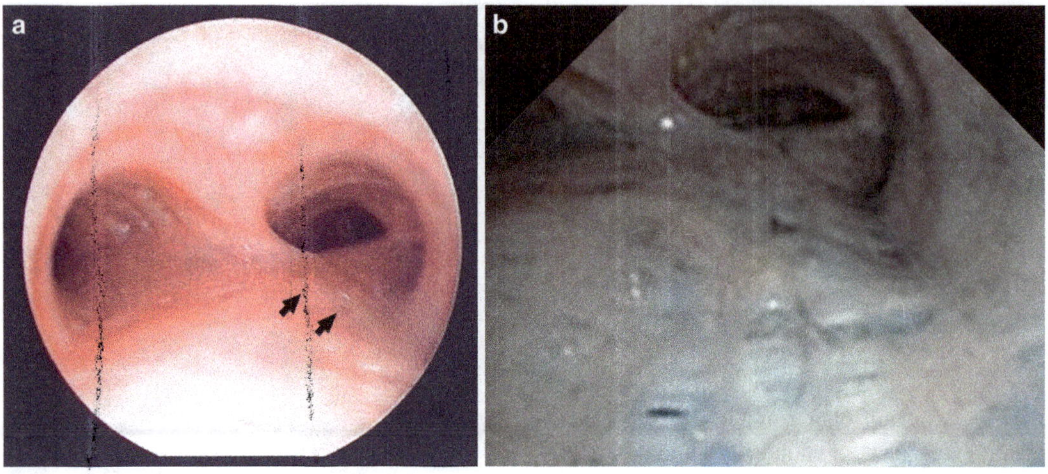

Fig. 7.14 (**a**, **b**) Endoscopic photograph of multiple small diverticula of distal airway (*arrows*) with and without methylene blue staining, respectively

performed in patients older than 10 years of age and in 1 % of autopsies [41, 42].

Heredity

Unknown.

Etiology

There are multiple theories to explain the aberranices in tracheal and bronchial segmentations [43]. It is thought that the development of a tracheal bronchus occurs after 32 days of gestation, at which point the bronchi branch and elongate [40]. The pig bronchus is believed to represent vestigial supernumerary lungs or aborted abnormally high divisions of the primary lung bud. If it is associated with surrounding lung tissue, it is properly referred to as "accessory tracheal bronchi" [42]. Tracheal diverticula can form iatrogenically following repair of a TEF.

Associated Malformations

An aberrant tracheal bronchus can be associated with other anomalies as described in two cases in which the patient had an azygos lobe ventilated by a displaced right aberrant bronchus, partial anomalous pulmonary venous return, displaced accompanying segmental arteries, and supernumerary lobe completely separated from adjacent lung by an accessory fissure [40].

Clinical Features

This anomaly may have no symptoms associated with it [40]. Several presentations have been thought to be associated with a symptomatic pig bronchus: recurrent pulmonary infections, cough, and shortness of breath [42]. In children with tracheal diverticulum who require intubation or ventilation through a tracheostomy tube, the pouch may become a source of distal airway obstruction.

Diagnosis

Bronchoscopy is the gold standard for visualization and evaluation of the trachea including pig bronchus and diverticulum (Figs. 7.12 and 7.14a, b). Computed tomography has been used to further define the anatomy of the bronchi. Characteristic CT findings include air-filled tubular structure, often located posteriorly and to the right of the trachea, and communicating with the trachea. Inflammatory changes around the diverticulum may also be appreciated [42]. Barium swallow studies can be performed in cases of a suspected associated TEF.

Treatment

Because tracheal diverticula are often asymptomatic, conservative observation is common. In situation wherein the diverticulum is affecting ventilation, an open excision of the pouch or an endoscopic fulgarisation of the pouch may ablate the tracheal anomaly.

Bronchogenic Cyst

Definition

Bronchogenic cysts are primary mediastinal cysts that are lined with bronchial epithelium and thought to represent a foregut duplication. These cysts are tightly adherent to the bronchial or bronchiolar wall, and vary in size, measuring a few millimeters to a few centimeters. They may be filled with fluid, blood, or air and usually do not have intraluminal communication with the airway. These cysts are more commonly unilocular.

History

Bronchogenic cysts were first described in the literature in 1948 by Maier [44]. The term broncho-pulmonary foregut malformation was defined by Gerle in 1968, explaining the pathophysiology leading to its formation.

Incidence

The true incidence of bronchogenic cysts is unknown since most of them are asymptomatic. The incidence of bronchogenic cysts in the neonatal period is extremely rare. These congenital anomalies are often recognized later in childhood or even in adulthood. There is a reported prevalence of 0.05 % in the neonatal period and 10 % of cases are recognized at birth [45].

Heredity

Unknown.

Etiology

Bronchogenic cysts arise due to aberrant budding of the embryonic foregut. If the remnant remains attached to the primitive tracheobronchial tree, the cyst may be found along the tracheobronchial tree, pulmonary sequestration or in the mediastinum. If the remnant separates, then the solitary cyst may migrate in the neck and could be found in the mediastinum, neck, pericardium, vertebrae, subpleural space, and any other aberrant sites. Lesions arising before or during the embryonic site separation are found in the mediastinum (30 %). Lesions arising after the separation are intrapleural (70 %) and are lined with respiratory epithelium and cartilage. This supports a hypothesis of erratic tracheobronchial separation as a more feasible etiology than foregut duplication [46].

Associated Malformations

Bronchogenic cysts may be associated with other broncho-pulmonary foregut malformations such as tracheoesophageal fistula, esophageal diverticulum, esophageal cyst, and lung sequestration. Vertebral abnormalities (hemivertebrae) are often associated with bronchogenic cyst of mediastinal origin [46].

Clinical Features

Patients with undiagnosed bronchogenic cysts may present at birth with severe respiratory distress or cardiovascular compromise. In the infant, compression of the airway or esophagus from an enlarged cyst may lead to recurrent cough, wheezing, pneumonia, or obstructive emphysema. Progressive enlargement of the cyst can lead to superior vena cava syndrome, atrial compression, pericardial compression, bronchial atresia, pulmonary artery stenosis, or pneumothorax if the cyst ruptures into the pleural space.

Diagnosis

Diagnosis of bronchogenic cysts is rarely made on prenatal ultrasonography. In these unusual circumstances, sonography would reveal an anechoic unilocular cystic lesion in the lung fields.

Symptomatic postnatal patients can be diagnosed by routine chest radiography or sometimes by bronchoscopy (Fig. 7.15). Definitive diagnosis is made by use of a chest CT or MRI. A conventional 2-view chest radiograph would typically show a sharply demarcated spherical mass most

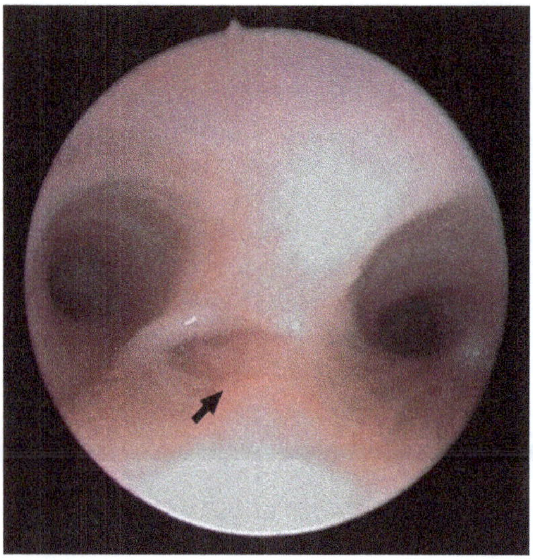

Fig. 7.15 Endoscopic photograph of a bronchial cyst near take off of carina (*arrow*)

commonly located around the carina. When the cyst is infected or contains secretions, it may appear as a solid tumor or may demonstrate an air fluid level. On a chest CT, bronchogenic cysts appear as lesions with smooth borders and thin walls and may contain secretions, pus, or blood. Sometimes calcification may be observed. MRI of the chest would reveal a homogeneous mass of moderate-to-bright intensity on T2-weighted MRI. On T1-weighted images, lesions may vary in their intensity because of their protein content. The finding on CT or MRI of a cystic lesion at the level of the carina is most frequently associated with a bronchogenic cyst [46].

Management

A prenatal diagnosis of bronchogenic cysts does not alter the indications for the mode of delivery. However, it is important to avoid significant positive pressure ventilation once the child is delivered in order to prevent possible progressive enlargement of the cyst. This could be fatal. Due to the unclear natural history of these lesions, with possible risks of pulmonary compression, infection, or malignant degeneration, it has been advocated to perform a complete excision of these lesions. If no prenatal diagnosis has been made, once symptoms ensue, a plain chest radiograph followed by a chest CT or MRI should be performed to evaluate the lesion. This will help solidify a diagnosis and allow for surgical planning. The two recommended surgical approaches for complete cyst excision are via a lobectomy or segmentectomy [44].

References

1. O'Rahilly R, Müller F. Chevalier Jackson lecture. Respiratory and alimentary relations in staged human embryos. New embryological data and congenital anomalies. Ann Otol Rhinol Laryngol. 1984;93(5 Pt 1):421–9.
2. Manoukian JJ, Tan AK. Embryology of the larynx. In: Tewfik TL, Der Kaloustian VM, editors. Congenital anomalies of the ear, nose, and throat. New York, NY: Oxford University Press; 1997.
3. Sprague H, Ernlund C, Albright F. Clinical aspects of persistent right aortic root. New Eng J Med. 1933;209:679–86.
4. Carden KA, Boiselle PM, Waltz DA, et al. Tracheomalacia and tracheobronchomalacia in children and adults: an in-depth review. Chest. 2005;127:984–1005.
5. Mitchell DB, Koltai P, Matthew D, et al. Severe tracheobronchomalacia associated with laryngeal cleft. Int J Pediatr Otorhinolaryngol. 1989;18(2):181–5.
6. Spitz L. Esophageal atresia and tracheoesophageal fistula in children. Curr Opin Pediatr. 1993;5(3):347–52.
7. Shah RK, Mora BN, Bacha E, et al. The presentation and management of vascular rings: an otolaryngology perspective. Int J Pediatr Otorhinolaryngol. 2007;71(1):57–62.
8. Altman KW, Wetmore RF, Mahboubi S. Comparison of endoscopy and radiographic fluoroscopy in the evaluation of pediatric congenital airway abnormalities. Int J Pediatr Otorhinolaryngol. 1998;44(1):43–6.
9. Jacobs IN, Wetmore RF, Tom LW, et al. Tracheobronchomalacia in children. Arch Otolaryngol Head Neck Surg. 1994;120(2):154–8.
10. Hockstein NG, McDonald-McGinn D, Zackai E, et al. Tracheal anomalies in Pfeiffer syndrome. Arch Otolaryngol Head Neck Surg. 2004;130:1298–302.
11. Scheid SC, Spector AR, Luft JD. Tracheal cartilaginous sleeve in Crouzon syndrome. Int J Pediatr Otorhinolaryngol. 2002;65:147–52.
12. Davis S, Bove KE, Wells TR, et al. Tracheal cartilaginous sleeve. Pediatr Pathol. 1992;12:349–64.
13. Inglis Jr AF, Kokesh J, Siebert J, et al. Vertically fused tracheal cartilage. An underrecognized anomaly. Arch Otolaryngol Head Neck Surg. 1992;118(4):436–8.
14. Mixter RC, David DJ, Perloff WH, et al. Obstructive sleep apnea in Apert's and Pfeiffer's syndromes: more than a craniofacial abnormality. Plast Reconstr Surg. 1990;86(3):457–63.

15. Noorily MR, Farmer DL, Belenky WM, et al. Congenital tracheal anomalies in the craniosynostosis syndromes. J Pediatr Surg. 1999;34:1036–9.
16. Lin SY, Chen JC, Hotaling AJ, et al. Congenital tracheal cartilaginous sleeve. Laryngoscope. 1995;105:1213–9.
17. Faust RA, Stroh B, Rimell F. The near complete tracheal ring deformity. Int J Pediatr Otorhinolaryngol. 1998;45(2):171–6.
18. Cohen SR, Landing BH. Tracheostenosis and bronchial abnormalities associated with pulmonary artery sling. Ann Otol Rhinol Laryngol. 1976;85(5 Pt. 1):582–90.
19. Janik JS, Nagaraj HS, Yacoub U, et al. Congenital funnel-shaped tracheal stenosis: an asymptomatic lethal anomaly of early infancy. J Thorac Cardiovasc Surg. 1982;83(5):761–6.
20. Idriss FS, DeLeon SY, Ilbawi MN, et al. Tracheoplasty with pericardial patch for extensive tracheal stenosis in infants and children. J Thorac Cardiovasc Surg. 1984;88(4):527–36.
21. Rutter MJ, Willging JP, Cotton RT. Nonoperative management of complete tracheal rings. Arch Otolaryngol Head Neck Surg. 2004;130:450–2.
22. Backer CL, Mavroudis C, Holinger LD. Repair of congenital tracheal stenosis. Semin Thorac Cardiovasc Surg Pediatr Card Surg Annu. 2002;5:173–86.
23. Bravo MN, Kaul A, Rutter MJ, et al. Down syndrome and complete tracheal rings. J Pediatr. 2006;148(3): 392–5.
24. Rutter MJ, Cotton RT, Azizkhan RG, et al. Slide tracheoplasty for the management of complete tracheal rings. J Pediatr Surg. 2003;38(6):928–34.
25. Haight C, Towsley HA. Congenital atresia of the esophagus with tracheoesophageal fistula. Surg Gynec Obstet. 1943;76:672.
26. Diaz LK, Akpek EA, Dinavahi R, et al. Tracheoesophageal fistula and associated congenital heart disease: implications for anesthetic management and survival. Paediatr Anaesth. 2005;15:862–9.
27. Hall BD. Vater/vacterl association. In: Cassidy SB, Allanson JE, editors. Management of genetic syndromes. Hoboken, NJ: John Wiley & Sons; 2010. p. 871–9.
28. Quan L, Smith DW. The VATER association: vertebral defects, anal atresia, tracheoesophageal fistula with esophageal atresia, radial dysplasia. Birth Defects. 1972;8:75–8.
29. Lander TA, Schauer G, Bendel-Stenzel E, et al. Tracheal agenesis in newborns. Laryngoscope. 2004;114:1633–6.
30. Payne WA. Congenital absence of the trachea. Brooklyn Med J. 1900;14:568.
31. Bercker S, Kornak U, Bührer C, et al. Tracheal atresia as part of an exceptional combination of malformations. Int J Pediatr Otorhinolaryngol. 2006;70(6):1137–9.
32. Evans JA, Reggin H, Greenberg C. Tracheal agenesis and associated malformations: a comparison with tracheoeso-phageal fistula and the VACTERL association. Am J Med Genet. 1985;21:21–34.
33. Wei JL, Rodeberg D, Thompson DM. Tracheal agenesis with anomalies found in both VACTERL and TACRD associations. Int J Pediatr Otorhinolaryngol. 2003;67(9):1013–7.
34. Sankaran K, Bhagirath CP, Bingham WT, et al. Tracheal atresia, proximal esophageal atresia, and distal tracheoesophageal fistula: report of two cases and review of literature. Pediatrics. 1983;71(5):821–3.
35. van Veenendaal MB, Liem KD, Marres HA. Congenital absence of the trachea. Eur J Pediatr. 2000;159:8.
36. Forsen Jr JW, Lusk RP, Huddleston CB. Costal cartilage tracheoplasty for congenital long-segment tracheal stenosis. Arch Otolaryngol Head Neck Surg. 2002;128(10):1165–71.
37. Cooper JD, Grillo HC. The evolution of tracheal injury due to ventilatory assistance through cuffed tubes: a pathologic study. Ann Surg. 1969;169(3): 334–48.
38. Wolpoe ME, Braverman N, Lin SY. Severe tracheobronchial stenosis in the X-linked recessive form of chondrodysplasia punctata. Arch Otolaryngol Head Neck Surg. 2004;130(12):1423–6.
39. Filler RM, Forte V, Chait P. Tracheobronchial stenting for the treatment of airway obstruction. J Pediatr Surg. 1998;33(2):304–11.
40. Ghaye B, Szapiro D, Fanchamps JM, et al. Congenital bronchial abnormalities revisited. Radiographics. 2001;21(1):105–19.
41. Frenkiel S, Assimes IK, Rosales JK. Congenital tracheal diverticulum. A case report. Ann Otol Rhinol Laryngol. 1980;89(5 Pt 1):406–8.
42. Early EK, Bothwell MR. Congenital tracheal diverticulum. Otolaryngol Head Neck Surg. 2002;127(1):119–21.
43. Evans JA. Aberrant bronchi and cardiac vascular anomalies. Am J Med Genet. 1990;35:46–54.
44. Tsunezuka Y, Shimizu Y, Tanaka N, et al. Progressive intraparenchymal bronchogenic cyst in a neonate. Ann Thorac Cardiovasc Surg. 2008;14(1):32–4.
45. Cooke FN, Blades B. Cystic disease of the lungs. J Thorac Surg. 1952;23:546–69.
46. Cuillier F, Bideault J, Daguindeau D, Alessandri JL, Cartault JF, Michel JL. Bronchogenic cyst. http://www.sonoworld.com/TheFetus/page.aspx?id=1504. Accessed 26 Sept 2012.

Congenital Malformations of the Neck

8

Jonathan A. MacLean and Steven E. Sobol

Abstract

This chapter includes embryologic and clinical descriptions, photographs, and illustrations of the more common congenital anomalies of the neck. The authors present the topics in sections based on the underlying pathology. These sections include descriptions of malformations resulting from abnormal development of (1) the branchial arches (branchial cleft cysts: first, second, third, and fourth branchial cleft fistulas; thymic cysts), (2) the thyroid gland (thyroglossal duct cysts), (3) the germ line tissue resulting in ecto/meso/endodermal anomalies (dermoids, teratomas, midline cervical cleft) and (4) the cervical vasculature and neural structures (lymphatic malformations, hemangiomas, neurofibromas).

Keywords

Branchial cleft cysts • Branchial fistula • Dermoid • Teratoma • Lymphatic malformation • Infantile hemangioma • Neurofibroma

J.A. MacLean, M.D.
Department of Otolaryngology – Head and Neck Surgery, Emory Children's Center, Emory University School of Medicine, 2015 Uppergate Drive, NE, Atlanta, GA 30322, USA

S.E. Sobol, M.D., M.Sc. (✉)
Division of Pediatric Otolaryngology, The Children's Hospital of Philadelphia, 1 Wood Center, 34th Street and Civic Center Boulevard, Philadelphia, PA 19104, USA

Department of Otolaryngology: Head and Neck Surgery, Perelman School of Medicine at the University of Pennsylvania, Philadelphia, PA, USA
e-mail: sobols@email.chop.edu

The diagnosis of a cervical lesion in a child can be a challenge, given the broad differential diagnosis and similarity between common and rare anomalies. Overall, pediatric neck masses can be categorized as congenital, inflammatory, or neoplastic. This chapter focuses on congenital cervical anomalies, providing a comprehensive review of both common and rare lesions. The pertinent embryology, clinical presentation, diagnostic work up, and treatment are presented, in order to help the practitioner develop strategies for managing these complex patients.

L.M. Elden and K.B. Zur (eds.), *Congenital Malformations of the Head and Neck*,
DOI 10.1007/978-1-4419-1714-0_8, © Springer Science+Business Media New York 2014

Branchial Cleft Anomalies

Embryology

A significant proportion of head and neck development is derived from the branchial apparatus. Development of this area begins between the fourth and sixth week of gestation. The embryo changes from a flattened tube to a more complex series of structures consisting of paired mesodermal branchial arches, endodermal lined pharyngeal pouches, ectodermal lined branchial clefts, and an unpaired ventral endodermal floor (Fig. 8.1) [1]. The branchial apparatus has four clefts on each side of the embryo at the level of the pharynx [2]. These are adjacent to five pharyngeal evaginations or "pouches." The interposed arches typically consist of a skeletal, ligamentous, muscular, vascular, and nervous components [3]. Arches ultimately develop to become the structures listed in Table 8.1.

In normal development, the first cleft will persist as the external auditory canal. The remaining three clefts develop into what is collectively known as the cervical sinus, which obliterates during the sixth and seventh weeks as the second arch grows inferiorly (Fig. 8.1).

The first pharyngeal pouch develops in to the middle ear and Eustachian tube, while the second pouch forms a portion of the pharynx including the palatine tonsil. The third pouch will later subdivide to become the thymus and the inferior parathyroid glands, whereas the fourth pouch derivative is the superior parathyroid gland. The fifth pouch is rudimentary and becomes part of the fourth pouch, ultimately developing into the parafollicular c-cells within the thyroid gland [3].

The first arch mesenchyme forms the majority of the malleus, incus and provides the framework for mandibular development. Muscle derivatives of the first arch correspond to those innervated by the trigeminal nerve. The first arch vascular structure becomes the internal maxillary artery. The second arch mesenchyme develops into the stapes suprastructure, styloid process, and portions of the hyoid. Muscle derivatives of the second arch correspond to those innervated by the facial nerve. The second arch artery is the stapedial, which typically obliterates but in rare cases can persist [4]. Third arch derivatives include the remainder of the hyoid bone, glossopharyngeal nerve, stylopharyngeus muscle as well as the common and internal carotid arteries. The fourth and sixth arches go on to form the framework of the larynx, its innervation and musculature. These arches also form the blood vessels within the mediastinum.

Definition

Branchial cleft anomalies can be divided into cysts, sinuses and fistulae. A cyst is an epithelial lined sac with no communication to the skin or the pharynx. A sinus has a connection to one surface (external or internal), and a fistula forms a communication between two epithelial surfaces (typically cutaneous and pharyngeal) [2].

History

Hunczowski has been credited with the first description of a cervical fistula in 1789; however, this anomaly was not attributed to the branchial apparatus until noted by Von Ascherson in 1832 [2]. Since the initial description, there have been extensive reviews in the literature regarding the embryology, diagnosis, and management of these conditions.

Heredity

Branchial cleft anomalies are most commonly sporadic but can be associated with inherited disorders such as branchio-oto-renal syndrome. This autosomal-dominant condition consists of hearing impairment, auricular anomalies, branchial cleft remnants, and renal abnormalities [5].

Table 8.1 Structures developed from branchial arch components

Arch	Artery	Nerve	Muscle	Skeletal	Ligament
First (mandibular, Meckel's)	Internal • Maxillary • Artery	Trigeminal	Muscles of mastication Mylohyoid Anterior belly of digastric Tensor tympani Tensor veli palatine	Malleus Incus	Anterior malleolar Sphenomandibular
Second (hyoid, Reichert's)	Stapedial	Facial	Muscles of facial expression Stapedius Stylohoid Posterior belly digastric	Stapes Styloid process Lesser cornu and upper body of hyoid	Stylohyoid
Third	Internal and Common Carotid arteries	Glossopharyngeal	Stylopharyngeus	Greater cornu and lower body of hyoid	
Fourth	Right: Subclavian Left: Aorta	Superior laryngeal	Cricothyroid Pharyngeal constrictors	Thyroid Cuneiform Epiglottis	
Sixth	Right: Right pulmonary artery Left: Left pulmonary artery, ductus arteriosus	Recurrent laryngeal	Intrinsic muscles of larynx	Cricoid Corniculate Arytenoid	

Adapted from Moore KL. *The Developing Human*: *Clinically Oriented Embryology*. 4th ed. Philadelphia, PA: W.B. Saunders; 1988

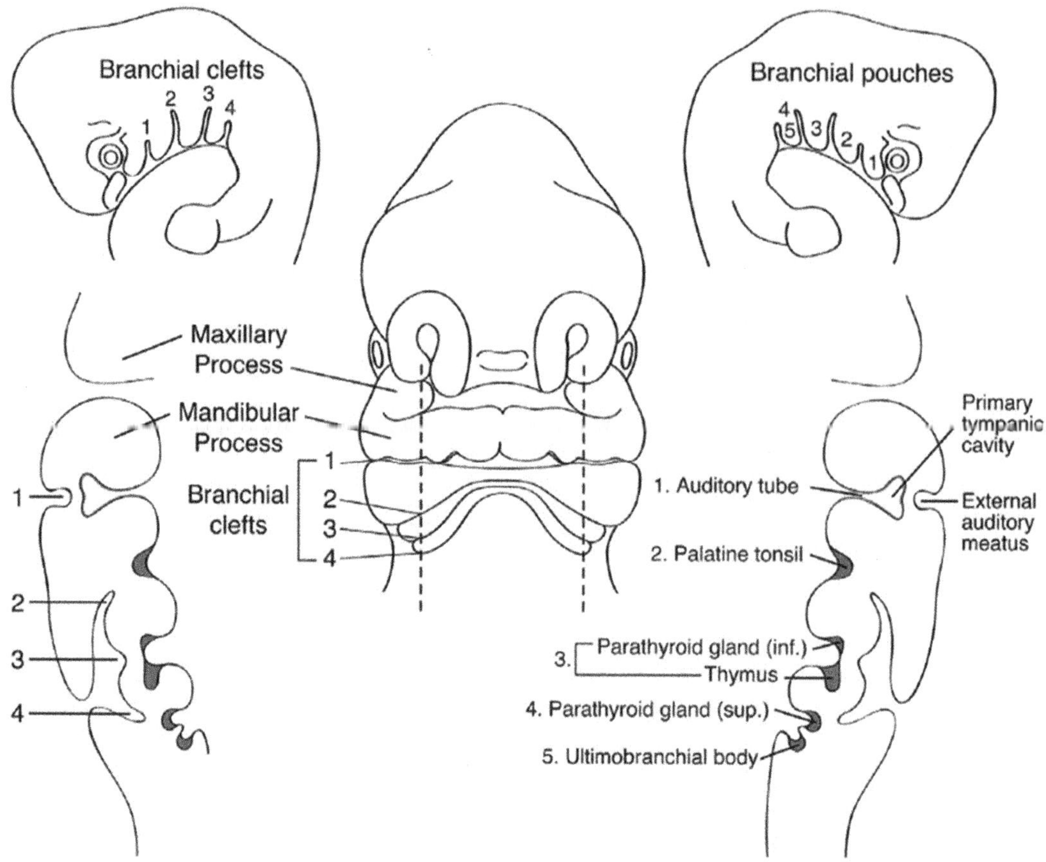

Fig. 8.1 A frontal schematic representation of a 5-mm human embryo at the fifth week of gestation. Sagital sections taken through the branchial apparatus demonstrate the anatomic relationship of external clefts and internal pouches as well as the derivation of important head and neck structures (Reprinted from *Seminars in Pediatric* Surgery, vol. 15, Waldhausen JHT, "Branchial cleft and arch anomalies in children," pp. 64–69, copyright 2006, with permission from Elsevier)

First Branchial Cleft Anomalies

Incidence

First branchial cleft anomalies are rare. They have an estimated incidence of 1 in 100,000 and account for less than 10 % of all branchial cleft anomalies [6, 7].

Etiology

Duplication or failure of obliteration of the embryologic tract is the likely etiology of these lesions. First branchial cleft anomalies are subdivided using the Work classification [8]. Type 1 anomalies are ectodermal in origin and consist of a duplication of the membranous portion of the auditory canal. They course medial to the conchal cartilage and can extend into the post-auricular crease. They pass anterior and deep to the lobule, stay superficial to the facial nerve and parallel to the normal external auditory canal. Type 2 anomalies have both ectodermal and mesodermal components. The external opening is near the angle of the mandible (Fig. 8.2), while the tract courses superiorly and can be closely associated to the facial nerve. The anomaly may present with a sinus inferior to the membranous ear canal or open into the canal itself, typically at the bony-cartilaginous junction [8].

Clinical Features

These lesions can present with findings attributable to the ear, parotid or neck regions. Otologic signs include otorrhea, which can be mucoid or purulent. Parotid signs generally include inflammation and can resemble primary parotitis with rapid gland enlargement and associated tenderness. Cervical signs include cellulitis, abscess, and drainage from a pit inferior to the mandible (Fig. 8.2).

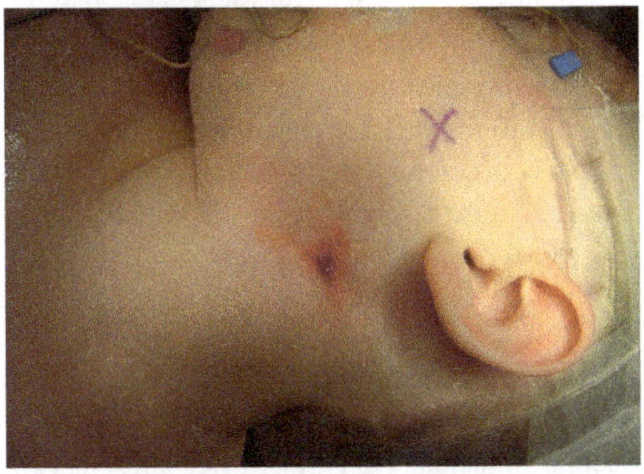

Fig. 8.2 Photo demonstrating the characteristic opening associated with a Type II, first branchial cleft anomaly

Diagnosis

First branchial cleft anomalies can be a diagnostic challenge and are often misdiagnosed and receive non-curative treatment (refer to Chap. 2). They must be differentiated from preauricular sinuses and tags, which have a different embryologic origin. A complete history and physical examination is the initial step in arriving at a diagnosis. Otoscopy should be performed to assess for any communication with the external auditory canal or attachment to the tympanic membrane. Facial nerve function should be recorded. Cervical skin should be closely examined for signs of a pit or sinus tract. Computed tomography (CT) or magnetic resonance imaging (MRI) scan can help delineate the course of the tract (Fig. 8.3).

Management

The treatment of first branchial cleft anomalies is surgical, and complete excision is necessary to prevent recurrence. In the majority of cases, definitive surgery requires a superficial parotidectomy approach with identification and preservation of the facial nerve. The nerve's relationship

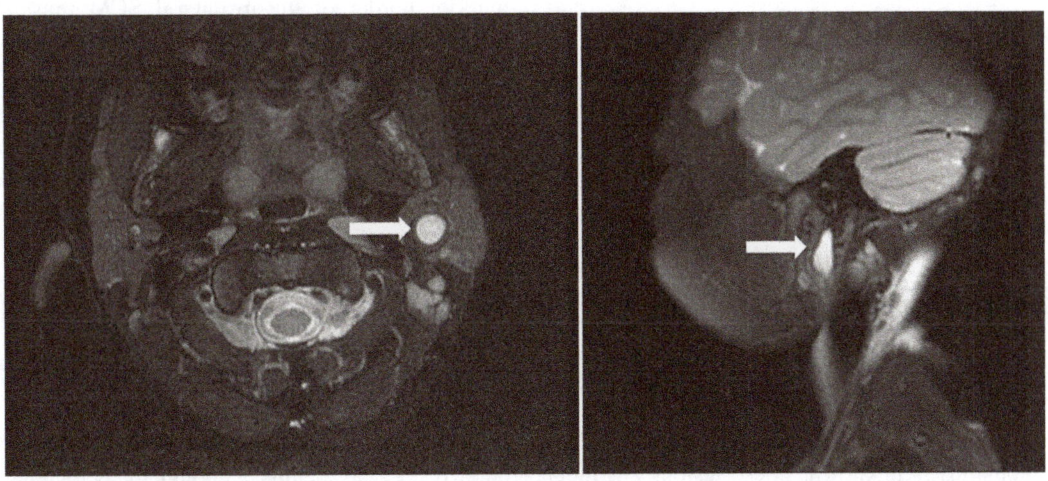

Fig. 8.3 Axial and sagital MRI images of a first branchial cleft anomaly (*arrows*). The lesion lies within the parotid gland and courses toward the ear canal

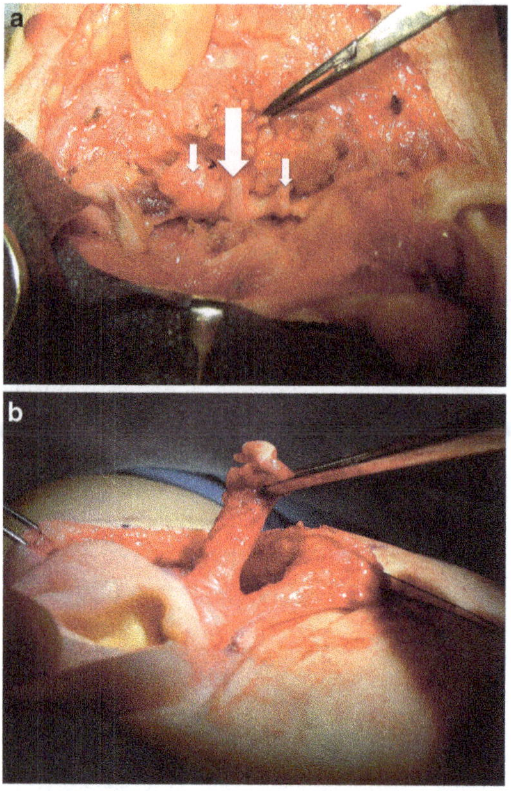

Fig. 8.4 (**a**) Intraoperative photograph demonstrating the close relationship between the first branchial cleft anomaly (*small arrows*) and the facial nerve (*large arrow*). The anomaly runs deep (*medial*) to the facial nerve. (**b**) Intraoperative photograph of another child with a branchial cleft anomaly that remained superficial (*lateral*) to the nerve, which has been dissected out from the parotid gland

to the lesion is variable and can be medial or lateral (Figs. 8.4a, b) [9]. In the case of abscess formation, incision and drainage is often required. Purulent material should be cultured to direct antimicrobial therapy, reserving full excision for after the resolution of infection.

Second Branchial Anomalies

Incidence

The true incidence of second branchial cleft anomalies is unknown. These lesions are much more common than other branchial anomalies, accounting for 90 % of these abnormalities. Overall, second branchial cleft anomalies are second only to thyroglossal duct cysts (TGDCs) as the most commonly diagnosed head and neck malformations.

Etiology

Failure of involution of the cervical sinus with or without connection to the pharynx is the most accepted theory for the development of second branchial anomalies. Second branchial fistulas pass between the second and third arch derivatives. Anatomically, the tract begins at the inferior aspect of the anterior border of the sternocleidomastoid (SCM) muscle, courses deep to the platysma, the stylohyoid and posterior belly of digastric muscles to the carotid sheath. It stays superficial to the glossopharyngeal nerve and travels between the internal and external carotid arteries before terminating in the tonsillar fossa (Fig. 8.5).

Clinical Features

Second branchial cleft cysts often present as a soft, mobile, painless, and slow growing mass in the lateral neck. They often present after a respiratory tract infection and can become abscessed requiring incision and drainage. The opening of a sinus or fistulous tract can be identified on the anterior border of the ipsilateral SCM muscle (Fig. 8.6) and may present with intermittent nonpurulent drainage.

Diagnosis

Lateral neck swelling in the pediatric age group has a broad differential diagnosis (Table 8.2). The diagnosis can be narrowed significantly when a presence of a pit is present on the surface of the neck, although differentiation from other branchial anomalies can be challenging. An infected branchial cleft cyst needs to be differentiated from suppurative cervical adenitis. Although many imaging modalities have been used in the diagnosis of branchial cleft anomalies, CT scan remains the study of choice in most circumstances.

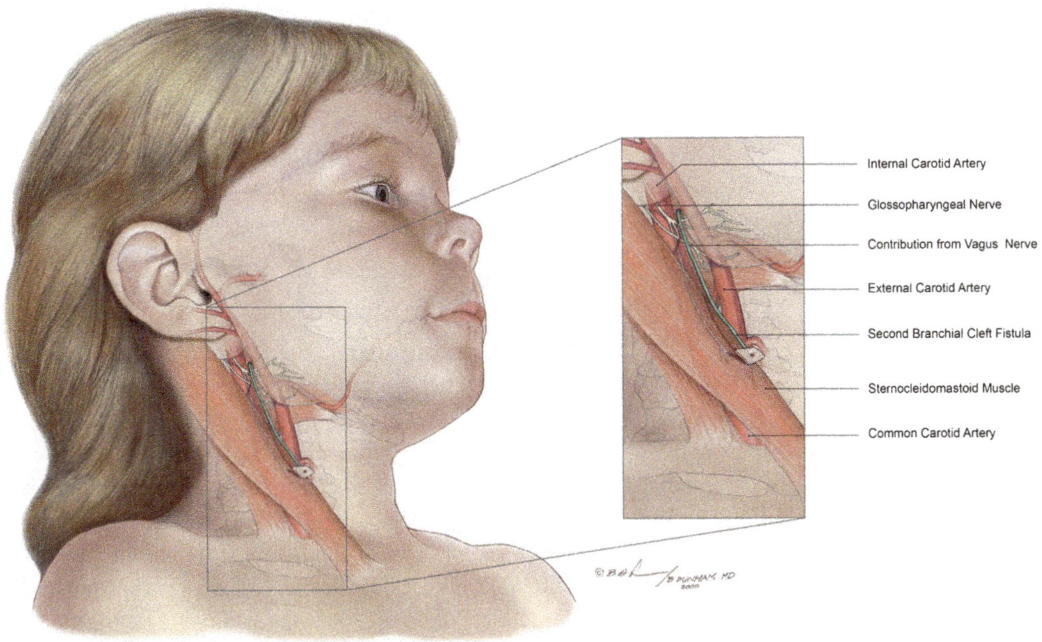

Fig. 8.5 Diagram of the right neck demonstrating the course of a second branchial cleft anomaly. The tract courses over the ninth cranial nerve (glossopharyngeal nerve) and between the bifurcation of the carotid artery (internal and external branches) to end in the inferior tonsillar fossa of the pharynx

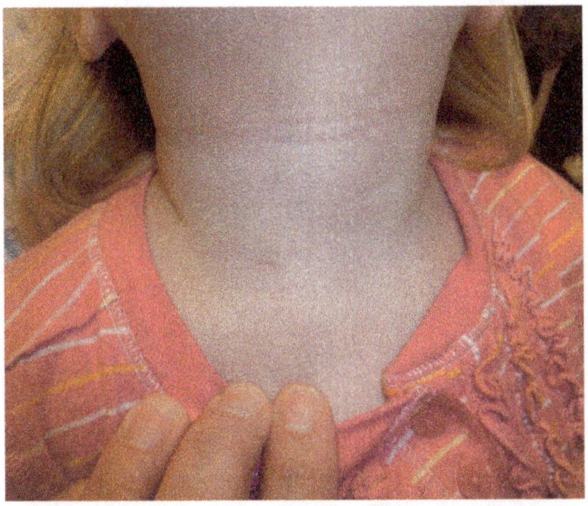

Fig. 8.6 External pit along the anterior border of the SCM muscle associated with a second branchial cleft anomaly

Table 8.2 Differential diagnosis of lateral neck mass in children

Branchial cleft anomaly
Lymph node
Vascular malformation
Sternocleidomastoid tumor of infancy
Thymic cyst
Laryngocele

Management

Treatment of second branchial anomalies requires complete surgical excision. When removing a cyst it is imperative that one attempts to identify and remove an associated tract if there is one present in order to minimize the risk of recurrence. For sinuses and fistulae, the tract must be completely excised. Some surgeons advocate removing the tonsil when the tract is excised to prevent recurrence within the lower tonsillar fossa. Identification and preservation of surrounding structures along the tract's path is essential. Gentle probing of the sinus/fistula with lacrimal probes can be helpful. Methylene blue injected into the tract is another commonly used technique to allow for tract delineation.

Third and Fourth Anomalies

Incidence

Third branchial cleft anomalies are rare with just over 200 cases reported in the literature [10]. Lesions involving the fourth cleft are extremely uncommon.

Etiology

As with other branchial cleft anomalies, failure of the tract to involute is accepted as the most likely cause. The path of these lesions is based on the embryology. Third cleft lesions will travel deep to the internal and common carotid arteries as well as the glossopharyngeal nerve. The tract will then course through the thyrohyoid membrane to enter the cranial portion of the pyriform fossa. A complete fistulous tract of the fourth branchial cleft or pouch has not been reported so the course of the lesion is speculative [2]. The suspected course of these anomalies will be different depending on the side of the lesion. On the right side, the tract will loop around the subclavian artery, course deep to the internal carotid artery, ascend superficial to the hypoglossal nerve, and then descend to enter the apex of the pyriform fossa. On the left side, the lesion travels around the arch of the aorta with the remainder of the course mimicking that seen on the right.

Clinical Features

These lesions can have a similar presentation to the more common second branchial anomalies with some important variations. Both can present as a slow growing lateral neck mass and have an external pit along the anterior border of the SCM muscle, similar to second cleft anomalies. A systematic review of the literature identified that 89 % of reported third arch anomalies were on the left side and often present with abscess formation or acute suppurative thyroiditis [10]. In the setting of infection, hypoglossal nerve palsy may be present. Fourth cleft anomalies can present with neck pain, thyroid abscess, and recurrent upper respiratory tract infections [5].

Diagnosis

Diagnosis is based on history and physical exam with imaging including contrast enhanced CT, MRI, and barium swallow being most useful [10]. High resolution scans can sometimes identify the course of the tract, allowing the type to be identified, although in many cases the diagnosis will often be made intraoperatively based on the course of the tract. Because of the possible communication of the sinus or fistula into the pyriform fossa, direct laryngoscopy can aid in the diagnosis. A sinus or fistulous opening may be identified (Fig. 8.7) and in the setting of acute infection, purulent drainage can be seen in the pyriform fossa. If not infected, gentle massage of the neck can allow saliva to be expressed from the sinus.

Management

Traditionally, the mainstay of treatment of third and forth branchial anomalies has been surgical excision. Knowledge of the relevant embryology guides the surgeon through the expected path of these lesions. Exposure of the laryngeal framework and possible removal of a cartilaginous window to access the pyriform sinus may be required. A fourth cleft anomaly requires an ipsilateral thyroidectomy to completely remove the tract [2]. Abscesses (Fig. 8.8) should be managed with incision and drainage and appropriate antimicrobial therapy, with definitive surgery delayed until resolution of inflammation. Recently, an alternative management strategy of third and forth anomalies has included identification of the fistula opening within the pyriform fossa with endoscopic cauterization (Fig. 8.9) [10, 11]. This approach has encouraging results without the potential morbidity of an open procedure.

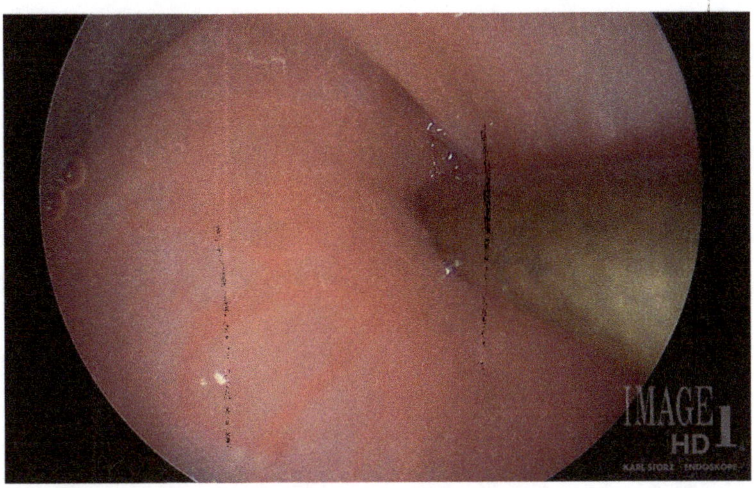

Fig. 8.7 View of the left pyriform fossa with sinus opening identified in a patient with recurrent neck abscesses. The probe is in the sinus

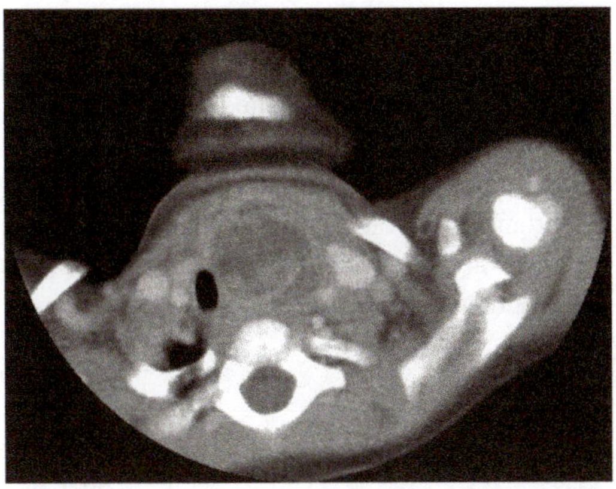

Fig. 8.8 CT scan image of a child with an abscessed third branchial cleft anomaly

Thyroid

Embryology

The thyroid gland begins to arise during the end of the third week of gestation. It is formed by a single medial anlage and paired lateral anlages [2]. The larger median anlage arises on the floor of the primordial pharynx. It begins as an evagination termed the thyroid diverticulum and lies caudal to the developing oral tongue. The lateral anlages are derivatives from the ventral portion of the fourth branchial pouch and fuse with the median portion during the fifth week. As the embryo grows the gland passes ventral to the developing hyoid bone and reaches its final position at the level of the second and third tracheal rings [3] (Fig. 8.10).

The thyroglossal duct is an epithelial lined tract that connects the tongue to the thyroid gland. The duct opens at the junction of the anterior two-thirds and the posterior third of the tongue at the foramen cecum. The duct typically obliterates and disappears by the fifth week of gestation. The inferior portion of the duct can often persist and is represented as the pyramidal lobe of the gland which can have fibrous stalk connected to the hyoid [2].

Definition

Thyroid tissue can be present anywhere along the duct. It can be in the form of the entire gland or small rests of cells. If the gland fails to descend, the thyroid tissue remains within the tongue base and is termed lingual thyroid. In 70–80 % of patients with this anomaly, this is the only functioning thyroid tissue present [12]. An epithelial lined cyst forming along the tract is termed a TGDC.

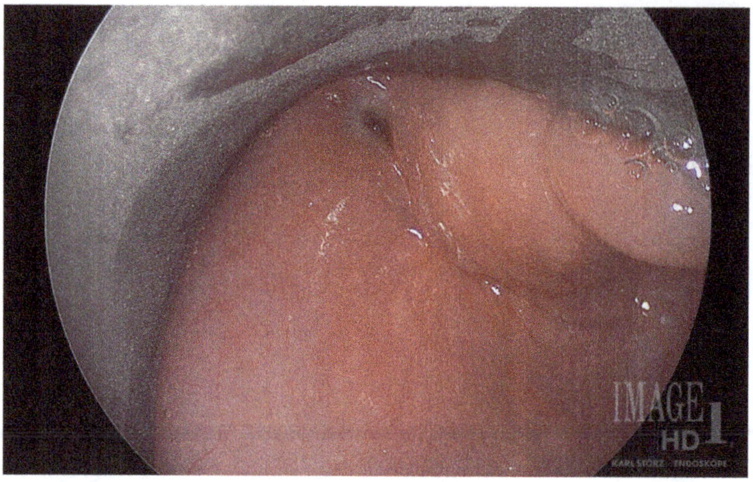

Fig. 8.9 View of sinus opening in pyriform fossa after being cauterized. Note the blanching of the mucosa around the opening of the sinus

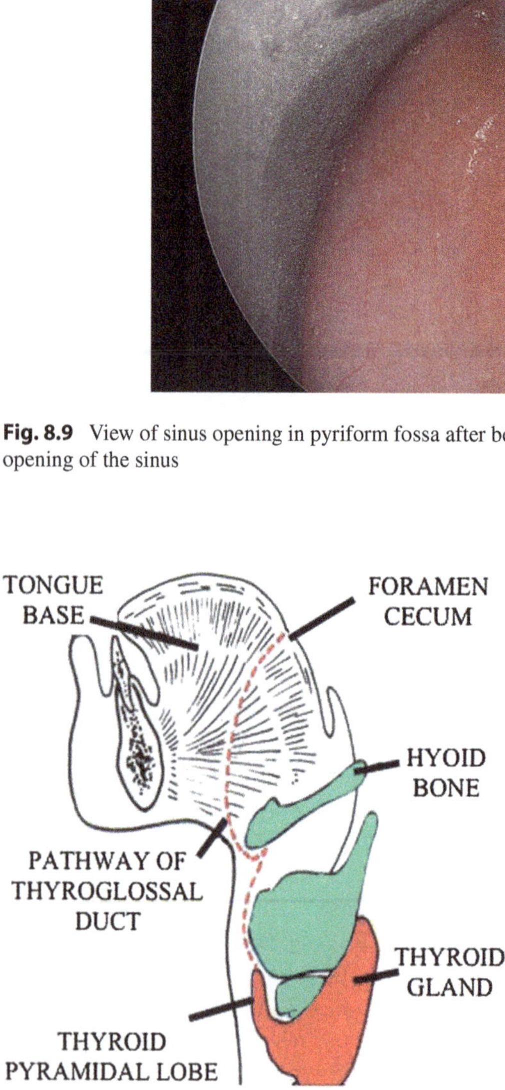

Fig. 8.10 Migratory course of the thyroglossal duct. Thyroglossal duct cysts may occur anywhere along the course of the duct if the duct fails to obliterate during development (From Moore KL, Persaud TVN. *The Developing Human: Clinically Oriented Embryology*, 5th ed. Philadelphia: W.B. Saunders; 1993:201. Copyright Elsevier 1993)

History

The historical aspects of TGDCs relate to their management. In 1893, Schlange first suggested resection of the hyoid bone with the cyst, which significantly reduced recurrence rates [13]. Walter E. Sistrunk is credited with developing today's surgical treatment based on his paper published in 1920 [14]. He too discussed the importance of hyoid removal and also advocated for removal of a core of tissue above the hyoid to the foramen cecum.

Incidence

TGDCs are the most common congenital neck mass, accounting for more than 75 % of pediatric midline neck masses [15, 16]. Although the incidence of clinically apparent TGDCs is unknown, autopsy specimens have revealed that 7 % of the population has a remnant of the thyroglossal duct tract [17].

Heredity

The majority of TGDCs occur sporadically without a positive family history. A very rare hereditary form of TGDC exists, with 29 cases in 9 families reported in the literature [18]. The transmission is thought to be autosomal dominant with a higher incidence in females [19].

Etiology

It is unclear what causes the thyroid not to descend normally. Failure of involution of the thyroglossal duct results in rests of cells remaining along the tract. Proliferating and secreting epithelium in response to inflammation along the tract is thought to result in a TGDC development [13].

Associated Malformations

Thyroid carcinoma can develop within TGDCs and lingual thyroid glands. The reported incidence of TGDC carcinoma is 1 % and is usually found incidentally after surgical excision [15]. This diagnosis is exceedingly rare in the pediatric age group with only 22 cases reported [20]. Lingual thyroid cancer is also rare with approximately 40 cases reported in the literature [21].

Clinical Features

A TGDC typically presents as a painless, slow growing midline neck mass. The cyst can become apparent at any age with the majority presenting before the age of five [22]. It can arise at any location along the tract, but is most commonly found below the hyoid bone. The mass is typically soft, mobile, non-tender and often moves with swallowing or protrusion of the tongue. Associated findings may include dysphagia, dysphonia, airway obstruction, and abscess formation. Although an infected TGDC may present with drainage or fistulization, it is never primarily associated with a communication to the skin because embryologically there is no communication with the surface of the neck [22]. A lingual thyroid will present as a solid mass within the posterior tongue and may be associated with feeding difficulties or airway obstruction.

Diagnosis

Although TGDC is the most common pediatric midline neck mass, there is a broad differential diagnosis (Table 8.3). History and physical exam consistent with the clinical features mentioned above are very important in the diagnosis of TGDC. An ultrasound can be useful, not only to characterize the lesion, but also to identify normal thyroid tissue within the neck and is the imaging modality of choice. Contrast enhanced CT and MRI can also be helpful, but are generally not necessary. These studies can be reserved for larger lesions, lesions presenting with a complication, or recurrent cases. Nuclear medicine studies can identify functional thyroid tissue within the lesion and the normal gland. If the thyroid gland appears to be normal on U/S, then a thyroid function scan is usually not warranted. Moreover, these investigations utilize an intravenously administered radiopharmaceutical compound and should be avoided if possible in the pediatric age group [23]. Thyroid function scans can be reserved for situations where the other diagnostic modalities are inconclusive or if the patient has signs and symptoms of hypothyroidism [16]. In rare cases where a lingual thyroid is suspected, diagnosis can be confirmed by ultrasound or thyroid function scans.

Table 8.3 Differential diagnosis for midline neck mass in children

Thyroglossal duct cyst
Epidermoid/dermoid/teratoma
Plunging ranula
Lymph node
Thyroid nodule
Sebaceous cyst
Thymic cyst
Vascular malformation
Third/fourth branchial cleft cyst

Management

The treatment of a TGDC is complete surgical excision. In his famous manuscript, Sistrunk described the surgical technique for dealing with these lesions. The procedure bears his name and has essentially not changed since 1920. The key to successful removal includes removal of the mid-portion of the hyoid bone in continuity with the cyst and a core of tissue up to the foramen cecum [14]. The recurrence rate using the Sistrunk procedure is estimated to be 4 %. Patients undergoing a cystectomy, without removal of the mid-portion of the hyoid bone, have an average recurrence rate of 50 % with some series reporting rates of 100 % [24]. For the rare occurrence of a TGDC arising in the tongue base, transoral endoscopic removal has been successful [25]. Management of a lingual thyroid is covered elsewhere in this text (Chap. 4).

Lymphangiomas

Embryology

During the third and fourth month of development two paired (jugular and posterior) and two unpaired (mesenteric and cysterna chili) endothelial sacs form the basis of the lymphatic system. These join with lymphatic channels by the end of the ninth week, with cervical lymph nodes forming around the same time [26].

Definition

Lymphangiomas are lymphatic malformations and do not represent neoplastic growths as their name implies. They are fluid filled, endothelial lined spaces derived from lymphatic vessels [26]. They can be subdivided into macrocystic, microcystic, or cavernous. The term "cystic hygroma" is a misnomer often used to describe macrocystic lesions.

History

Redenbacher first described these lesions in 1828, with Wehrner coining the term "cystic hygroma" in 1834 [26]. Although not widely supported initially, Wehrner's theory of the lesion being a neoplasm was later supported by Virchow in 1863 [27].

Incidence

The reported incidence of lymphatic malformations is 1.2–2.8 per 1,000 newborns [28]. Lymphangiomas constitute 5.6 % of all benign lesions of childhood with no reported sex predilection [29]. Although they can occur anywhere within the lymphatic system, more than 80 % of lymphatic malformations arise in the neck [26].

Heredity

Lymphatic malformations most commonly arise as sporadic lesions. They can rarely be associated with other anomalies in patients with Turner or Noonan syndrome.

Etiology

Lymphangiomas are hamartomas—an overgrowth or expansion of normal lymphatic tissue. The precise embryologic origin of their occurrence is unknown.

Associated Malformations

Macrocystic lymphangiomas are known to be associated with Turner and other syndromes [26]. Aborted fetuses with Turner syndrome have been found to have these lesions in the posterior neck. If resolution by spontaneous drainage occurs in utero, the characteristic webbing of the neck in patients with Turner syndrome remains [29].

Clinical Features

The most common presentation of a lymphatic malformation is that of a soft, ill defined mass in the posterior triangle of the neck, which can be quite large (Fig. 8.11) [28]. Common-associated symptoms include respiratory and feeding difficulties. Lymphatic malformations can swell rapidly, typically in the setting of infection or with

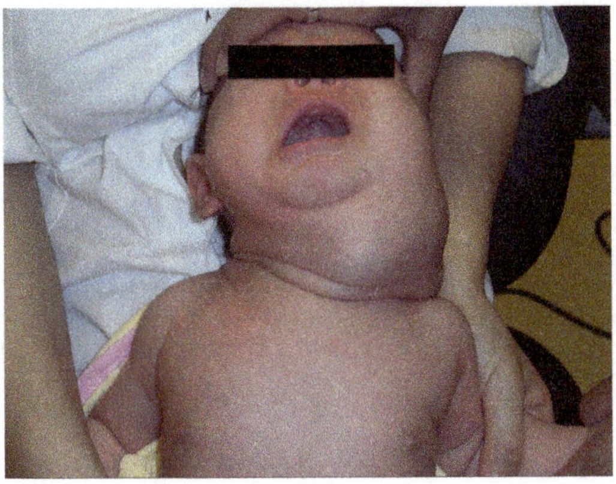

Fig. 8.11 Large neck mass in a newborn identified as a lymphatic malformation. The patient also had significant intrathoracic involvement

intracystic bleeding, and can occasionally present with life-threatening airway compromise. Microcystic malformations typically arise from the area above the mylohyoid muscle and in the region of the oral cavity.

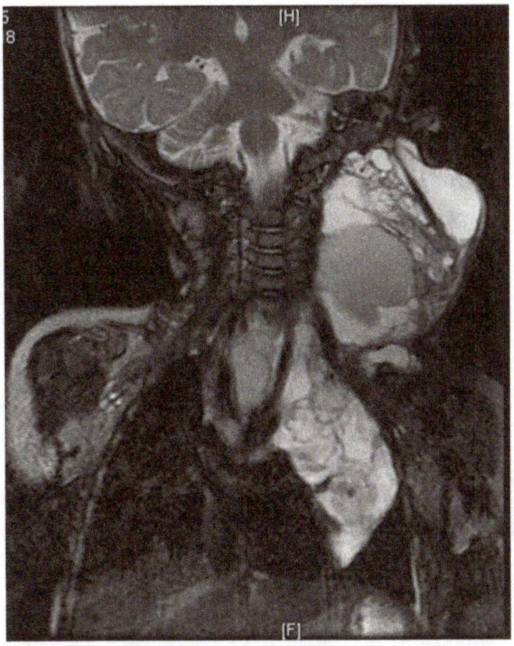

Fig. 8.12 MRI image demonstrating massive lymphatic malformation involving both the neck and chest. Note the large fluid filled spaces within the lesion

Diagnosis

The clinical presentation of a lymphatic malformation is characteristic and differs from hemangiomas in that they do not have proliferative and involutionary phases. Ultrasound is a useful initial investigation establishing size and flow characteristics and can diagnose lesions prenatally [30]. MRI is the preferred imaging modality with lesions appearing hypointense on T1-weighted and hyperintense on T2-weighted images (Fig. 8.12).

Management

Asymptomatic lymphatic malformations can be observed. Treatment is controversial and typically involves surgical removal, sclerotherapy or a combination of the two. There are proponents of both as a primary therapeutic modality. Sclerotherapy with agents such as bleomycin and OK-432 is advocated for unicystic or macrocystic lesions, but is not appropriate or microcystic lesions. In these cases surgery is recommended. Complete surgical removal is required to prevent recurrence but in most cases is not possible without risk of injury to vital structures. Some authors advocate surgery as the primary therapy with sclerosing agents reserved for recurrences [28].

Infantile Hemangiomas

Definition

Hemangiomas are benign neoplasms caused by proliferation of endothelial cells. History: In 1938, Lister published the first review of the natural history of hemangiomas (termed "strawberry naevi" in his manuscript) [31]. His recommendations were based on 93 lesions on 77 patients. He described the typical proliferation and involution of these lesions and suggested observation and conservative measures as the treatment of choice.

Incidence

Infantile hemangiomas are the most common neonatal neoplasm with an incidence of 12 % in term infants and higher in cases of prematurity [32].

Heredity

Hemangiomas usually occur sporadically, and studies involving twins do not suggest a genetic basis [33]. However 10 % of cases may occur secondary to an autosomal-dominant transmission [32].

Etiology

Current theory suggests that hemangiomas arise through hormonally driven vessel growth, but the exact cause remains controversial. Two popular theories include revival of dormant embryonic angioblasts and neogenesis [32].

Associated Malformations

Cervical hemangiomas can be associated with coexisting lesions elsewhere in 20 % of patients. Hemangiomas within the airway can prove to be a life-threatening problem. The child will present with progressive stridor and can be misdiagnosed as having croup, reactive airway disease, or feeding difficulties [34]. However, 1–10 % of patients who have cutaneous lesions also have airway lesions. The location is typically in the subglottis, most commonly arising posteriorly on the left side. Fifty percent of children with airway hemangiomas will have cutaneous lesions [34]. Airway lesions should be suspected in patients who present with large cutaneous hemangiomas in the so-called "beard" distribution [35] (Fig. 8.13).

Large segmental hemangiomas on the face can also be associated with PHACES syndrome. This represents a constellation of findings including posterior fossa abnormalities, hemangiomas, arterial anomalies, cardiac defects, eye anomalies, and sternal defects [35].

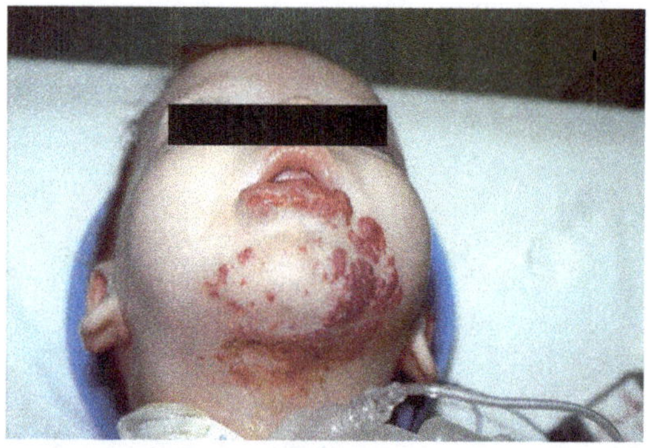

Fig. 8.13 Cutaneous hemangioma that occurs in a "beard" distribution. Note that the child has a tracheotomy in place because he also has a large, obstructing airway hemangioma

Kasabach-Merritt phenomenon is often *incorrectly* associated with infantile hemangiomas. This consumptive coagulopathy is actually related to a more aggressive lesion known as kaposiform hemangioendothelioma [36].

Clinical Features

Hemangiomas are rarely present at birth [35]. They usually become apparent in the first few weeks of life and then undergo rapid proliferation in the first year. Lesions can appear red or violaceous depending on their depth. After the proliferative stage, hemangiomas typically begin to involute with 50 % of lesions resolved by 5 years and 70 % by 7 years of age. They can become symptomatic, usually during the proliferative phase. Rapid growth can lead to ulceration and bleeding. Depending on location of the lesion compressive symptoms of the upper aerodigestive tract can occur.

Diagnosis

The diagnosis is predominantly based on the history and physical examination. Ultrasound (U/S) can help characterize the lesion as well as demonstrate flow. For complex lesions or when the diagnosis is in question, MRI is the imaging modality of choice.

Management

Treatment in the absence of complications is observation. As most hemangiomas will spontaneously involute, reassurance and education are important. In the setting of complications, medical and surgical therapy may be indicated. The mainstay of medical treatment has been systemic steroids. Other therapies for recalcitrant cases include interferon and vincristine. These medications are associated with potentially serious side effects. More recently there has been promising literature supporting the used of propranolol for the treatment of hemangiomas [37, 38]. Long-term data regarding safety and efficacy for this has yet to be published. Surgical excision or debulking is required in rare cases when the patient has functional compromise unresponsive to medical management or if the lesion fails to resolve during childhood. Given the favorable natural history of hemangiomas, preservation of vital structures is imperative when surgery is considered.

Dermoids and Teratomas

Definition

Dermoid cysts are congenital lesions comprised of ectodermal and mesodermal derivatives. They are lined with epithelium and can contain hair, hair follicles, and sebaceous glands. These mesodermal elements differentiate dermoids from the more common epidermoid cysts, which contain only epithelial tissue. Teratomas contain ectoderm, mesoderm, and endodermal tissue.

History

Virchow first used the term teratoma in 1869 but similar lesions were described as far back as 1658 [39].

Incidence

The incidence of dermoids in the neck is unknown. Cervical teratomas are rare and account for 3 % of all teratomas [39].

Heredity

Both dermoids and teratomas are thought to be inherited sporadically.

Etiology

Dermoid cysts arise because of the entrapment of epithelial elements during development. This often occurs along embryonic fusion planes, both midline and paramedian. Theories regarding the embryogenesis of teratomas include entrapment of primordial cells between endoderm and ectoderm, as well as the lesion being the remnant of a "failed twin." [39]

Associated Malformations

Malignant transformation of cervical teratomas in the infants is rare; however, an overall incidence of 10 % has been reported in older children and adults [40]. Tumor location outside the head and neck is associated with a higher rate of malignancy [39]. Teratomas are also associated with prematurity, polyhydramnios, and respiratory distress in the neonatal period.

Clinical Features

Cervical dermoids present as soft, smooth subcutaneous lesions, often in the anterior neck. They can extend deep and can cause airway obstruction. Because they are often located in close proximity to the hyoid bone, they can mimic TGDCs (Fig. 8.14). Cervical teratomas are often quite large and often have a more irregular appearance (Fig. 8.15). In the neonate, they can be associated with significant airway obstruction.

Diagnosis

A complete history and physical exam aids in the diagnosis of dermoid cysts. A superficial lesion, which does not move with swallowing can help differentiate a dermoid from a TGDC. However,

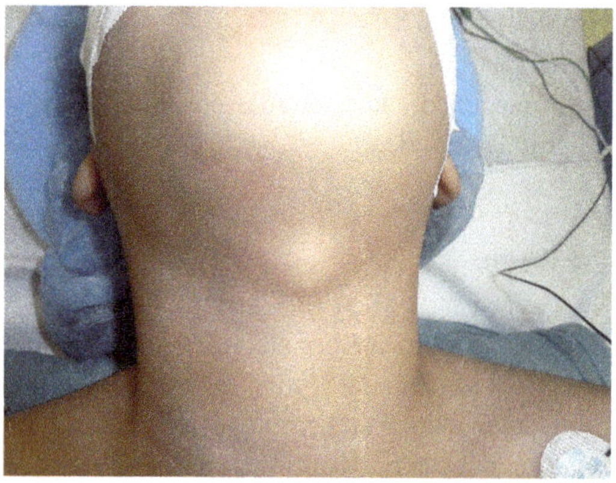

Fig. 8.14 Anterior neck mass in a child that was initially thought to be a thyroglossal duct cyst. Pathologic examination identified the lesion as a dermoid cyst. Both lesions present similarly on physical exam

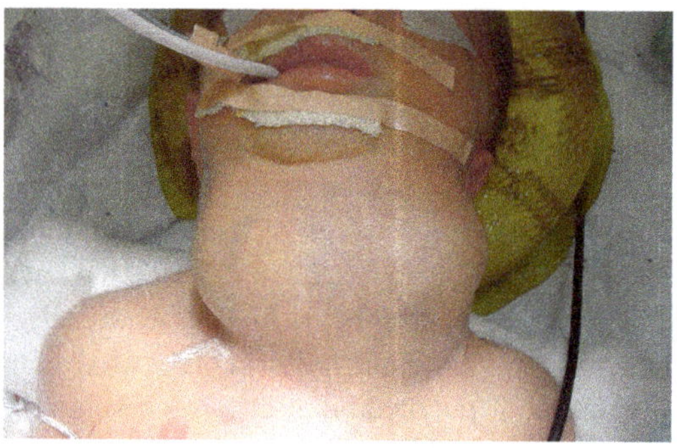

Fig. 8.15 Large teratoma in a newborn. The child was intubated prior to being fully delivered (see Fig. 8.13) (Photo courtesy of Dr. Bruce Korman)

as mentioned they can mimic other lesions and often times diagnosis requires pathologic examination demonstrating epidermal and mesodermal elements. Ultrasound or CT can provide additional information regarding these lesions prior to excision. Teratomas should be imaged with MRI to aid in preoperative planning [41].

Management

The treatment for a dermoid cyst is complete surgical excision (Figs. 8.16a, b). Inadequate removal or spillage of the cyst contents is associated with a higher rate of recurrence. Teratomas also require surgical removal. Cervical teratomas diagnosed by in utero by ultrasound may require immediate intubation at the time of delivery due to airway obstruction. In these instances an EXIT (ex utero intra-partum therapy) procedure can be performed to secure the airway via intubation or tracheostomy while the fetus is being oxygenated via the maternal circulation (Fig. 8.17).

Midline Cervical Cleft

Definition

Congenital midline cervical cleft (CMCC) is a superficial, vertical defect in the anterior neck skin (Fig. 8.18a).

History

A congenital midline cervical cleft was first described by Luscka in 1848 with Bailey describing the lesion in the English literature in 1924 [42]. Since then numerous case reports and series have been published describing the etiology and management of this anomaly.

Incidence

This anomaly is rare with fewer than 100 cases reported in the literature [42].

Heredity

Congenital midline cervical clefts present sporadically with no associated hereditary form of transmission. The lesion, however, is more common in Caucasian females [43].

Etiology

The exact embryologic development of a congenital midline cervical cleft is not known, but most authors agree that failure of fusion of the lateral branchial arches is the likely cause.

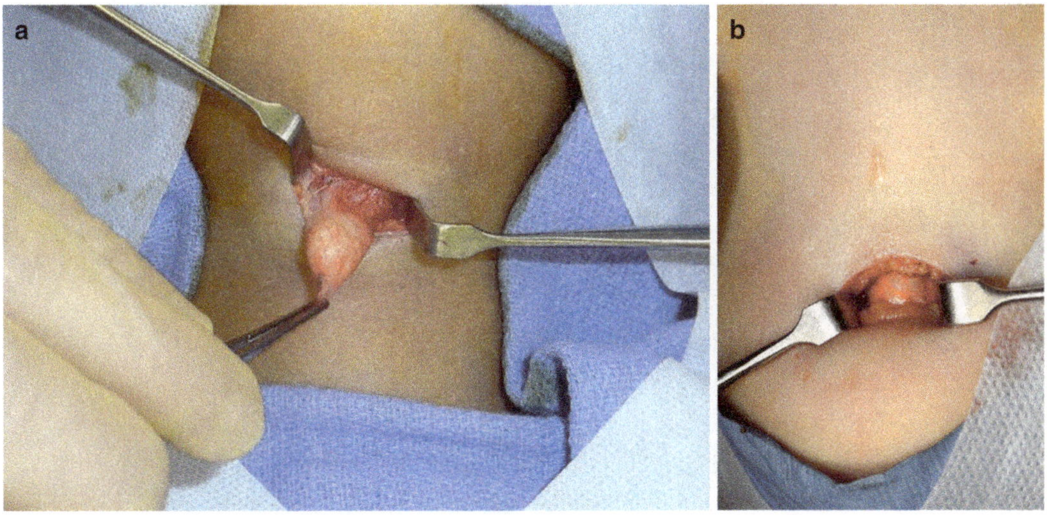

Fig. 8.16 (**a**) Intraoperative photograph of the patient in Fig. 8.14 demonstrating the *yellow-colored* cyst partially dissected from the surrounding tissues. No tract was identified in keeping with the diagnosis of a dermoid cyst. (**b**) Intraoperative photograph of another patient with a thyroglossal duct cyst. This cyst is *pink* in color and has a tract that attaches to the hyoid bone

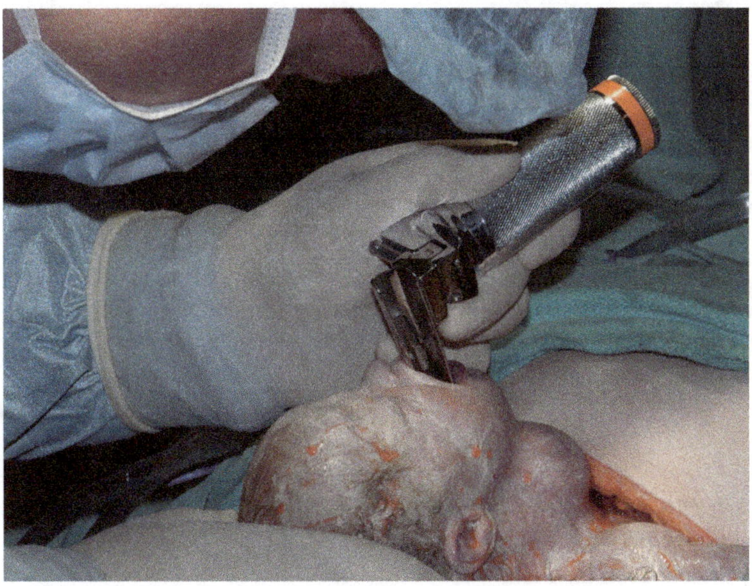

Fig. 8.17 Direct laryngoscopy being performed on a child with a large anterior neck mass still being oxygenated via the placental circulation. The child was successfully intubated (Photo courtesy of Dr. Bruce Korman)

Associated Malformations

There is an increased incidence of additional anomalies in patients with CMCC. In their review of the literature, Mlynarek, et al. found that dermoid, bronchogenic, and TGDCs were identified during pathologic examination of CMCCs [43].

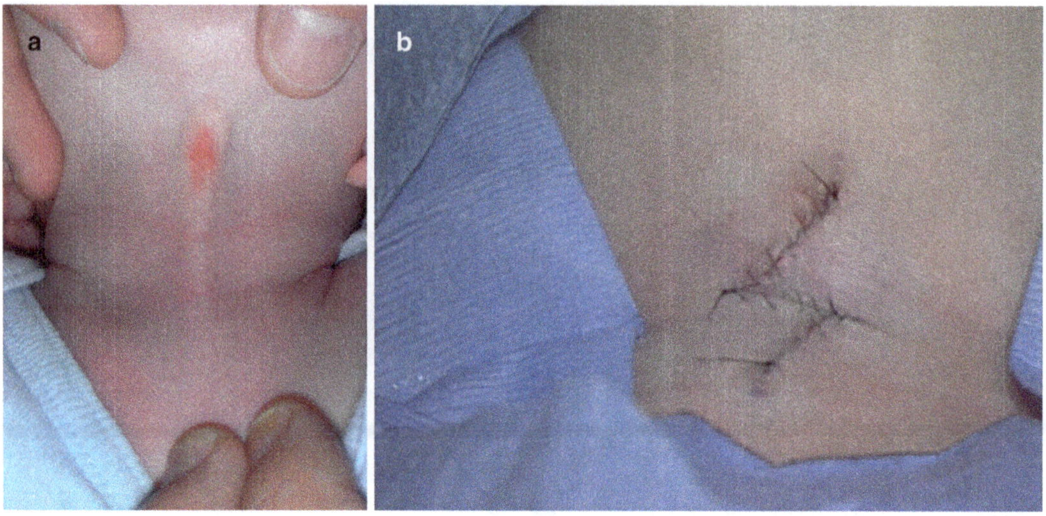

Fig. 8.18 (**a**) Congenital midline cervical cleft. Note the appearance of the fibrous cord extending inferiorly. (**b**) Intraoperative photograph demonstrating the "Z-plasty" used to close the excised defect

Clinical Features

The cleft typically has a nipple-like protuberance at the superior aspect and a sinus at the inferior portion of the lesion. It can extend anywhere from the lower lip to the sternal notch. The epithelium is typically erythematous and there can be associated mucoid drainage. With time the cleft will epithelialize and form a fibrous cord. If left uncorrected the lesion can limit neck extension and restrict mandibular movement.

Diagnosis

Diagnosis is generally made by physical examination. The lesion is superficial with no connection to the deep structures of the neck.

Management

The treatment for congenital midline cervical cleft is complete surgical excision. Because it is oriented vertically, the defect can be significant if excising using a horizontal ellipse in a natural skin crease. A Z-plasty (single or multiple) is a convenient way to excise the defect allowing for a closure with much less tension (Fig. 8.18b) [43].

Thymic Cysts

Embryology

During the sixth week of development, the third branchial pouch expands creating a solid dorsal and hollow ventral portion. The hollow portion forms the thymopharyngeal duct. The connection to the pharynx degenerates and cellular proliferation causes the formation of two lateral masses by the eighth week. The lateral masses descend and fuse in the midline forming a bilobed gland [2].

Definition

Cervical thymic cysts can be subdivided into unilobular and multilobular. The unilobular cysts are most commonly found in the neck and are thought to be congenital. The multilobular cysts are typically seen in the neck and mediastinum and can be congenital or inflammatory. In addition to cysts, there can also be ectopic thymic tissue in the neck. This is common and often found incidentally during pathologic examination of surgical specimens or at autopsy [44].

History

The first description of cervical thymic cyst excision was by Polloson and Piery in 1901, and the first successful removal was described by Hyde in 1944 [45]. Since then there have been numerous case reports and case series documenting this rare entity.

Incidence

Cervical thymic cysts are rare with approximately 150 cases reported in the literature [46].

Heredity

There is one reported case of familial thymic cyst in the literature. It describes two brothers aged 5 and 8 with multilobular cysts involving the lower neck and mediastinum [47].

Etiology

There are two current theories regarding the development of cervical thymic cysts. The first is the persistence of the thymopharyngeal duct and the second is degeneration of Hassal's corpuscles in ectopic thymic tissue [48].

Clinical Features

Cervical thymic cysts are soft, unilocular or multilocular, non-tender and can taper to a palpable tract or cord. They can be found both in the lateral and anterior neck and can feel similar to a branchial cleft cyst. While these lesions typically present as a painless swelling, they can present with infection and abscess formation in addition to compressive symptoms of the trachea, esophagus, or both [44, 49].

Diagnosis

Cervical thymic cysts present a diagnostic challenge and are often misdiagnosed as branchial cleft anomalies, lymphadenitis, dermoids, epidermoids, and neoplasms. In a series of 20 patients with cervical thymic remnants, only 15 % had a correct preoperative diagnosis based on physical examination and imaging [49]. A similar diagnostic accuracy rate of 11 % was cited in a smaller series of nine patients [48]. Histopathology reveals Hassal's corpuscles, which are pathognomonic for thymic tissue. These are concentric epithelioreticular cells with characteristic keratinized centers.

Management

Complete surgical excision is the treatment of choice. This can be accomplished via a transcervical approach but may require partial sternotomy to access lesions with significant mediastinal extension.

Sternocleidomastoid Tumor of Infancy

Definition

Sternocleidomastoid tumor of infancy (STOI) and congenital muscular torticollis (CMT) are often described as the same clinical entity related to a fibrotic change in the sternocleidomastoid muscle. This causes shortening and resultant tilting of the head to the affected side. Although no strict definition describing differences between STOI and CMT is identified within the literature, the general consensus is STOI occurs more frequently in younger infants than does CMT [50].

Incidence

STOI is present in 0.4 % of newborns. CMT is the third most common congenital musculoskeletal anomaly after hip dislocation and clubfoot [50].

History

Sternocleidomastoid tumor was first described in the German literature by Heusinger in 1812. The first surgical treatment for torticollis was a tenotomy performed by Dutch surgeon Minneus in 1685 [51].

Heredity

STOI and CMT appear to be sporadic with no reported hereditary relationship.

Etiology

For over 200 years there has been debate regarding the etiology of STOI and CMT. Most agree that there is a fibrotic change within the SCM but the cause for this is uncertain. Ischemia, birth trauma, hematoma formation have all been cited as potential causes. Anoxic injury to the muscle was first theorized by Miculicz in 1895 and is still the most widely accepted theory [52].

Associated Malformations

In a large review, 6.8 % of 515 patients with STOI had developmental dysplasia of the hip (DDH) [53]. Other studies report variable association rates ranging from 2 to 29 % [54]. This is more than the typical 1–3 % incidence of DDH and therefore more rigorous screening is warranted in patients with STOI.

Clinical Features

STOI presents as an isolated lateral neck swelling along the SCM muscle, typically noted in the first 8 weeks of life. The vast majority of cases are unilateral; however, bilateral cases have been reported [55]. The mass is typically firm, mobile, and non-tender. The overlying skin is normal and there is no associated pathologic lymphadenopathy. If there is associated torticollis there will be rotation of the chin to the contralateral side and tilting of the head to the ipsilateral side. Deformities can develop if the infant always lays on one side of the head, including plagiocephaly, facial asymmetry (because the SCM chronically pulls on the growing facial structures), and ocular abnormalities (because the child compensates for facial asymmetry). These generally resolve with treatment of the torticollis.

Diagnosis

The diagnosis of STOI is usually made based on the clinical features alone. In addition to physical exam, various imaging modalities can help differentiate the STOI from other lateral neck masses such as branchial cleft anomalies and lymphadenopathy. Ultrasound is a safe, cost effective, and noninvasive way to assess these lesions and is regarded as the modality of choice.

Management

There are multiple treatment modalities available for STOI. Fifty to seventy percent resolve spontaneously with no intervention. The key to successful treatment is to start therapy as soon as a problem is identified. Physical therapy in the form of stretching exercises is initiated if there is restricted mobility. This can be carried out by the caregiver after a supervised instruction period with a trained therapist. In a large prospective study, 90.7 % of patients resolved with these measures alone [53]. Other treatment modalities are reserved for failed conservative management. Botulism toxin type A has been shown to be effective in small series [56]. This may prevent the need for surgery; however, there is still a need for general anesthesia, as well as a potential for complications associated with Botulism toxin in this area, including allergic reactions, neck weakness, and dysphagia. Surgery is often required when other treatment options fail, most commonly in patients who did not undergo any therapy prior to 1 year of age or in cases when more severe torticollis was present at initial presentation [53]. Common surgical options include tenotomy and/or muscle release.

Neurofibroma

Definition

Neurofibromas are benign lesions arising from the Schwann cells that surround peripheral nerves and can occur anywhere in the peripheral nervous system. They are separated into plexiform and cutaneous types and can arise in isolation; however, they are most commonly associated with Neurofibromatosis type 1 (NF1).

Incidence

The incidence of isolated neurofibroma is unknown. NF1 occurs in 1 in 4,000 live births, although 50 % of cases are believed to be from new mutations [57].

History

Descriptions of patients believed to have neurofibromatosis date back hundreds of years. A thirteenth century drawing by a Cistercian monk of a disfigured man is thought to represent a patient with neurofibromatosis (NF). Akenside first described NF in English in 1768. Later, Rudolph Virchow developed classification systems for neuromas and fibromas, and it was his student Friedrich Daniel von Recklinghausen, who coined the term *neurofibroma*, describing a lesion containing neural and connective tissue elements [58].

Heredity

NF1 is inherited in an autosomal-dominant manner with complete penetrance and variable expression. Almost one half of all affected individuals have de novo mutations.

Etiology

A defect in a tumor suppressor gene on chromosome 17 causes individuals with NF1 to develop a variety of benign and malignant tumors [57].

Clinical Features

Plexiform neurofibromas are often congenital with approximately 50 % arising in the head and neck. They frequently arise along nerve bundles (especially nerve plexuses and dorsal root ganglia). These benign tumors can be locally invasive and there is a 4–5 % incidence of malignant degeneration [59]. Cutaneous neurofibromas typically arise in the prepubescent period and have no malignant potential [57].

Diagnosis

The diagnosis of an isolated neurofibroma is confirmed after pathologic examination which reveals the presence of Schwann cells, fibroblastic elements, and embedded axons. Solitary neurofibromas are well-delineated, firm lesions that are white and shiny. Plexiform neurofibromas are multifocal myxoid lesions often described as having the appearance of "a bag of worms." Multiple neurofibromas are strongly suggestive of NF1. The diagnostic criteria for NF1 are based on the National Institute of Health (NIH) Consensus Conference in 1987. Diagnosis can be made if the individual has two of the following features in the absence of another diagnosis: (1) Six or more café-au-lait spots >5 mm in prepubertal individuals and >15 mm in post pubertal individuals; (2) Two or more neurofibromas of any type or one plexiform neurofibroma; (3) Axillary or inguinal freckling; (4) Optic glioma; (5) Two or more Lisch nodules; (6) A distinctive osseous lesion such as sphenoid wing dyplasia or tibial pseudoarthrosis; or (7) A first degree relative with NF1 [60].

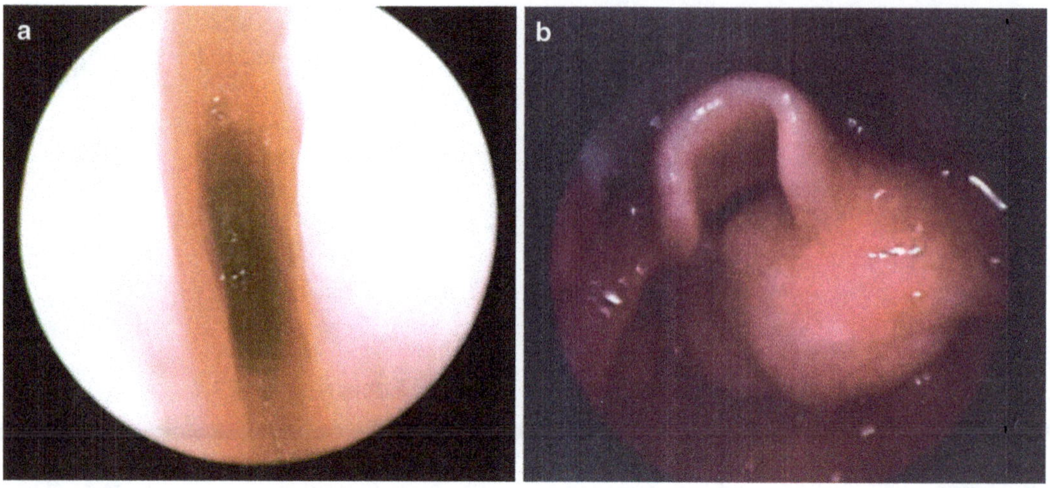

Fig. 8.19 (**a**) Endoscopic photograph of a child with external airway compression from bilateral vagal neurofibromas that have caused bilateral tracheal narrowing in the subglottis. (**b**) Endoscopic photograph of the larynx in the same child demonstrating a neurofibroma that causes distortion and displacement of the right arytenoid cartilage in to the lumen of the airway

Figures 8.19a to 8.20b demonstrate the extent of disease that may occur in the head and neck of a child with NF1. Multiple nerve bundles may be affected including dorsal root ganglia and cranial nerves (including the vagus nerve, as occurred in this child).

Associated Malformations

Patients with NF1 often have visual impairment, learning disabilities and skeletal abnormalities resulting from lesions associated with the syndrome. The learning disabilities can range from global developmental delays to learning disabilities, especially hyperactivity or speech problems. Many of the children with larger head and neck lesions complain of chronic neurogenic pain and headaches related to their lesions. Hydrocephalus can develop from intracranial lesions and lead to seizures. Hypertension in these patients can be the result of an associated renal artery stenosis or pheochromocytoma [61].

Management

The treatment of neurofibromas is surgical with little benefit from radiotherapy or chemotherapy. Large plexiform lesions can create a considerable cosmetic deformity as well as compressive symptoms including airway obstruction [62]. The timing of surgical management is controversial because there is a significant recurrence rate, especially in young children with head and neck neurofibromas [59]. Therefore, regular clinical follow up with serial imaging (usually with MRIs of the head and neck) can be helpful in determining when to intervene surgically. Children with NF1 should be regularly monitored for progression of their disease with annual ophthalmologic exams, developmental assessments using screening questionnaires, blood pressure evaluations, and examinations to identify scoliosis or other long bone changes. Referral to specialists should be considered when the masses rapidly expand to rule out malignancy or

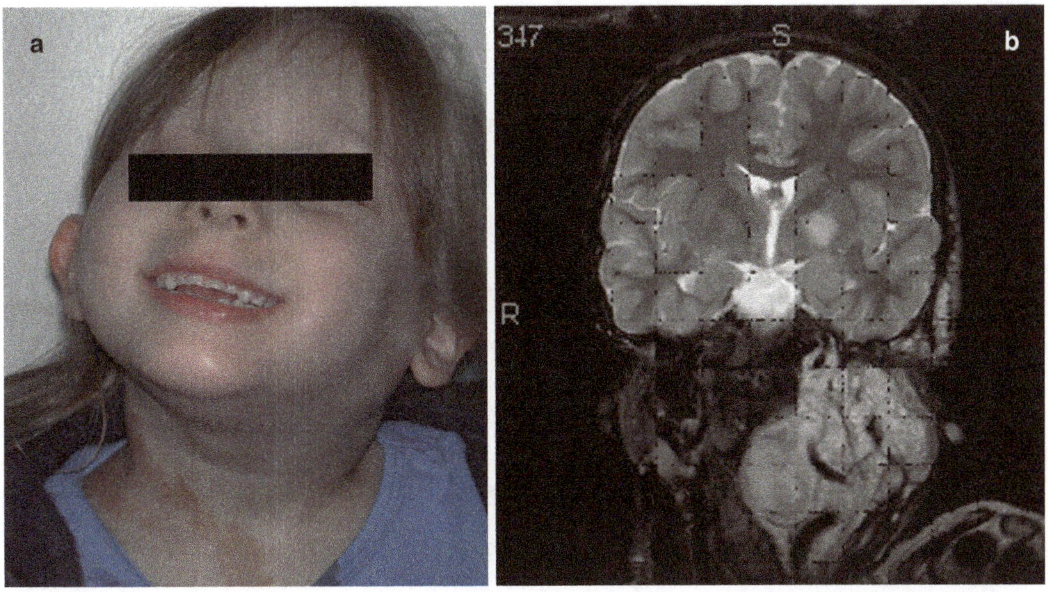

Fig. 8.20 (**a**) Six-year-old girl with a large left-side neck mass and café-au-lait spots on her neck. (**b**) MRI of head and neck with section taken in the coronal plane demonstrating the massive enhancing vagal plexiform mass within the carotid sheath space that extends to the skull base. The mass appears as a heterogeneous intensely enhancing mass on the T2-weighted image

when the child develops neurogenic pain or weakness, develops symptoms of airway compression, or when the tumors cause disfiguring changes in the child's appearance.

References

1. Waldhausen JHT. Branchial cleft and arch anomalies in children. Semin Pediatr Surg. 2006;15:64–9.
2. Skandalakis JE, Gray SW, Todd NW. Pharynx and its derivatives. In: Skandalakis JE, Gray SW, editors. Embryology for surgeons. 2nd ed. Baltimore, MD: Williams and Wilkins; 1994. p. 17–64.
3. Moore KL. The branchial apparatus and the head and neck. In: Moore KL, editor. The developing human. 4th ed. Philadelphia, PA: W.B. Saunders Co.; 1988. p. 170–206.
4. Silbergleit R, Quint DJ, Mehta BA, Patel SC, Metes JJ, Noujaim SE. The persistent stapedial artery. AJNR Am J Neuroradiol. 2000;21(3):572–7.
5. Acierno SP, Waldhausen JHT. Congenital cervical cysts, sinuses and fistulae. Otolaryngol Clin North Am. 2007;40:161–76.
6. Arndal H, Bonding P. First branchial cleft anomaly. Clin Otolaryngol Allied Sci. 1996;12:203–7.
7. Olsen KD, Maragos NE, Weiland LH. First branchial cleft anomalies. Laryngoscope. 1980;90:423–35.
8. Work WP. Newer concepts of first branchial cleft defects. Laryngoscope. 1972;82:1581–93.
9. Solares CA, Chan J, Koltai P. Anatomical variations of the facial nerve in first branchial cleft anomalies. Arch Otolaryngol Head Neck Surg. 2003;129:351–5.
10. Nicoucar K, Giger R, Jaecklin T, et al. Management of congenital third branchial arch anomalies: a systematic review. Otolaryngol Head Neck Surg. 2010;142:21–8.
11. Chen EY, Inglis AF, Ou H, et al. Endoscopic electrocauterization of pyriform fossa sinus tracts as definitive treatment. Int J Pediatr Otorhinolaryngol. 2009;73:1151–6.
12. Rahbar R, Yoon MJ, Connolly LP, et al. Lingual thyroid in children: a rare clinical entity. Laryngoscope. 2008;118:1174–9.
13. Mondin V, Ferlito A, Muzzi E, et al. Thyroglossal duct cyst: personal experience and literature review. Auris Nasus Larynx. 2008;35:11–25.
14. Sistrunk WE. The surgical treatment of cysts of the thyroglossal tract. Ann Surg. 1920;71:121–2.
15. Motamed M, McGlashan JA. Thyroglossal duct carcinoma. Curr Opin Otolaryngol Head Neck Surg. 2004;12:106–9.
16. Tunkel DE, Domenech EE. Radioisotope scanning of the thyroid gland prior to thyroglossal duct excision. Arch Otolaryngol Head Neck Surg. 1998;124:597–9.

17. Ellis PD, van Nostrand AW. The applied anatomy of thyroglossal tract remnants. Laryngoscope. 1997;87:765–70.
18. Ayache S. A hereditary case of thyroglossal duct cyst. Ann Otolaryngol Chir Cervicofac. 2009;126:61–4.
19. Schader I, Robertson S, Maoate K, et al. Hereditary thyroglossal duct cysts. Pediatr Surg Int. 2005;21:593–4.
20. Peretz A, Leiberman E, Kapelushnik J, Hershkovitz E. Thyroglossal duct carcinoma in children: case presentation and review of the literature. Thyroid. 2004;14:777–85.
21. Kennedy TL, Riefkohl WL. Lingual thyroid carcinoma with nodal metastasis. Laryngoscope. 2007; 117(11):1969–73.
22. Organ GM, Organ CH. Thyroid gland and surgery on the thyroglossal duct: an exercise in applied embryology. World J Surg. 2000;24:886–90.
23. Ahuja AT, Wong KT, King AD, et al. Imaging for thyroglossal duct cyst: the bare essentials. Clin Radiol. 2005;60:141–8.
24. Josephson GD, Spencer WR, Josephson JS. Thyroglossal duct cyst: the New York eye and ear infirmary experience and a literature review. Ear Nose Throat J. 1998;77:642–7.
25. Burkart CM, Richter GT, Rutter MJ, Myer III CM. Update on endoscopic management of lingual thyroglossal duct cysts. Laryngoscope. 2009;119:2055–60.
26. Skandalakis JE, Gray SW, Ricketts RR. The lymphatic system. In: Skandalakis JE, Gray SW, editors. Embryology for surgeons. 2nd ed. Baltimore, MD: Williams and Wilkins; 1994. p. 877–97.
27. Brooks JE. Cystic hygroma of the neck. Laryngoscope. 1973;83:117–28.
28. Grasso DL, Pelizzo G, Zocconi E, et al. Lymphangiomas of the head and neck in children. Acta Otorhinolaryngol Ital. 2008;28:17–20.
29. Zadvinkis DP, Benson MT, Kerr HH, et al. Congenital malformations of the cervicothoracic lymphatic system: embryology and pathogenesis. Radiographics. 1992;12:1175–89.
30. Graesslin O, Derniaux E, Alanio E, et al. Characteristics and outcome of fetal cystic hygroma diagnosed in the first trimester. Acta Obstet Gynecol Scand. 2007;86:1442–6.
31. Lister WA. The natural history of strawberry naevi. Lancet. 1938;1:1429–34.
32. Beck DO, Gosain AK. The presentation and management of hemangiomas. Plast Reconst Surg. 2009;123:181–91.
33. Cheung DS, Warman WL, Mulliken JB. Hemangioma in twins. Ann Plast Surg. 1997;38:269–74.
34. O-Lee TJ, Messner A. Subglottic hemangioma. Otolaryngol Clin North Am. 2008;41:903–11.
35. Tucci FM, De Vincentiis GC, Sitzia E, et al. Head and neck vascular anomalies in children. Int J Ped Otorhinolaryngol. 2009;73S:S71–6.
36. Sarkar M, Mulliken JB, Kozakewich HPW, et al. Thrombocytopenic coagulopathy (Kasabach-Merritt Phenomenon) is associated with kaposiform hemangioendothelioma and not with common infantile hemangioma. Plast Reconst Surg. 1997;100:1377–86.
37. Maturo S, Hartnick C. Initial experience using propranolol as the sole treatment for infantile airway hemangiomas. Int J Ped Otorhinolaryngol. 2010;74:323–5.
38. Buckmiller LM, Munson PD, Dyamenahalli U, et al. Propranolol for infantile hemangiomas: early experience at a tertiary vascular anomalies center. Laryngoscope. 2010;120:676–81.
39. Ricketts RR, Gray SW, Skandalakis JE. Teratomas. In: Skandalakis JE, Gray SW, editors. Embryology for surgeons. 2nd ed. Baltimore, MD: Williams and Wilkins; 1994. p. 1060–5.
40. Hasiotou M, Vakaki M, Pitsoulakis G, et al. Congenital cervical teratomas. Int J Ped Otolaryngol. 2004;68: 1133–9.
41. Green JS, Dickinson A, Rickett A, et al. MRI in the assessment of a newborn with a cervical teratoma. Ped Radiol. 1998;28:709–10.
42. Renukaswamy GM, Soma MA, Hartley BEJ. Midline cervical cleft: a rare congenital anomaly. Ann Otol Rhinol Laryngol. 2009;118:786–90.
43. Mlynarek A, Hagr A, Tewfik TL, et al. Congenital mid-line cervical cleft: case report and review of literature. Int J Ped Otorhinolaryngol. 2003;67:1243–9.
44. Sturm-O'Brien AK, Salazar JD, Byrd RH, et al. Cervical thymic anomalies – the Texas Children's Hospital experience. Laryngoscope. 2009;119:1988–93.
45. Jensen JH, Larsen JL, Asschenfeldt P. Congenital thymic cysts in the neck. Int J Ped Otorhinolaryngol. 1983;6:95–100.
46. Khariwala SS, Nicollas R, Triglia JM, et al. Cervical presentations of thymic anomalies in children. Int J Ped Otorhinolaryngol. 2004;68:909–14.
47. Joshua BZ, Raveh E, Saute M. Familial thymic cyst. Int J Ped Otorhinolaryngol. 2004;68:573–9.
48. Cigliano B, Baltogiannis N, De Marco M, et al. Cervical thymic cysts. Pediatr Surg Int. 2007;27:1219–25.
49. Statham MM, Mehta D, Willging JP. Cervical thymic remnants in children. Int J Ped Otorhinolaryngol. 2008;72:1807–13.
50. Wei JL, Schwartz KM, Weaver AL, et al. Pseudotumor of infancy and congenital muscular torticollis: 170 cases. Laryngoscope. 2001;111:688–95.
51. Lidge RT, Bechtol RC, Lambert CN. Congenital muscular torticollis: etiology and pathology. J Bone Joint Surg Am. 1957;39:1165–82.
52. Bradenkamp JK, Hoover LA, Berke GS, et al. Congenital muscular torticollis. Arch Otolaryngol Head Neck Surg. 1990;116:212–6.
53. Cheng JCK, Tang SP, Chen TMK, et al. The clinical presentation and outcome of treatment of congenital muscular torticollis in infants – a study of 1086 cases. J Pediatr Surg. 2000;35:1091–6.
54. Von Heideken J, Green DW, Burke SW, et al. The relationship between developmental dysplasia of the hip and congenital muscular torticollis. J Pediatr Orthop. 2006;26:805–8.
55. Kumar V, Prabhu BV, Chattopadhayay A, et al. Bilateral pseudotumor of infancy. Int J Pediatr Otorhinolaryngol. 2003;67:673–5.

56. Oleszek JL, Chang N, Apkon SD, et al. Botulinum toxin type A in the treatment of children with congenital muscular torticollis. Am J Phys Med Rehabil. 2005;84:813–6.
57. Wise JB, Cryer JE, Belasco JB, et al. Management of head and neck plexiform neurofibromas in pediatric patients with neurofibromatosis type 1. Arch Otolaryngol Head Neck Surg. 2005;131:712–8.
58. Morse RP. Neurofibromatosis type 1. Arch Neurol. 1999;56:364–5.
59. Needle MN, Cnaan A, Dattilo J, et al. Prognostic signs in the surgical management of plexiform neurofibroma: the Children's Hospital of Philadelphia experience, 1974-1994. J Pediatr. 1997;131: 678–82.
60. NIH Consensus Development Conference. Neurofibromatosis. Arch Neurol. 1998;45:575–8.
61. Zografos GN, Vasiliadis GK, Zagouri F, et al. Pheochromocytoma associated with neurofibromatosis type 1: concepts and current trends. World J Surg Oncol. 2010;8:14.
62. Sobol SE, Tewfik TL, Ortenberg J. Otolaryngologic manifestations of neurofibromatosis in children. J Otolaryngol. 1997;26:13–9.

Abbreviations

22q11.2 DS	22q11.2 Deletion syndrome
ABG	Air bone gap
ABR	Auditory brainstem response
ACM	Arnold-Chiari malformation
AVM	Arterial venous malformations
BMP	Bone morphogenic protein
BOR	Branchio-oto-renal syndrome
CA	Cochlear aplasia
CAA	Congenital aural atresia
CC	Congenital cholesteatoma
CCM	Common cavity malformation
CGH	Comparative genomic hybridization
CHAOS	Congenital high airway obstruction syndrome
CHARGE	Coloboma, heart defects, atresia of the chonae, retarded growth or development of the central nervous system, genito-urinary anomalies, and ear anomalies
CHL	Conductive hearing loss
CLA	Complete labyrinthine aplasia
CL/P	Cleft lip with or without cleft palate
CLUFT	Cranial nerve, lower limb, upper limb, face, and thorax
CMCC	Congenital midline cervical cleft
CMT	Congenital muscular torticollis
CNPAS	Congenital nasal piriform aperture stenosis
COL2A1	Collagen, type II, alpha I gene
CP	Cleft palate
CPAP	Continuous positive airway pressure
CR	Crown-rump stage
CS	Cartilaginous sleeve
DDH	Developmental dysplasia of the hip
DML	Distal motor latencies
EA	Esophageal atresia
EAC	External auditory canal
ECMO	Extracorporeal membrane oxygenation
EVA	Enlarged vestibular aqueduct
EXIT	Ex utero intrapartum treatment
FEES	Functional endoscopic evaluation of swallowing

L.M. Elden and K.B. Zur (eds.), *Congenital Malformations of the Head and Neck*,
DOI 10.1007/978-1-4419-1714-0, © Springer Science+Business Media New York 2014

FGFR2	Fibroblast growth factor receptor 2
GERD	Gastroesophageal reflux disease
IAC	Internal auditory canal
LM	Lymphatic malformation
LTEC	Laryngotracheoesophageal clefts
MLPA	Multiplex ligation-dependent probe amplification
MM	Mondini malformation
MUAP	Motor unit action potentials
NAM	Nasoalveolar molding
NF	Neurofibromatosis
NF1	Neurofibromatosis type 1
NICH	Non-involuting congenital hemangioma
NIH	National Institutes of Health
OAVS	Oculo-auriculo-vertebral spectrum
PDA	Patent ductus arteriosus
PEEP	Positive end expiratory pressure
PHACE	Posterior cranial fossa malformations, large cervicofacial or laryngeal hemangiomas, arterial anomalies of the head and neck, coarctation of the aorta and cardiac defects, and eye anomalies
RICH	Rapidly involuting congenital hemangioma
SCM	Sternocleidomastoid (muscle)
SF	Stapes fixation
SGS	Subglottic stenosis
SNHL	Sensorineural hearing loss
SNP	Single nucleotide polymorphism
STOI	Sternocleidomastoid tumor of infancy
TACRD	Tracheal agenesis, complex congenital cardiac anomalies, radial ray defects, and duodenal atresia
TBX1 gene	T box transcription factor
TCS	Tracheal cartilaginous sleeve
TEF	Tracheoesophageal fistula
TGDC	Thyroglossal duct cyst
TM	Tympanic membrane
VATER/VACTERL	Vertebral, anal, cardiac, trachea-esophageal fistula, esophageal atresia, renal, radial dysplasia
VCFS	Velocardiofacial syndrome
VEGF	Vascular endothelial growth factor
VSS	Video swallow study

Index

L.M. Elden and K.B. Zur (eds.), *Congenital Malformations of the Head and Neck*,
DOI 10.1007/978-1-4419-1714-0, © Springer Science+Business Media New York 2014

T

www.ingramcontent.com/pod-product-compliance
Lightning Source LLC
Chambersburg PA
CBHW080735150926
51501CB00005B/167
* 9 7 8 1 4 4 1 9 1 7 1 3 3 *